LATENT HERPES VIRUS INFECTIONS IN VETERINARY MEDICINE

W0050592

CURRENT TOPICS IN VETERINARY MEDICINE AND ANIMAL SCIENCE

LATENT HERPES VIRUS INFECTIONS IN VETERINARY MEDICINE

A Seminar in the CEC Programme of Coordination of Research on Animal Pathology, held at Tübingen, Federal Republic of Germany, September 21–24, 1982

Sponsored by the Commission of the European Communities, Directorate-General for Agriculture, Coordination of Agricultural Research

Edited by

G. Wittmann
Bundesforschungsanstalt für Viruskrankheiten der Tiere
Tübingen, Federal Republic of Germany

Rosalind M. Gaskell
University of Bristol, Department of Veterinary Medicine
Bristol, United Kingdom

H.-J. Rziha
Bundesforschungsanstalt für Viruskrankheiten der Tiere
Tübingen, Federal Republic of Germany

1984 **MARTINUS NIJHOFF PUBLISHERS**
a member of the KLUWER ACADEMIC PUBLISHERS GROUP
BOSTON / THE HAGUE / DORDRECHT / LANCASTER
for
THE COMMISSION OF THE EUROPEAN COMMUNITIES

Distributors

for the United States and Canada: Kluwer Boston, Inc., 190 Old Derby Street, Hingham, MA 02043, USA
for all other countries: Kluwer Academic Publishers Group, Distribution Center, P.O.Box 322, 3300 AH Dordrecht, The Netherlands

Library of Congress Cataloging in Publication Data

Main entry under title:

Latent herpes virus infections in veterinary medicine.

(Current topics in veterinary medicine and animal
science)
    Subtitle: A seminar in the CEC Programme of Coordina-
tion of Research on Animal Pathology, held in Tubingen,
Federal Republic of Germany, September 21-24, 1982, spon-
sored by the Commission of the European Communities,
Directorate-General for Agriculture, Coordination of the
Agricultural Research."
    1. Herpesvirus diseases in animals--Congresses.
I. Wittmann, G. (Günther), 1926-   . II. Gaskell,
Rosalind M.   III. Rziha, H.-J.   IV. Commission of the
European Communities. Coordination of Agricultural
Research. V. Series. [DNLM: 1. Herpesvirus infections--
Veterinary--Congresses. SF 809.H47 L351 1982]
SF809.H47L38 1984   636.089'6925   83-23663
ISBN 0-89838-622-5

ISBN-13: 978-94-010-8998-2   e-ISBN-13: 978-94-009-5662-9
DOI: 10.1007/978-94-009-5662-9

Book information

Publication arranged by: Commission of the European Communities, Directorate-General Information Market and Innovation, Luxembourg

Copyright/legal notice

PREFACE

This seminar referred to latent herpes virus infections in veterinary medicine, with emphasis on the domestic animals. The phenomenon of latency is of particular importance in veterinary medicine because it can jeopardize the successful control and eradication of diseases such as Aujeszky's disease and infectious bovine rhinotracheitis, diseases which are often the cause of great economic losses.

For this reason, the Commission of the European Communities (CEC) realized the importance of summarizing the present state of knowledge on latent herpes virus infections in veterinary medicine. A seminar was therefore organized by the Federal Research Institute for Animal Virus Diseases in Tübingen, Federal Republic of Germany, from September 21 to 23, 1982, as a part of the 'Animal Pathology Programme' of the CEC. The seminar was attended by 50 participants not only from the countries of the CEC, and 38 papers were selected for presentation.

In veterinary medicine, more intensive investigations on the latency of animal herpes viruses have only relatively recently been initiated. In contrast, great efforts have been made for many years to elucidate latency in human and primate herpes viruses, and consequently the most considerable advances have been made in this field. Some of the most experienced scientists working on both systems were therefore invited. As a result, this seminar was the first occasion on which scientists from different countries and faculties investigating herpes virus latency had the opportunity to present and exchange their latest results. The establishment, maintenance, and reactivation of latency were discussed including considerations of the virology, pathology, pathogenesis, immunology and molecular biology of the diseases. Comparisons could be made between the results obtained with herpes viruses which are usually not investigated in their natural host, e.g. herpes simplex virus, and herpes viruses which allow experiments in their natural host. In this respect, veterinary medicine has the edge on human medicine. The seminar comprehensively reflected the present state of research on herpes virus latency and revealed some future trends and perspectives.

We would like express our appreciation of all the participants who contributed to the success of the seminar. In addition we would thank to the chairmen and co-chairmen for their help and for formulating the summary of each session. We are especially indebted to Mrs. Loraine E. Goddard for helping to improve the English in a part of the papers, and Mrs. Marie-Luise Donner and Mrs. Christel Roming for their great efforts in typing the "Proceedings". We also thank the CEC for financing the seminar from its budget for the Coordination of Agricultural Research.

CONTENTS

SESSION I

HUMAN, SIMIAN AND MURINE HERPESVIRUSES

Part 1

Chairman: H. Openshaw

Co-chairlady: Marianne Scriba

HERPES SIMPLEX VIRUS TYPE 1 THYMIDINE KINASE GENE ACTIVITY
CONTROLS VIRUS LATENCY AND NEUROVIRULANCE IN MICE

Y. Becker*, D. Gilden**, Y. Shtram, Y. Asher, E. Tabor,
M. Wellish**, M. Devlin**, D. Snipper, J. Hadar, Y. Gordon[+]
Department of Molecular Virology and Ophthalmology
The Hebrew University-Hadassah Medical Center,
Jerusalem, Isreal
[+]Present address: Dept.of Ophthalmology, Univ.of Pittsburg,
School of Medicine, Pittsburgh, PA., U.S.A
**Present address: Dept.of Neurology, The Univ.of Pennsylvania,
School of Medicine, Philadelphia, PA., U.S.A.
*To whom all correspondence should be addressed.

ABSTRACT
    The neurovirulence and latency of herpes simplex virus
type 1 (HSV-1) was investigated using three virus strains
originally isolated on the basis of plaque morpholgy. These
included a large plaque strain (LP(TK[+])) with a high level of
thymidine kinase (TK) activity, a small plaque strain (SP(TK[+]))
with 25% of the TK activity of the LP(TK[+]) strain was highly
virulent in mice, and after inoculation into the eyes invaded
the trigeminal ganglia and then migrated to, and replicated in,
the brain, killing most of the mice. The SP(TK[+]) strain also
replicated in the eyes, invaded the trigeminal ganglia and
established latency, but did not reach the brain or kill the
mice. The LP(TK[-]) strain (with no TK activity) replicated in
the inoculated eyes but did not invade the trigeminal ganglia,
and therefore was unable to establish latency in mice.
Increasing the virus doses of the SP(TK[+]) strain tenfold, and
therefore the amount of TK expression, enhanced virus
pathogenicity. Thus the degree of virulence of HSV-1 is
dependent on the level of expression of the viral TK gene.
Infection with the LP(TK[-]) and SP(TK[+]) strains protected the
mice against infection with the LP(TK[+]) virulent virus strain.

INTRODUCTION

    Studies on the mechanism of herpes simplex virus (HSV)

infections in animals have indicated that the virus requires

the activity of the thymidine kinase (TK) gene for infection of

nerve tissue (Marcialies et al., 1975; Field and Wildy, 1978;

Field and Darby, 1980; Tenser et al., 1979; Tenser and Dunstan,

1979; Tenser et al., 1981; Price, 1979; Price and Schmitz,

1979; Price and Kahn, 1981; Kleine et al., 1981). These

studies, summarized in Table 1, showed that an iododeoxyuridine

(IUdR)-resistant mutant of HSV type 1 (HSV-1) lost its

virulence for rabbits when inoculated into the eye, and

TABLE 1: Published studies on the pathogenicity of TK$^+$ HSV strains and lack of pathogenicity of the TK$^-$ mutants.

Reference	Experimental system	Virus	Results
Marcialis et al., 1975 (1)	a) Keratitis in rabbit eye b) I.p. or i.c. injection Swiss male mice	1. wt HSV-1 (NIH) 2. IUdR-resistant variant	IUdR-mutant virus lost virulence and protected against challenge by wt virus
Field & Wildy, 1978 (2)	a) Injection into the left pinna of 3-week old mice to infect dorsal root ganglia	1. HSV-1 strain C1(101) 2. TK$^-$ mutant of C1(101) (BUdR selection) 3. HSV-2 Bry strain 4. HSV-2 Bry-strain TK mutant (BUdR selection)	Mutants less virulent than parent strains; following large inoculum in the ear, type 1 mutant established in dorsal root ganglia; mice inoculated i.c. with mutant viruses solidly immune to challenge with lethal dose of parent strain.
Field & Darby, 1980 (3)	Injection into mouse skin	1. Parental isolates: 1-4 as above and HSV-1 SC16 2. Mutant strains producing various levels of TK derived by passage in presence of acyclovir	Mutant producing low TK level multiplied better in nervous system than TK virus

continue TABLE 1

Reference	Experimental system	Virus	Results
Tenser, Miller & Rapp, 1979 (4)	Corneal infection of guinea pig eyes	1. TK$^+$ (KOS) 2. TK$^-$ (KOS) (ara-T selection) 3. TK$^-$ (Glasgow 17)	Incidence of trigeminal ganglion infection with HSV-1 TK mutants markedly reduced as compared to TK$^+$; TK$^-$ mutants replicated well in ocular tissues but not in trigeminal ganglion.
Tenser & Dustan, 1979 (5)	Corneal infection of CD-1 mice	1-3. as above 4. TK$^+$ revertant of TK$^-$ virus	Ocular replication of TK$^-$ virus; TK$^+$ virus replicated in trigeminal ganglia, but not TK$^-$ virus; TK$^+$ revertant of TK$^-$ virus replicated in ganglia as parental TK$^-$ virus.
Tenser, Ressel & Dunstan (1981) (6)	Infection of trigeminal ganglion by corneal infection in mice	1. 8 TK$^-$ mutants of HSV-1 2. Some TK$^-$ mutants were intermediate for TK activity (TK$^\pm$) based on thymidine phosphorylation	TK$^-$, TK$^\pm$ and TK$^+$ virus replicated in ocular tissue TK$^-$ mutants were rarely isolated from trigeminal ganglia.

continue TABLE 1

Reference	Experimental system	Virus	Results
		TK^+ 60-100% or greater (KOS$^+$, Pat_4^+, C1 101$^+$) TK^- 5-15% (Pat_{4-2}, Pat_5, C1 101 S_{30}^-, C1 101 S_5^-) TK^- <5% (KOS$^-$, Pat_{4-1}^-, Glas$^-$, B2006$^-$)	TK^+ and to a lesser degree TK^- viruses were frequently isolated.
			Relationship was found between the virus titer in the trigeminal ganglia and the ability of the virus to produce TK. The highest titer with TK^+ (10^4 pfu/mg tissue) Pat_{4-2}^- (10^3 pfu/mg tissue) Pat_5^+ (10^2 pfu/mg tissue) C1 101 S_{30}^+ (10^{05} pfu/mg tissue) B2006$^-$, KOS_1^-, Glas, Pat_{4-1}^- (10 pfu/mg tissue).
			TK^- HSV may be complemented by TK^+ and TK^- HSV to permit trigeminal ganglion infection.
Price, 1979 (7)	Superior cervical ganglion (SCG) in mice after intraocular infection		6-hydroxydopamine potentiates acute HSV infection.

continue TABLE 1

Reference	Experimental system	Virus	Results
Price & Schmitz, 1979 (8) Price & Kahn, 1981 (9)	SCG in mice after intra-ocular infection.	1. TK^+ (KOS) 2. TK^- (KOS) 3. TK^+ (C1 101) 4. TK^- (B2006)	Replication of TK^- strains at the site of inoculation; little, if any, virus replication occurred in SCG. Cyclophosphamide immunosuppression did not induce TK^- infection.
Klein, Friedman-Kien & DeStefano, 1981 (10)	Orofacial skin inoculation of hairless mice.	1. Strains of HSV-1 2. ACV resistant mutant	ACV resistant virus is latency negative.

protected the animals against challenge by the virulent wild
type (wt) virus strain (Marcialis et al., 1975). By means of
injection of HSV-1 into the left pinna of mice (Field and
Wildy, 1978), it was shown that TK$^-$ mutants of HSV-1 and HSV-2,
selected by bromodeoxyuridine (BUdR), were less virulent than
the parental TK$^+$ virus strains and immunized mice against
challenge by a lethal dose of the parent strain. Not only TK$^-$
mutants of HSV-1, but also a mutant producing a low level of
TK, were able to cultiply in the nervous system (Field and
Darby, 1980). It was also reported that TK$^-$ mutants of HSV-1
resembled TK$^+$ parental strains in their ability to cause
infections in the eyes of guinea pigs or mice, but were unable
to infect the trigeminal ganglion (Tenser et al., 1979; Tenser
and Dunstan, 1979).

In a detailed study, it was reported (Tenser et al., 1981)
that TK$^-$, TK$^{\pm}$ and TK$^+$ HSV-1 strains replicated in ocular
tissue, but the TK$^-$ mutants were rarely isolated from the
trigeminal ganglia. A relationship was found between the virus
titre in the trigeminal ganglia and the ability of the virus to
produce TK (Table 1).

In studies on the behavior of a TK$^-$ HSV-1 mutant during
infection of the superior cervical ganglia (SCG) it was found
that TK$^-$ mutants of HSV-1 did not infect the SCG, while the TK$^+$
strains did (Price, 1979; Price and Schmitz, 1979; Price and
Kahn, 1981). It was not possible to reactivate the HSV-1 TK$^-$
mutant from SCG after explantation to in vitro conditions.
Virus strains resistant to acyclovir (ACV) were found to be
latency negative (Klein et al., 1981).

We investigated infection of the eye, trigeminal ganglion
and the central nervous system (CNS) of mice, using mutants of
HSV-1 (NIH strain) originally isolated on the basis of plaque
morphology: a highly virulent large plaque strain, producing a
high level of TK in the infected cells (LP(TK$^+$)), a TK$^-$ mutant
of this strain (LP(TK$^-$)) and a small plaque mutant that
produced 25% of the TK activity of the large plaque virulent
strain (SP(TK$^+$)). The results of our experiments confirmed that
the viral TK gene is essential for the infection of the

trigeminal ganglion and for the establishment of latency, since the virus mutant that produced a low level of TK was able to establish latency but the TK$^-$ mutant was not able to do so.

MATERIALS AND METHODS
Virus strains and cells

The NIH wt strain No. 11124 of HSV type 1 was propagated in BSC-1 cell monolayers grown in Dulbecco's modified Eagle's medium (DMEM; GIBCO) containing 10% calf serum. The wt virus that produced a heterogeneous population of 79% large plaque and 21% small plaque morphology was diluted to yield about 10 plaque-forming units (pfu)/plate, and from these large (2 mm diameter) and small (0.5 mm diameter) plaques were isolated for plaque purification. The process was repeated many times until a small plaque strain was obtained that could be purified three times with 100% small plaque purity; the large plaque derivative showed about 95% plaque purity. The large plaque strain, designated LP(TK$^+$), and the small plaque strain, designated SP(TK$^+$), each required about 20 hr to reach a virus titre of 2-4x10^7 pfu/ml in vitro.

A TK$^-$ mutant, designated LP(TK$^-$), was isolated from the large plaque strain by incubating about 100 pfu/plate in the presence of 20 µg/ml of BUdR in the agar overlay (Dasgupta and Summers, 1978). Virus plaques were isolated, passaged in the presence of BUdR and tested for TK activity.

L(TK$^-$) cells were received from Dr. H. Cedar (Department of Molecular Biology, The Hebrew University-Hadassah Medical School, Jerusalem) and propagated in DMEM plus 10% calf serum.

TK assay

L(TK$^-$) cells were infected with the HSV-1 mutants at the same titre and incubated at 37°C. At 10 hr postinfection (p.i.), the cells were harvested in 10 mM Tris-HCl, pH 7.8 and 2 mM 2-mercaptoethanol and sonicated for 1 min at 15 sec intervals. Each homogenate was centrifuged for 30 min at 10,000 rpm in the Sorvall ultracentrifuge at 4°C, and the supernatant fluid was mixed with the TK reaction mixture which

consisted of 0.2 M sodium phosphate, pH 6.0, 25 mM NaF,
50 µCi/ml of ³H-thymidine methyl-T (5000 mCi/mmol, Nuclear
Research Center, Negev, Israel) and 4 mM ATP. The cell
homogenate and TK reaction mixture in the proportion of 1:2
were incubated at 37°C for 30 min. Each mixture was separated
by thin layer chromatography (TLC) on PEI paper (0.1 mm
cellulose MN 300 polyethyleneimine impregnated; Macherey-Nagel
& Co., Germany) to separate the thymidine monophosphate (TMP)
from the di- and triphosphates. The specific activity of the TK
was calculated from the amount of radioactivity in the TMP/µg
protein/hr.

The V_{max} and K_m of the TK coded by the various strains of
HSV-1 in L(TK⁻) cells were determined by standard procedures.

Infection of mice

Outbred albino mice, four weeks of age, were infected with
the HSV-1 strains by inoculation on to scarified corneas
(Pavan-Langston et al., 1979). At different time intervals,
mice were sacrificed, and eyes, trigeminal ganglia, pons and
brain were removed. The tissues were kept at -20°C until
processed by Dounce homogenization in 1 ml of phosphate
buffered saline (PBS). After centrifugation, tenfold dilutions
of the supernatant fluid were made in DMEM and were titrated in
BSC-1 monolayers using the plaque assay. Results are expressed
as pfu/ml for each tissue sample. To determine latency, ganglia
were cocultivated with BSC-1 cells by placing a piece of tissue
on the cell monolayer, and the appearance of CPE indicated the
reactivation of the virus from the ganglia. The pathogenicity
of the different virus strains in mice was determined by
corneal infection as above, and the number of animals that
survived was determined.

RESULTS
Studies on TK expression by the HSV-1 strains

The ability of the LP(TK⁺) and SP(TK⁺) isolates of the NIH
strain to produce TK in L(TK⁻) mouse cells was studied. In the
control experiment, uninfected L(TK⁻) mouse cells were shown to

have no TK activity, whereas infection of the cells with the HF
strain of HSV-1 produced an active TK enzyme. Both the LP(TK$^+$)
and SP(TK$^+$) virus isolates produced TK, although far less TK
activity was induced by the SP(TK$^+$) strain. Determination of
the K_m of the enzyme of the two virus isolates revealed that
the enzymes are identical (Table 2), but the V_{max} of the TK
induced by SP(TK$^+$) was 25% of that induced by LP(TK$^+$).

TABLE 2   Thymidine kinase activity in L(TK$^-$) cells
infected with HSV-1 strains

Virus strain	V_{max}	K_m
LP(TK$^+$)	8.44×10^{-6} M/Min	9.47×10^{-7} M
SP(TK$^+$)	2.07×10^{-6} M/Min	9.68×10^{-7} M

Indeed, the specific activity of the TK induced in L(TK$^-$)
cells by LP(TK$^+$) was 4.1 pmol of ^{3}H-TMP/µg protein/hr, as
opposed to 0.96 for the SP(TK$^+$) strain. Thus the SP(TK$^+$) mutant
produces only 25% of the TK produced by the LP(TK$^+$) strain. The
nature of the mutation in SP(TK$^+$) is currently under study.

Infection of mouse eyes

Mice were inoculated into the eyes with the three virus
isolates, using a standard virus inoculum with a titre of
10^6 pfu/ml. Groups of 10 mice were sacrificed each day for six
days after the infection, and the virus titre in the eyes,
trigeminal ganglia and brain was determined. The results of a
typical experiment (Table 3) show that all three virus strains
replicated in the eyes, with the highest virus titres occurring
at days 1 and 2 postinfection (p.i.). The virus strains LP(TK$^+$)
and LP(TK$^-$) infected 100% of the eyes by day 2, while the virus
strain SP(TK$^+$) infected only 90% of the eyes (Table 3). On the
second day p.i., the mean virus titre in the eyes was about the
same for all three virus strains.

Keratitis was scored and was found to be maximal on day 2
in mice infected with all three virus strains, although

TABLE 3: Kinetics of centripetal spread of HSV-1 virus mutants

	Day post infection						
	1	2	3	4	5	6	10
	MEAN PFU/ml a						
LP(TK+)							
Eyes	165 (90)b	153 (100)	53 (70)	17 (30)	12 (80)	105 (70)	0
Ganglia	0	0	27 (20)	98 (40)	1512 (70)	900 (90)	0
Brain	0	0	6 (20)	1 (20)	120 (40)	3200 (90)	20 (40)
SP(TK+)							
Eyes	27 (80)	148 (90)	64 (90)	20 (30)	32 (60)	18 (60)	0
Ganglia	0	0	<1 (20)	<1 (10)	<1 (10)	2 (20)	0
Brain	0	0	2	0	0	0	0
LP(TK−)							
Eyes	2010 (100)	161 (100)	32 (60)	29 (60)	5 (60)	9 (20)	0
Ganglia	0	0	0	0	0	0	0
Brain	0	0	0	0	0	0	0

a Mean Pfu/ml of tissues from mice: two eyes, two ganglia and one brain constituted three samples processed from each mouse.

b Percent samples with virus calculated from number of mice (out of ten) whose tissues yielded virus.

differences were noted in the severity of keratitis occurred in eyes infected with LP(TK$^+$), with low scores being noted in eyes infected with the LP(TK$^-$) or SP(TK$^+$) strains. The inability of the LP(TK$^-$) strain to produce TK, or the lower TK activity induced by SP(TK$^+$), did not prevent infection of the eyes, but the keratitis caused by these two virus strains was milder than that caused by the LP(TK$^+$) virus strain.

Infection of the trigeminal ganglia

Replication of the three virus strains in the trigeminal ganglia is shown in Table 3. The LP(TK$^+$) strain replicated in the ganglia, reaching a maximal titre on day 5, followed by a gradual decrease in the virus titre at day 6, and no detectable virus at day 10. On day 6, 90% of the mice were infected and harbored the LP(TK$^+$) virus. The SP(TK$^+$) virus strain differed markedly, and only 10-20% of the mice showed signs of virus infection with a very low virus titer (Table 3). The LP(TK$^-$) virus strain was not detected in the ganglia. The only virus strain able to replicate consistently with trigeminal ganglia was the LP(TK$^+$) virus strain, which produces a high level of TK. Virus that produces no TK, namely the LP(TK$^-$) strain cannot replicate in the trigeminal ganglia and cause ganglionitis, and low level TK produces virus, the SP(TK$^+$) strain, shows only minimal replication at this site.

Invasion of the central nervous system by the three virus strains

Following the invasion of the trigeminal ganglia, the LP(TK$^+$) virus strain migrated to the brain. The virus replicated in the brain, in the pons and in the cerebrum, reaching a maximum titre at day 6 p.i. (Table 3). 90% of the mice infected with the LP(TK$^+$) strain showed active virus replication in the brain. The LP(TK$^-$) virus strain that did not invade the trigeminal ganglia, and the SP(TK$^+$) virus strain that reached the trigeminal ganglia but did not cause ganglionitis, were unable to infect the brain (Table 3).

14

These results indicate that the level of expression of the TK gene of the HSV-1 virus strain determines the sequence of virus infection: high TK expression allows the virus to cause ganglionitis; in the absence of TK activity, or when the virus mutant is a low producer of TK, the virus loses its neurovirulence.

Pathogenicity of the three virus strains in mice

The virulence of the virus strains after inoculation into the eyes was determined by the number of mice that survived (Fig. 1). The $LP(TK^+)$ strain was highly virulent and killed 85% of the infected mice, whereas the wt virus was slightly less virulent. However, the $LP(TK^-)$ and $SP(TK^+)$ strains hardly killed any mice after infection of the eyes. These results are compatible with those of the replication of $LP(TK^+)$ in the brain. The $LP(TK^-)$ and $SP(TK^+)$ strains have lost their virulence for mice.

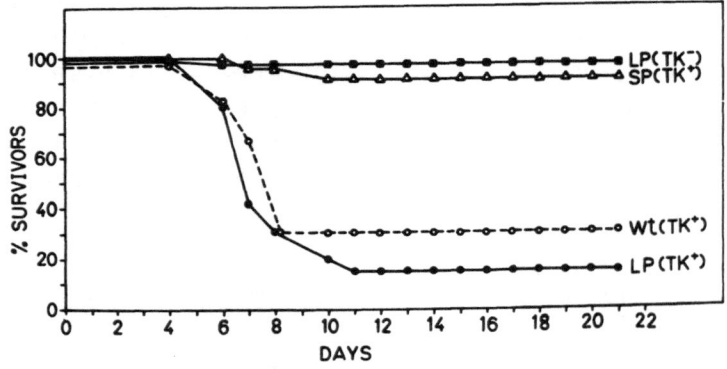

Fig. 1   Survival of mice after inoculation with 10^8 pfu/ml of the three HSV-1 virus isolates and the wt virus.

The relationship between the virus dose used for infecting the eyes and virus pathogenicity is shown in Table 4. The $LP(TK^-)$ strain was avirulent at doses of 10^6 and 10^7 pfu/ml, whereas the $SP(TK^+)$ was avirulent at a dose of 10^6 pfu/ml but became virulent at a dose of 10^7 pfu/ml.

These results provide additional evidence that the amount

of TK produced by the herpes virus strain determines its
pathogenicity for mice.

TABLE 4   Survival of mice inoculated with different
            doses of the various strains of HSV-1

Virus strain	% Survivors	
	Inoculum dose (pfu/ml)	
	10^6	10^7
LP(TK$^+$)	29 (30/104)[a]	14 (3/22)
LP(TK$^-$)	93 (105/113)	95 (19/20)
SP(TK$^+$)	90 (112/125)	57 (17/30)
wt(TK$^+$)	46 (31/68)	20 (1/5)
Mock-infected control 93 (70/75)		

[a] No. of survivors/total mice inoculated

Role of the viral TK in the establishment of latent infections
in the trigeminal ganglia

In the above experiments, it was noted that the LP(TK$^-$)
mutant did not replicate in the ganglia, while the SP(TK$^+$)
strain infected the ganglia in 20% of the mice, but with a very
low virus titre. It was of interest to determine whether these
two avirulent virus strains were able to establish latent
infections. For this purpose, each of the two trigeminal
ganglia from each mouse infected with the different virus
strains was cocultivated with BSC-1 cells. Table 5 shows that
the virulent strain LP(TK$^+$) could be recovered from at least
one ganglion in 75% of the mice that survived infection with
the wt virus. With the avirulent strain SP(TK$^+$), virus was
recovered from 80% of the survivors. However, no virus was
recovered from ganglia of mice infected with strain LP(TK$^-$)
(Table 5), and it was concluded that the TK$^-$ strain was unable
to establish latency in the mice. A follow-up study of the

TABLE 5   Recovery of latent virus from trigeminal ganglia

Virus recovery	Virus recovery (%)			
	21 days p.i.		116 days p.i.	
	Positive mice	Positive ganglia	Positive mice	Positive ganglia
LP(TK$^+$)	75 (6/8)[a]	56 (9/16)[b]	ND[c]	ND
LP(TK$^-$)	0 (0/27)	0 (0/54)	0 (0/9)	0 (0/18)
SP(TK$^+$)	80 (24/30)	65 (39/60)	25 (2/8)	19 (3/16)
wt	100 (9/9)	67 (12/18)	ND	ND

[a] No. of survivors with at least one positive ganglion/no. of mice

[b] Total positive ganglia/no. tested

[c] Not done

TABLE 6   Correlation between HSV-1 TK gene activity and virus pathogenicity

Virus	Virus inoculum pfu/ml	TK gene activity	Kera-titis	Penetration to ganglia	Latency	Encepha-litis
LP(TK$^+$)	10^6	High	++++	++++	++++	++++
SP(TK$^+$)	10^7	High	++++	+++	++++	++++
SP(TK$^+$)	10^6	Low	++++	++	++++	--
LP(TK$^-$)	10^6	None	++++	--	--	--

++++	high
++	intermediate
--	none

state of latency in mice infected with the SP(TK$^+$) strain
revealed that the virus could be reactivated in fewer mice 116
days after infection (Table 5). The reason for this is not
known.

DISCUSSION

The original object of this study was to investigate the
pathogenicity of HSV-1 mutants isolated on the basis of plaque
morphology. A large plaque variant highly virulent for mice and
a small plaque variant that was less virulent were isolated.
Investigation of these mutants showed that the large plaque
LP(TK$^+$) strain was an effective producer of TK, while the small
plaque SP(TK$^+$) strain produced only 25% of the TK activity of
the large plaque strain. We also isolated a large plaque mutant
(LP(TK$^-$)) with no TK activity.

In the present study, the relationship between HSV-1
pathogenicity and TK expression was investigated in mice by
using the eyes as the site of inoculation. The course of
infection in the eyes, trigeminal ganglia and mouse brain was
followed on a daily basis after corneal inoculation of the
three virus isolates that differed in their TK activity. We
have shown that a virus strain that cannot induce TK (the
LP(TK$^-$) mutant) is unable to invade the trigeminal ganglion and
establish latency, whereas a virus strain able to produce a low
level of TK (the SP(TK$^+$) mutant) can invade the trigeminal
ganglia and establish latency, but does not reach the pons or
the cerebrum. The LP(TK$^+$) virus strain with a high livel of TK
activity invaded the ganglia, replicated and caused
ganglionitis, and afterwards reched the brain, causing
encephalitis (Table 6).

This study confirms and extends the results of Marcialis
et al. (1975), Field and Wildy (1978), Tenser and Dunstan
(1979) and Price and Khan (1981), who reported that the TK$^-$
strains of HSV-1 had lost their pathogenicity, as compared to
the TK$^+$ parent strains, and that the mutant virus strains were
unable to cause latent infections. Nevertheless, the TK$^-$
mutants did immunize the infected animals against challenge by
the virulent parent strain.

18

Our study showed that the SP(TK$^+$) strain which produces 25% of the TK activity found with the LP(TL$^+$) strain, can penetrate the ganglia and cause a latent infection at a virus dose of 10^6 pfu/ml. However, by increasing the virus dose to 10^7/pfu/ml and thus increasing the amount of TK produced, the pathogenicity of the virus was enhanced and the virus reached the brain and killed the mice (Table 6). These results suggest that there is a relationship between the level of TK expression and HSV-1 pathogenicity, as well as between the viral TK gene and the ability of the virus to establish a latent infection.

Another aspect of the studies summarized in Table 1 is the demonstration that avirulent strains of HSV-1 (mostly HSV-1 TK$^-$ mutants) do exist that are able to protect against infection with anturally occurring virulent strains. For an avirulent strain to render maximum protection, it must have lost the ability to invade the trigeminal ganglion and cause a latent infection (Klein et al., 1981), while being able to immunize the eye.

ACKNOWLEDGMENT

This study was supported in part by a grant from the chief Scientist, Ministry of Health, Israel, and by a grant from the Israel Academy Commission for Basic Research of the Sciences and Humanities. Y. Gordon was supported by a grant from the Hebrew University-Hadassah Research Fund. D. Gilden was a visiting professor from the Department of Neurology, University of Philadelphia, and the recipient of a Fogarty Senior International Fellowship from the National Institutes of Health, Bethesda, Maryland.

REFERENCES

DasGupta, U.B. and Summers, W.C. 1978. Ultraviolet reactivation of herpes simplex virus is mutagenic and inducible in mammalian cells. Proc. Natl. Acad. Sci. USA, 75, 2378-2381.

Field, H.J. and Wildy, P. 1978. The pathogenicity of thymidine kinase-deficient mutants of herpes simplex virus in mice. J. Hyg. Camb., 81, 267-277.

Field, H.J. and Darby, G. 1980. Pathogenicity in mice of strains of herpes simplex virus which are resistant to acyclovir in vitro and in vivo. Antimicrob. Ag. Chemother., 17, 209-216.

Klein, R.J., Friedman-Kien, A.E. and Destefano, E. 1981.
    Pathogenesis of experimental skin infections induced by
    drug resistant herpes simplex virus mutants. Infec.
    Immun., 34 693-701.
Marcialies, M.A., La Colla, P., Schivo, M.L., Flore, O.,
    Firinu, A. and Loddo, B. 1975. Low virulence and
    immunogenicity in mice and in rabbits of variants of
    herpes simplex virus resistant to 5-iodo-2-deoxyuridine.
    Experientia, 31, 502-503.
Pavan-Langston, D., Park, N.H. and Lass, J.H. 1979. Herpetic
    ganglionic latency. Acyclovir and vidarabine therapy.
    Arch. Ophthalmol., 97, 1508-1510.
Price, R.W. 1979. 6-Hydroxydopamine potentiates acute herpes
    simplex virus infection of the superior cervical ganglion
    in mice. Science, 205, 518-520.
Price, R.W. and Schmitz, J. 1979. Route of infection, systemic
    host resistance and integrity of ganglionic axon influence
    in acute and latent herpes virus infection of the superior
    cervical ganglion. Infec. Immun., 23, 373-383.
Price, R.W. and Kahn, A. 1981. Resistance of peripheral
    autonomic neurons to in-vivo productive infection by
    herpes simplex virus mutants deficient of TK activity.
    Infec. Immun., 34, 571-580.
Tenser, R.B., Miller, R.L. and Rapp, F. 1979. Trigeminal
    ganglion infection by thymidine kinase-negative mutants of
    herpes simplex virus. Science, 205, 915-917.
Tenser, R.B. and Dunstan, M.E. 1979. Herpes simplex virus
    thymidine kinase expression in infection of the trigeminal
    ganglion. Virology, 99, 417-422.
Tenser, R.B., Ressel, S. and Dunstan, M.E. 1981. Herpes simplex
    virus thymidine kinase expression in trigeminal ganglion
    infection: correlation of enzyme activity with ganglion
    virus titre and evidence for in vivo complementation.
    Virology, 112, 328-341.

LATENCY OF HERPES SIMPLEX VIRUS IN TREE SHREW; GENERATION OF INTERTYPIC RECOMBINANTS OF HERPES SIMPLEX VIRUS IN VIVO

G. Darai, H.J. Scholz

Institut für Medizinische Virologie
der Universität Heidelberg
Im Neuenheimer Feld 324
6900 Heidelberg, F.R.G.

ABSTRACT

The susceptibility of juvenile and adult Tupaias to infection with herpes simplex virus (HSV) was investigated in detail. It was found that HSV type 1 and 2 were highly pathogenic for juvenile and adult Tupaias. The state of viral latency was studied using the co-cultivation technique in those animals which had survived an acute infection. Infectious virus was recovered from the ganglia of chronically infected tree shrews. The susceptibility of juvenile Tupaias to several strains of temperature-sensitive mutants of HSV type 1 and 2 was also investigated. These experiments revealed that the animals survived an infection of different ts-mutants of HSV 1 and 2 and were protected against a superinfection of a lethal dose of wild-type HSV-1 and/or 2. The state of viral latency in these surviving animals was studied. It was found that infectious virus could only be recovered from the spleen of these animals. Genomic analysis of these newly recovered viruses showed significant changes as compared to their parental viruses. This finding led to the development of a model system for the generation of intertypic recombinants in vivo.

INTRODUCTION

Plummer and his co-workers succeeded in 1970 in recovering infectious virus from the ganglia of rabbits which were inoculated previously with herpes simplex virus. Therefore the hypothesis on the "neurotropic potential of HSV and the properties of this virus for remaining in a persistent state within the nervous system" was confirmed, which was first postulated by Goodpasture in 1923. The pathogenicity and latency of HSV has been studied in a variety of laboratory animals, especially rodents (Plummer et al., 1970; Stevens et

al., 1971; Scriba et al., 1977). We have been investigating
the pathogenicity and latency of HSV in tree shrews. The
reason why we chose this animal (Tupaia belangeri) for the
study of HSV latency and tropism was based on the fact that,
firstly, the tree shrew is highly susceptible to HSV (Darai et
al., 1979, 1980), and, secondly, that this animal
phylogenetically belongs to higher developed species when
compared to rodents, and is placed nearer to prosimians.

MATERIALS AND METHODS

The experimental approach for this study (e.g. animals,
HSV-1 and 2, ts-mutants of HSV-1 and 2, virus propagation, and
titration, cells, media, neutralization test, co-cultivation
assay and DNA restriction enzyme analysis) was carried out as
described previously (Darai et al., 1978, 1980, and 1983).

RESULTS

Pathogenicity of wild types and temperature-sensitive mutants
of HSV type 1 and 2 in tree shrew

Whilst testing the susceptibility of juvenile Tupaias to
several strains of HSV type 1 and 2 it was found that HSV type
1 and 2 are highly pathogenic for these animals. The
administration of 1.0×10^2 PFU of HSV type 1 and/or 2 per
animal led to 100% lethality during two to eight days after
inoculation (Darai et al., 1978, 1980). The clinical picture
was manifested as a state of herpetic hepatitis when the
animals were inoculated intravenously, intraperitoneally, and
subcutaneously. The cause of death was generalized herpesvirus
infection with liver necrosis. The highest titre of virus was
found in the liver indicating that the centre for HSV
production is the liver cells. These results confirm the
observation of Mogensen et al. (1974). In contrast, a necrosis
of stomach and intestine was found when the animals were
inoculated orally (Darai et al., 1980, 1982). The animals died
two to six days after oral infection. They were dissected

after death and/or sacrificed when moribund. The pathological examination revealed that only stomach and intestine were affected. Determination of virus production in different organs of these animals revealed that the highest virus titre was found in stomach and intestine (Darai et al., 1980, 1982). The pathogenicity of HSV in the adult Tupaia is similar to that in the juvenile Tupaia with the exception that the percentage of lethality is far lower when compared to the percentage for juvenile animals (100% lethality by 10^2 PFU/animal). Table 1 summarizes the results of these experiments.

TABLE 1   Sensitivity of juvenile and adult Tupaia to infection with HSV-1 and 2

No. of animals juvenile adult		Virus	No. of animals dead/No. of animals tested	Lethality (%)
18			18/18	100
		HSV-1		
	57		46/57	80.7
19			19/19	100
		HSV-2		
	47		34/47	72.3

Following HSV type 1 and 2 strains were used:
HSV-1: 17, F. Thea, ANG, WAL
HSV-2: HG-52, G, Müller

The sensitivity of juveline tree shrews to infection with different temperature-sensitive mutants of HSV type 1 strain 17 and HSV type 2 strain HG-52 (kindly provided by Dr. John Subak-Sharpe, University of Glasgow) was investigated. It was found that in all cases the animal survived an infection of intravenously administered ts-mutants (Darai et al., 1980, 1983). The results of these studies are summarized in Table 2.

The development of antibodies against inoculated
ts-mutants of HSV type 1 and 2 was determined using
neutralization assay as described previously (Darai et al.,
1980). A value of 1:40 to 1:80 of neutralizing antibodies was
found in the inoculated animals 15 days after infection.

TABLE 2   Sensitivity of juvenile Tupaia to infection
with tempreature-sensitive mutants of HSV-2
HG-52, and HSV-1/17.

No.of ani-mals*	Virus*	PFU/ animal***	No.of animals dead/ No.of animals
4	HSV-2 HG-52 (wild-type) HSV-2 HG-52	1.0×10^4	4/4 (4 days p.i.)
4	ts: 1		0/4
4	2		0/4
4	5		0/4
4	9	1.0×10^7	0/4
4	10		0/4
4	12		0/4
2	13		0/2
1	HSV-1/17 (wild-type) HSV-1/17	1.0×10^3	1/1 (4 days p.i.)
1	ts: D^+	5.0×10^6	0/1
1	G^+	5.0×10^6	0/1
1	H^+	5.0×10^6	0/1
1	H^+	1.0×10^8	0/1
2	H	1.0×10^8	0/2
1	H_{syn}	5.0×10^6	0/1

*   Average values of weight (g) / age (days) = 15/118
**   ts = temperatur-sensitive mutants
***   The animals were inoculated intravenously

The susceptibility of those animals which had initially been infected with ts-mutants to infection with a lethal dose of wild-type HSV type 1 and 2 was tested. These studies revealed that the animals were protected against a superinfection of a fatal dose of wild-types HSV-1 and/or 2. The state of viral latency in these surviving animals was of special importance and was studied in detail. With this goal the animals which were infected with ts-mutants and/or challenged with wild-types of HSV; those animals which survived an acute infection of wild-type HSV-1 and 2 were sacrificed several months after infection and/or after superinfection. A variety of different specimens including brain, spinal cord, blood, thymus, spleen, kidney, liver, secretory glands, muscle, and skin were used for virus recovery using the co-cultivation technique with different susceptible cell cultures for HSV (Tupaia embryonic kidney cells) at different incubation temperatures ($32^{\circ}C$, $37^{\circ}C$, and $39^{\circ}C$). Each experimental approach was observed over a period of 6 to 8 weeks. The summary of these results is given in Table 3.

The results presented here demonstrate clearly that the state of viral latency in those animals which had initially been infected with ts-mutants of HSV-2 and superinfected with wild-type HSV-1 is different when compared to those animals which survived an acute HSV (wild-type) infection. In this case infectious virus was recovered from co-cultivated ganglia of the animals only. In contrast it was found that under these conditions the target organ responsible for the persistence of latent viruses was the spleen of those animals which were previously infected with ts-mutants and challenged with wild-type virus. Genomic analysis of these newly recovered viruses showed significant changes as compared to their parental viruses.

This finding led to the development of a model system for the generation of intertypic recombinants in vivo, in agreement with the generation of intertypic recombinants of HSV in vitro previously reported by Morse et al. (1977) and

Preston et al. (1978). The intertypic recombinants of HSV-1
and 2 were generated in tree shrews using a variety of

TABLE 3   Recovery of Herpes simplex virus during
            chronic latent infection of tree shrew.

No.of animals	Inoculated 1st infect.	Virus 2nd infect.	Time of sacrifice (days after 2nd infection	Virus organs	recovered no.of isolation/no. of animals
4	HSV-1	–	75-105	spinal cord	4/4
13	HSV-2	–	120-240	spinal cord	11/13
5	ts-2HSV-2*	–	180-280	spinal cord	1/5
4**	ts:2,5,9,10 12,and 13 HSV-2*	–	240	NR	0/4
2**	ts:D$^+$,G$^+$,H$_{syn}$ HSV-1/17	–	90-120	NR	0/2
4	ts H$^+$HSV-1/17	–	90-120	NR	0/4
4	HSV-2	HSV-1	240	spinal cord	1/4
4	HSV-1	HSV-2	240	spinal cord	4/4
16	ts 2 HSV-2*	HSV-1+*	14-240	SPLEEN	16/16
8	ts 2 HSV-2*	HSV-1+*	240	SPLEEN	8/8
4	ts10 HSV-2*	HSV-1+*	240	SPLEEN	4/4

*	HSV-2 HG52
**	for each ts-mutant
NR	not recovered
*	following HSV-1 strains were used: 17, F, KOS, and
+	Thea.

ts-mutants of HSV-2 HG-52 and wild-type of HSV-1 (strains 17,
KOS, F) which served as superinfecting virus. The intertypic
recombinants of HSV can also be generated in vivo using
ts-mutants of HSV type 1 and 2 administered simultaneously or
reciprocally. The infected animals were sacrificed at various
times after inoculation and/or superinfection and it was found
that latent HSV could be recovered only from the spleen as

shown in Table 4.

TABLE 4   Determination of the time necessary for intertypic interaction of HSV type 1 and 2 in vivo (in tree shrew)

No.of animals	Inoculated Virus 1st infection*	2nd infection* (14 days after 1st)	Time+ of sacrifice (days p.i.)	Virus recovered*** from:
1		HSV-1/17** 5.0×10^6 p.f.u.	animal dead	
2		HSV-1/17	4	SPLEEN
3	tsm 2 HSV-2 HG52 1.0×10^7	HSV-1/17 1.0×10^7 p.f.u.	20-34	SPLEEN
3	p.f.u.	HSV-1/F 1.0×10^7 p.f.u.	14-33	SPLEEN
2		HSV-1/KOS 4.3×10^7 p.f.u.	20-34	SPLEEN

*   Route of infection = intravenously
+   after second infection
**   simultaneous administration with first inoculum
***   all other organs including brain, spinal cord, blood, thymus, liver, muscle, and skin which were screened were negative.

The results presented in Table 4 demonstrate clearly that a minimum time of 4 days is necessary for intertypic interaction of HSV type 1 and 2 in vivo which is responsible for a shift of target organs for the persistence of latent HSV to spleen.

The analysis of plaque-purified reisolated viruses using a variety of restriction endonucleases revealed significant alterations in the genome structure of newly recovered viruses (Table 5). These results indicate that an intertypic

28

interaction between HSV-1 and 2 occurred in vivo which is
responsible for the observed shift in organotropism of latent
virus in tree shrew.

TABLE 5   Genomic alterations which were detected in a
            variety of reisolated HSV from the spleen of
            infected tree shrews.

Group	Enzyme	Arrangement of cleavage pattern of DNA of reisolated HSV from the spleen of Tupaia	
		HSV-1	HSV-2
I	Bam HI	−B	+F and +P
	Hind III		+0 and +J
II	HpaI	−K and −U	
	Kpn I		+L
	Bam HI		+Q
III	Bam HI	−A	+Q and +D
		M	
IV	Eco RI	−K	+M
		additional to II	
V	Eco RI	−K	+M
		additional to III	
VI	group I and II together		

−   not present
+   present

PATHOGENICITY AND LATENCY OF RECOVERED VIRUSES IN TREE SHREW
     The biological properties of the different reisolated
viruses from ganglia or spleen of tree shrew were studied in
vivo. Different animals (juvenile Tupaias) were inoculated
with a variety of recovered viruses and the results are shown
in Table 6. It is apparent that only those virus strains which
were recovered from the spleen of the tree shrew lost their
pathogenicity in the tree shrew and required new attentuated
properties.

CONCLUSION

Our data presented here demonstrate that intertypic interactions between temperature-sensitive mutants of HSV in vivo are experimentally inducible. Although the mechanism of this complex process is not completely understood at this stage of investigation, and for its understanding many detailed

TABLE 6   Sensitivity of tree shrew to infection with different reisolated HSV from the spleen of Tupaia.

Virus	No. of animals	PFU/ animal	Route of application	Time of death (days)	No. of animals dead/No.of animals
HSV-T-HD- O/R3	4	1.5×10^7	i.p.		0/4
	1	3.0×10^7	i.v.		0/1
HSV-T-1469	2	2.0×10^7	s.c.		0/2
HSV-T-1618	1	3.1×10^7	s.c.		0/1
HSV-T-1628	1	6.3×10^7	s.c.		0/1
HSV-T-1475	4	7.0×10^7	i.v.		0/4
	1	7.0×10^7	s.c.		0/1
HSV-T-1489	1	3.0×10^7	s.c.		0/1
HSV-1/17	2	1.0×10^3	i.v.	34	2/2
HSV-1 Thea	8	1.0×10^3	s.c.	45	8/8
HSV-1 F	2	1.0×10^5	i.p.	45	2/2

biological and molecular-biological investigations will be necessary, we can emphasize that the established Tupaia model system (see Figure 1) is of great help for a study of gene and gene function of HSV responsible for the tropism, pathogenicity and latency of this virus.

ACKNOWLEDGEMENTS

The authors are greatly indebted to Professor Dr. John Subak-Sharpe for his generosity in providing temperature-sensitive mutants of HSV and HSV wild-type strains, which were

30

used in this study.

This research was supported by Deutsche Forschungsgemein-
schaft, Schwerpunktprogramm "Persistierende Virusinfektionen:
Molekulare Mechanismen und Pathogenese", Teilprojekt
II B 6 - Da 142/1-1.

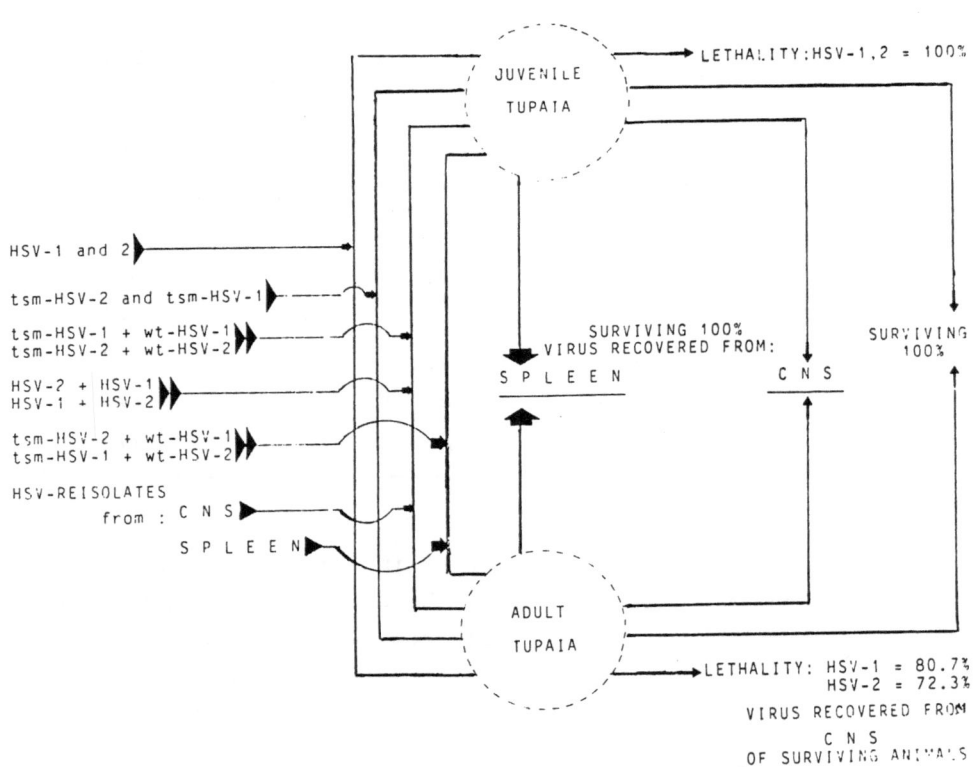

Fig. 1   Diagram of pathogenic and latent pathways of
herpes simplex virus in tree shrew.

REFERENCES

Darai, G., Schwaier, A., Komitowski, D. and Munk, K. 1978.
Experimental infection of Tupaia belangeri (tree shrews)
with Herpes Simplex Virus types 1 and 2. J. infect. Dis.,
137, 221-226.

Darai, G., Zöller, L., Matz, B., Schwaier, A., Flügel, R.M.
and Munk, K. 1980. Experimental infection and the state
of viral latency of adult Tupaia with Herpes Simplex
Virus type 1 and 2 and infection of juvenile Tupaia with
temperature-sensitive mutants of HSV type 2. Arch.
Virol., 65, 311-318.

Darai, G., Scholz, J., Kurz, W. and Koch, H.G. 1983. Inter
typic superinfection with Herpes Simplex Virus of Tupaia
leads to reisolation of latent viruses with newly
acquired lymphotropic properties. In "Herpes Virus of Man
and Animal, Developments in Biological Standardiza
tion". (Karger, Basel).

Goodpasture, E.W. and Teague, O. 1923. Transmission of herpes
febrilis along nerves in experimentally infected rabbits.
J. med. Res., 44, 139-184.

Mogensen, S.C., Teisner, B., Kerzel Andersen, H. 1974. Focal
necrotic hepatitis in mice as a biological marker for
differentiation of herpesvirus hominis type 1 and 2. J.
gen. Virol., 25, 151-155.

Morse, L.S., Buchman, T.G., Roizman, B. and Schaffer, P.A.
1977. Anatomy of Herpes Simplex Virus DNA. IX. Apparent
exclusion fo some parental DNA arrangements in the
generation of intertypic (HSV1 x HSV2) recombinants. J.
Virol., 24, 231-248.

Plummer, G., Hollingsworth, D.C., Phuangsab, A. and Bowling,
C.P. 1970. Chronic infections by herpes simplex viruses
and by the horse and cat herpesviruses. Infect. Immunol.,
1, 351-355.

Preston, V.G., Davison, A.J., Marsden, H.S., Timbury, M.C.,
Subak-Sharpe, J.H. and Wilkie, N.M. 1978. Recombinants
between Herpes Simplex Virus types 1 and 2: Analyses of
genome structures and expression of immediate early
polypeptides. J. Virol., 28, 499-517.

Scriba, M. 1977. Extraneural localisation of Herpes Simplex
Virus in latently infected guinea pigs. Nature, 267,
529-531.

Stevens, J.G. 1975. Latent herpes simplex and the nervous
system. Current Topics in Microbiology and Immunology,
70, 31-50.

Subak-Sharpe, J.H., Brown, S.M., Ritchie, D.A., Timbury, M.C.,
MacNab, J.C.M., Marsden, H.S. and Hay, J. 1974. Genetic
and biochemical studies with herpesvirus. Cold Spring
Harbor Symposium Quant. Biol., 39, 717-730.

A REVIEW OF HSV LATENCY IN EXPERIMENTAL ANIMALS

H. Openshaw
Department of Neurology
University of California at Davis
Davis, California 95616

INTRODUCTION

Of the five herpesviruses that infect man, only herpes simplex viruses 1 and 2 (HSV) are not strongly species specific. Therefore animal models can be used in an attempt to clarify the pathogenesis of the natural infection in man. Neural spread of HSV has been appreciated since the 1920' s (Goodpasture and Teague, 1923; Johnson, 1964; Wildy, 1967; Cook and Stevens, 1972), but it was not until the 1970' s that latency in sensory ganglia was documented first in an animal model and then in man (Plummer et al., 1970; Stevens and Cook, 1971; Bastian et al., 1972; Baringer and Swoveland, 1973). Latency occurs only in neurons in vivo with usually only 1% of the neurons involved in sensory ganglia (Cook et al., 1974; Galloway et al., 1979; McLennan and Darby, 1981; Galloway et al., 1982; Tenser et al., 1982).

There are comprehensive reviews of the human herpesviruses in a recent volume (Nahmias et al., 1981). The present brief review concerns selected aspects of HSV latency in animal models. Emphasis is placed on maintenance of the latent state and virus reactivation.

HSV LATENCY AND SPONTANEOUS REACTIVATION IN ANIMAL MODELS

Open discussion of HSV latency often leads to conflicting views. The problem, in part is lack of agreement in terminology. Most investigators consider latency as a block in transcription of HSV DNA (Puga, et al., 1978). This block may be complete or partial (i.e., transcripts present from only a limited part of the genome) (Yamamoto et al., 1977; Galloway et al., 1982). In agreement with the static state hypothesis (Roizman, 1965), viral replication does not occur. Reactivation refers to the reversal of the transcriptional block to the

point where full transcripts appear and viral replication
resumes. Such reactivation may be clinically manifest as
recurrent skin lesions or may be subclinical with or without
HSV shedding at the skin.

There are some discrepant observations that suggest the
dynamic state hypothesis of latency (i.e., a low level of virus
replication) (Baringer and Swoveland, 1974; Scriba, 1975; Hill
and Blyth, 1976; Schwartz et al., 1978). However, these
observations may correspond to the detection of spontaneous,
subclinical reactivations. Such reactivations are very common
in the rabbit model of HSV infection occurring at some time in
100 percent of animals followed for six months (Nesburn et al.,
1967). Similarly frequent asymptomatic as well as symptomatic
shedding occurs in some selected human population (Douglas and
Couch, 1970). In the guinea pig model, clinical recurrences and
subclinical shedding are so frequent that it is arguable
whether the concept of latency as used in this review fits this
model at all (Scriba, 1975; Donnenberg et al., 1980). In
contrast, spontaneous reactivation is rare in most mouse models
occurring in less than 10 percent of animals followed for three
months (Sekizawa et al., 1980).

As a working hypothesis, it is reasonable to suppose a
varying degree of "leakiness" in HSV transcription in various
species with the greatest degree of "leakiness" in the guinea
pig and the least in the mouse. The question remains which of
these models most closely parallels the natural infection in
man. As a model of recurrent skin lesions, the guinea pig is
certainly preferable. But to study the phenomenon of latency,
the mouse model with its low background of spontaneous
reactivation is preferable.

INDUCED REACTIVATION OF LATENT HSV

The basis for the species difference in spontaneous
reactivation is unknown. Probably related is the question in
man why certain individuals with a latent infection tend to
have frequent recurrences; whereas, others have few or no
recurrences. The question comes down to a discussion of what is

needed to maintain latency (i.e., maintain the virus transcriptional block). Suggested answers concern differences in the virus, the number of ganglion cells infected, the immune response, or some poorly defined feature of the latently infected neuron. An experimental approach to determine what maintains latency involves the study of stimuli that induce reactivation in latently infected animals.

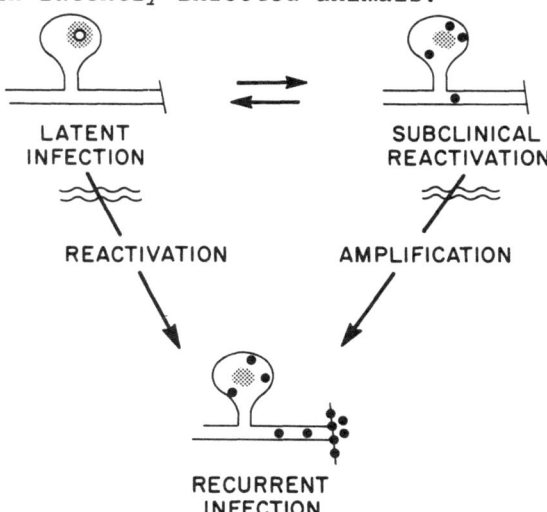

Fig. 1   Recurrent herpetic infection produced either by reactivation of latent HSV or by amplification of a pre-existing reactivation. The schematic drawing shows a bipolar sensory neuron with axons projected distally to the skin surface and proximally into the central nervous system. The wavy double lines indicate a test stimulus that is known to induce recurrent herpes: e.g., fever in man (Greenberg et al., 1969). Without knowing the incidence of spontaneous reactivation in the study population, it is not possible to tell whether the test stimulus induced a reactivation or amplified a pre-existing, subclinical reactivation.

Induced reactivation has been detected by scoring skin lesions or detecting HSV shedding at the skin (Underwood and Weed, 1974; Blyth et al., 1976; Hurd and Robinson, 1977; Hill et al., 1978), by culturing infectious virus in cell-free ganglionic homogenates (Walz et al., 1974; Stevens et al., 1975; Openshaw et al., 1979), and by demonstrating a serum antibody rise in antibody negative latently infected Animals

(Sekizawa et al., 1980). Only the first method can be used in man. However, as the figure shows, this method is badly confounded if there is a high background of spontaneous, subclinical reactivation. Under this circumstance, it is not possible to tell whether the test stimulus actually triggers reactivation (i.e., affects viral gene expression in neurons) or merely makes a pre-existing reactivation clinically manifest.

This objection is minimized by doing reactivation studies in the mouse, an animal model with a low level of spontaneous reactivation. Particular stimuli shown to reactivate HSV in the mouse include (1) axotomy done close to the ganglia (Walz et al., 1974), (2) epithelial irritants applied to those nerve terminals that correspond to the latently infected ganglion cells (Blyth et al., 1976; Hill et al., 1978; Sekizawa et al., 1980), and (3) treatment with the cytotoxic agents cyclophosphamide or x-irradiation (Kurata et al., 1978; Openshaw et al., 1979).

Clearly only the third method would be expected to have an effect on the host immune response. A role for anti-HSV IgG in the maintenance of latency has been suggested (Stevens and Cook, 1974). Yet in experimental studies, reactivation occurred in mice given cyclophosphamide at a time when the serum antibody titer to HSV was still high (Openshaw et al., 1979). Moreover, it has been shown that latency is maintained in certain mice in the absence of detectable neutralizing serum antibody (Sekizawa et al., 1980).

We favor the hypothesis that individual neurons have a varying degree of permissiveness for HSV replication (Openshaw et al., 1981). Ordinarily, neurons are non-permissive (i.e., there is a tight transcpritional block). But the same neurons become permissive under certain circumstances: e.g., transfer of the ganglion to explant culture, axotomy or other axonal injury, epithelial trauma, and treatment with cytotoxic agents. One of these stimuli (axonal injury) has been shown to alter neuronal gene expression (Levine et al., 1981). Perhaps associated with this alteration, critical HSV transcripts appear and eventually virus replication resumes. In summary, understanding the relationship between neuronal and viral gene expression may ultimately provide a clue to the mechanism of HSV latency.

REFERENCES

Baringer, J.R. and Swoveland, P. 1973. Recovery of herpes simplex virus from human trigeminal ganglions. New Eng. J. Med., 288, 648-650.
Baringer, J.R. and Swoveland, P. 1974. Persistent herpes simplex virus infection in rabbit trigeminal ganglia. Lab. Invest., 30, 230-240.
Bastian, F.O., Rabson, A.S. and Lee, C.L. 1972. Herpesvirus hominis: isolation from human trigeminal ganglion. Science, 178, 306-307.
Blyth, W.A., Hill, J.T., Field, H.J. and Harbour, D.A. 1976. Reactivation of herpes simplex virus infection by ultra-violet light and possible involvement of prostaglandins. J. Gen. Virol., 33, 547-549.
Cook, M.L., Bastone, V.B. and Stevens, J.G. 1974. Evidence that neurons harbor latent herpes simplex virus. Infect. Immun., 9, 946-951.
Cook, M.L. and Stevens, J.G. 1973. Pathogenesis of herpetic neuritis and ganglionitis in mice: evidence of intra-axonal transport of infection. Infect. Immun. 7, 272-288.
Donnenberg, A.D., Chaikof, E. and Aurelian, L. 1980. Immunity to herpes simplex virus type 2: cellmediated immunity in latently infected guinea pigs. Infect. Immun., 30, 99-109.
Douglas, R.G. and Couch, R.B. 1970. A prospective study of chronic herpes simplex virus infections and recurrent herpes labialis in humans. J. Immunol., 104, 289-295.
Galloway, D.A., Fenoglio, C.M. and McDougall, J.K. 1982. Limited transcription of herpes simplex virus genome when latent in human sensory ganglia. J. Virol., 41, 686-691.
Galloway, D.A., Fenoglio, C., Shevchuk, M. and McDougall, J.K. 1979. Detection of herpes simplex RNA in human sensory ganglia. Virology, 95, 265-268.
Goodpasture, E.W. and Teague, O. 1923. Experimental production of herpetic lesions in organs and tissues of the rabbit. J. Med. Res., 44, 121-138.
Green, M.T., Courtney, R.J. and Dunkel. 1981. Detection of an immediate early herpes simplex virus type 1 poly-peptide in trigeminal ganglia from latently infected animals. Infect. Immun., 34, 987-992.
Greenberg, M.S., Brightman, V.J. and Ship, I.I. 1969. Clinical and laboratory differentiation of recurrent intraoral herpes simplex virus infection following fever. J. Dent. Res., 48, 385-371.
Hill, T.J. and Blyth, W.A. 1976. An alternative theory of herpes simplex recurrence and possible role for prosta-glandins. Lancet, 1, 397-399.

Hill, T.J., Blyth, W.A. and Harbour, D.A. 1978. Trauma to the skin causes recurrence of herpes simplex in the mouse. J. Gen. Virol., 39, 21-28.

Hurd, J. and Robinson, T.W.E. 1977. Herpes virus reactivation in a mouse model. J. Antimicrobiol. Agents Chemother., 3, (Suppl. A): 99-106.

Johnson, R.T. 1964. The pathogenesis of herpes virus encephalitis. I. Virus pathway to the nervous system of suckling mice demonstrated by fluorescent antibody staining. J. Exp. Med., 119, 343-356.

Kurata, T., Kurata, K. and Aoyama, Y. 1978. Reactivation of herpes simplex virus (type 2) infection in trigeminal ganglia and oral lips with cyclophosphamide treatment. Jpn. J. Exp. Med., 48, 427-435.

Levine, J., Skene, P. and Willard, M. 1981. GAPs and fodrin: novel axonally transported proteins. TINS, 4, 273-277.

McLennan, J.L. and Darby, G. 1981. Herpes simplex virus latency: the cellular location of virus in dorsal root ganglia and the fate of the infected cell following virus activation. J. Gen. Virol., 51, 233-243.

Nahmias, A.J., Dowdle, W.R. and Schinazi, R.F. (eds). 1981. "The Human Herpesviruses: An Interdisciplinary Perspective". (Elsevier, New York).

Nesburn, A.B., Elliot, J.H. and Leibowitz, H.M. 1967. Spontaneous reactivations of experimental herpes simplex keratitis in rabbits. Arch. Ophthalmol., 78, 523-529.

Openshaw, H., Asher, L.V.S., Wohlenberg, C., Sekizawa, T. and Notkins, A.L. 1979. Acute and latent herpes simplex virus ganglionic infection: immune control and viral reactivation. J. Gen. Virol., 44, 205-215.

Openshaw, H., Sekizawa, T., Wohlenberg, C. and Notkins, A.L. 1981. The role of immunity in latency and reactivation of herpes simplex virus. In "The Human Herpesviruses: An Interdisciplinary Perspective" (Ed. A.J. Nahmias, W.R. Dowdle, R.F. Schinazi). (Elsevier, New York). pp. 289-296.

Plummer, G., Hollingworth, D.C., Phuangsab, A. and Bowling, C.P. 1970. Chronic infections by herpes simplex viruses and by the horse and cat herpesviruses. Infect. Immun., 1, 351-355.

Puga, A., Rosenthal, J.D., Openshaw, H. and Notkins, A.L. 1978. Herpes simplex virus DNA and mRNA sequences in acutely and chronically infected trigeminal ganglia of mice. Virology, 89, 102-111.

Roizman, B. 1965. An inquiry into the mechanisms of recurrent herpes infections in man. In "Perspectives in Virology" (Ed. M. Pollard). (Harper and Row, New York). pp. 283-301.

Schwartz, J., Whetsell, W.O. and Elizan, T.W. 1978. Latent herpes simplex virus infection of mice: infectious virus in homogenates of latently infected dorsal root ganglia. J. Neuropathol. Exp. Neurol., 37, 45-55.

Scriba, M. 1975. Herpes simplex virus infection in guinea pigs: an animal model for studying latent and recurrent herpes simplex virus infection. Infect. Immun., 12, 162-165.

Sekizawa, T., Openshaw, H., Wohlenberg, C. and Notkins, A.L. 1980. Latency of herpes simplex virus in absence of neutralizing antibody: model for reactivation. Science, 210, 1026-1028.

Stevens, J.G. and Cook, M.L. 1971. Latent herpes simplex virus in spinal ganglia of mice. Science, 173, 843-845.

Stevens, J.G. and Cook, M.L. 1974. Maintenance of latent herpetic infection: an apparent role for antiviral IgG. J. Immunol., 133, 1685-1693.

Stevens, J.G., Cook, M.L. and Jordan, M.C. 1975. Reactivation of latent herpes simplex virus after pneumococcal pneumonia in mice. Infect. Immun., 11, 635-639.

Tenser, R.B., Dawson, M., Ressel, S.J. and Dunstan, M.E. 1982. Detection of herpes simplex virus mRNA in latently infected trigeminal ganglion neurons by in situ hybridization. Ann. Neurol., 11, 285-291.

Underwood, G.E. and Weed, S.D. 1974. Recurrent cutaneous herpes simplex in hairless mice. Infect. Immun., 10, 471-474.

Walz, M.A., Price, R.W. and Notkins, A.L. 1974. Latent ganglionic infection with herpes simplex virus types 1 and 2: viral reactivation in vivo after neurectomy. Science, 184, 1185-1187.

Wildy, P. 1967. The progression of herpes simplex virus to the central nervous system of the mouse. J. Hyg., 65, 173-192.

Yamamoto, H., Walz, M.A. and Notkins, A.L. 1977. Viral specific thymidine kinase in sensory ganglia of mice infected with herpes simplex virus. Virology, 76, 866-869.

THE INFLUENCE OF IMMUNITY, NATURAL RESISTANCE AND VIRULENCE ON THE PERSISTENCY OF HERPES SIMPLEX VIRUS FOLLOWING THE INFECTION OF THE NON-INJURED MUCOUS MEMBRANES OF MICE

K. E. Schneweis

Institute of Medical Microbiology and
Immunology, University of Bonn,
Federal Republic of Germany

ABSTRACT

Using the vaginal route of infection in mice, we could show that the latency of Herpes simplex virus (HSV) in the lumbosacral ganglia correlated with the extent and the duration of the peripheral disease:
1. Mice which had been pre-immunized by infection with HSV type 1 (HSV-1) were rarely protected from the take of a vaginal challenge. Accordingly, protection from latent infection was moderate, whereas the mice were well protected against the lethal outcome of the disease. Immunization with killed vaccine from purified HSV-1 had even less protective effect on the take of infection and correspondingly on viral latency, but the low rate of lethal outcome was similar to that of mice immunized with the live vaccine.
2. The marked genetic resistance of intraperitoneally (i.p.) infected C57 Bl mice was only poorly developed in vaginally infected mice. The course of the vaginal disease was not reduced and the incidence of latency was not diminished. Resistance manifested itself in reduced viral titre and spread in acute ganglionic infection, and in decreased lethality.
3. Whereas wild virus strains of HSV-1 differed considerably in their neuro-virulence following intracerebral inoculation, only minor differences could be detected with respect to the vaginal disease. They did not lead to different rates of persistent infection. On the other hand, persistence of the virus was either not established or was rare respectively, in the case of TK⁻ and syn mutant strains of HSV-1 and HSV-2, which proved avirulent in vaginal infection.

INTRODUCTION

Whenever selected factors of pathogenesis are studied, it is often useful to choose experiments with artificial conditions. The relevance of the factors in the course of disease, however, becomes clearer, if the natural conditions are simulated. In an experimental model of vaginal herpes simplex virus (HSV) infection of mice, it was shown that this is also true for the influence of immunity (Schneweis et al., 1981), natural resistance (Schneweis et al., 1982), and virulence on the latent persistent virus infection.

MATERIALS AND METHODS

Mice: Outbred NMRI mice and - in some experiments - inbred C57 Bl mice were used. The mice were purchased from Zentralinstitut für Versuchstiere, Hannover, Federal Republic of Germany, and were infected when 6 to 8 weeks old.

Viruses: Herpes simplex virus type 1 (HSV-1): Strains MF (Sturn and Schneweis, 1978); Thea syn (Schneweis et al., 1972); Hof syn (Munk and Donner, 1963); ANG syn path (Kaerner et al., 1981); Kit and Dubbs TK$^-$ (Dubbs and Kit, 1964). Herpes simplex virus type 2 (HSV-2): Strains EP (Sturn and Schneweis, 1978); Lux syn (derived from a penile isolate in our laboratory); Bry TK$^-$ (Thouless, 1972).

Cell cultures: Human Embryo Fibroblasts (HEF) for cocultivation of the ganglion explants, Vero cells for virus propagation and titration.

Infection of mice: We used cotton pellets soaked with 10^6 TCID$_{50}$ (if not indicated otherwise) to infect the mice vaginally, carefully avoiding any injury to the mucous membranes. The take of infection and the virus titre produced in the vagina were tested by swabs, squashed in 1 ml Eagle's MEM supplemented with 10% newborn calf serum (Eagle 10).

Acute and persistent infection in the lumbosacral ganglia: Latency was ascertained by explantation of the lumbosacral ganglia (L4 to S3) 4 weeks or later post infection (p.i.). The ganglia of one side were pooled, explanted in plastic tissue culture flasks (50 ml) and cocultivated with HEF for 4 weeks. In the phase of acute infection the virus in the ganglia was titrated in homogenates of the ganglia, removed at the 3rd and 4th d.p.i. and - left and right ganglia separately - homogenized in 1.5 ml Eagle 10. In one additional experiment the ganglia were removed on days 2, 4, 6 and 8 p.i. and explanted separately in 24-well tissue culture cluster dishes.

RESULTS

Immunity and latency

Mice which experienced an oral infection with HSV-1
(strain MF) 4 weeks previously, were moderately protected
against vaginal infection with the same strain: Although the
number of takes was only scarcely diminished, virus elimination
from the vagina was clearly accelerated (Fig. 1). Immunization
by a killed vaccine made from purified HSV-1 (Hilfenhaus et
al., 1981), was even less effective. Nevertheless, both
experimental groups were protected equally well against the
lethal outcome of infection: lethality was only 4% in contrast
to 55% in the controls.

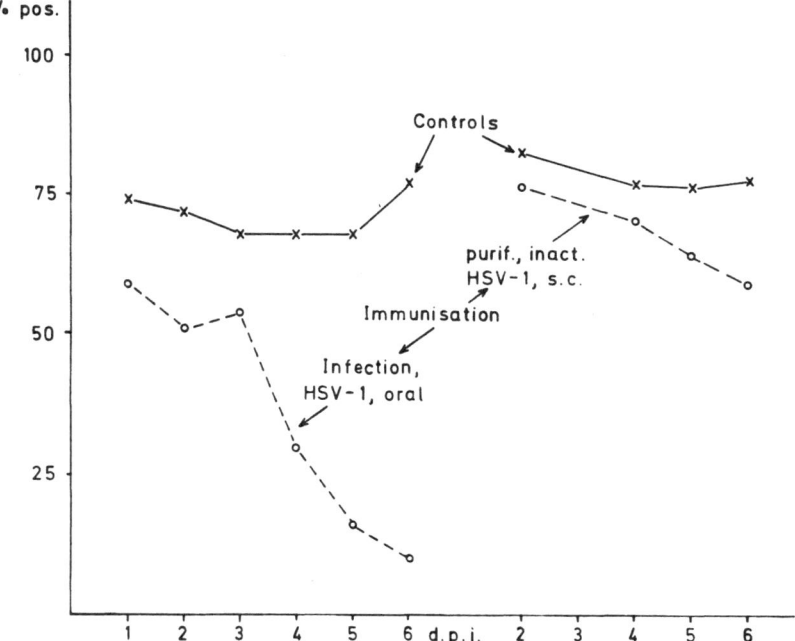

Fig. 1   The course of the genital challenge infection
with HSV-1 in mice, which were immunized (o --- o) either
by previous oral infection with HSV-1 (97 mice) or by
application of a heat-killed vaccine from purified HSV-1
virions (59 mice). The control animals (x———x) had oral
mock infection (79 mice) or s.c. application of PBS (40
mice) resp. The percentage of positive swabs following
the genital challenge is indicated.

The ratio and the extent of latent infection correlated
with the duration of vaginal infection (Table 1). The number of
latently infected mice was significantly reduced only in the
group immunized with live virus, whereas the extent of latency
was reduced in both groups. (For this purpose, resistant C57 Bl
mice are more relevant controls than NMRI mice, since the group
of surviving NMRI controls is selected in respect of an
attenuated course of infection).

TABLE 1   Latency following vaginal challenge with
HSV-1 after immunization with live and killed HSV-1.
* see text.

Immunization		Latency ascertained	Left and right gangl. affected
None	NMRI*	$\frac{23}{53}$ (43 %)	52 %
	C57Bl*	$\frac{47}{67}$ (70 %)	72 %
2 s.c. doses of inact.,purif.HSV-1		$\frac{47}{81}$ (58 %)	45 %
Oral infection with HSV-1		$\frac{15}{46}$ (33 %)	33 %

The correlation between latency and peripheral infection
was affirmed by the data in table 2: The frequency of latent
infection decreased proportionally with the number of positive
swabs.

TABLE 2   Incidence of latency in dependence on virus
elimination from the vagina. Swabs were taken 2, 4, 5
and 6 days p.i.

Number of pos. swabs	4	3	2	1
Latency ascertained	$\frac{23}{30}$ (77)	$\frac{15}{25}$ (60)	$\frac{6}{12}$ (50)	$\frac{3}{14}$ (21)

Natural resistance and latency

Since the finding of Lopez (1975) it is well known that
C57 Bl mice resist intraperitoneal infection of 10^6 $TCID_{50}$,
whereas the LD_{50} of sensitive mice is 10^2 to 10^3 $TCID_{50}$.

Surprisingly, the course of vaginal infection in resistant
(C57 Bl) and sensitive (NMRI) mice was identical (Fig. 2). The
viral titre produced in the vagina was also similar in both
strains of mice (Table 3). Accordingly, the numbers of latently
infected animals were equal in both experimental groups.
Looking for a difference in the early infectious cycle, which
could be the reason for reduced lethality in C57 Bl mice, we
found that the viral titer produced in the ganglia of C57 Bl
mice was below that of the sensitive mice.

In order to obtain more evidence for limited virus
production in the ganglia of resistant mice, a number of
infected ganglia were tested. For this purpose, mice were
inoculated in the right foot pad. The ganglia were removed at
days 2, 4, 6 and 8 p.i. and explanted separately. Fig. 3 shows
that resistant mice had less infected ipsilateral ganglia and
contralateral ganglia were infected only in sensitive mice.

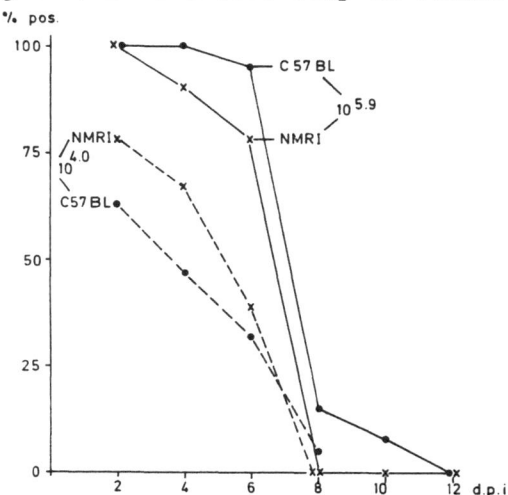

Fig. 2   Course of the vaginal infection with HSV-1 in
sensitive and resistant mice. Sensitive (NMRI) (x) and
resistant (C57 Bl) (o) mice were inoculated in the vagina
with $10^{5,9}$ (———) or $10^{4,0}$ (----) $TCID_{50}$/0,05 ml. The
extent of the local infection was calculated as percentage of positive swabs from the vagina.

TABLE 3   Course of infection after vaginal inoculation
of HSV-1 in sensitive and resistant mice.

Parameter of infection	Strain of mice	
	NMRI	C57 Bl
Titer of vaginal swab, 4th d.p.i.	2,48	2,35
Titer of acute inf. in lumbos. ganglia	2,83	2,09
Latent ganglionic inf. ascertained	$\frac{18}{25}$ (72 %)	$\frac{14}{18}$ (77 %)
Deaths per inf. mice (lethality)	$\frac{67}{75}$ (89 %)	$\frac{33}{61}$ (54 %)

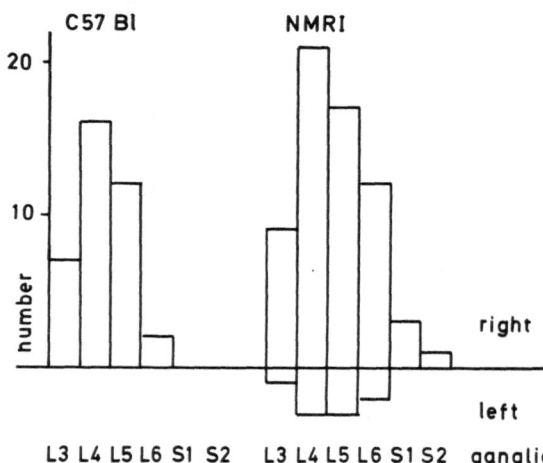

Fig. 3   Infected lumbosacral ganglia, which were
removed 2 to 8 days after subcutaneous HSV-1 infection
into the right foot pad of resistant (C57 Bl) and
sensitive (NMRI) mice.

Virulence and latency

It was observed that freshly isolated wild virus strains
differed very much in virulence when inoculated intracerebrally
(Table 4).

TABLE 4   High virulent (hv) and low virulent (lv) ocular
HSV-1 isolates, tested by i.c. inoculation (Neumann-
Haefelin, 1979).

hv strains	$\dfrac{TCID_{50}}{LD_{50}}$	lv strains	$\dfrac{TCID_{50}}{LD_{50}}$
281	10^{-1}	309	$10^{3,1}$
342	$10^{0,1}$	317	$10^{3,1}$
391	$10^{0,2}$	401	$10^{2,9}$

In the vaginal infection, however, the strains showed no
striking differences. The only difference we could find in the
course of the peripheral infection was the diminished titre of
the avirulent strains in the vagina towards the end of acute
infection. The slight difference did not result in a reduced
incidence of latency. Lethality, however, was also decreased in
this experimental group (Table 5).

TABLE 5   Vaginal infection with ocular HSV-1 isolates:
3 strains with high intracerebral virulence (hv) and
3 strains with low intracerebral virulence (lv).

	hv strains	lv strains
Number of takes	$\dfrac{102}{120}$ (85 %)	$\dfrac{96}{120}$ (80 %)
Viral titer in the vagina, 2nd d.p.i.	$10^{3,78}$	$10^{3,55}$
Viral titer in the vagina, 5th d.p.i.	$10^{3,88}$	$10^{3,11}$ $p< 0,001$
Latency established	$\dfrac{21}{29}$ (72 %)	$\dfrac{26}{38}$ (68 %)
Lethality	$\dfrac{58}{102}$ (57 %)	$\dfrac{37}{96}$ (39 %) $p< 0,05$

In contrast to the wild virus strains avirulent mutant
strains (syn and TK$^-$ strains of HSV-1 and HSV-2) produced weak
peripheral infection. The virus disappeared from the vagina
early (Fig. 4), and the viral titres, which developed in the

48

vagina, were low (Table 6). Consequently, latency was very rare and no mice died (Table 6).

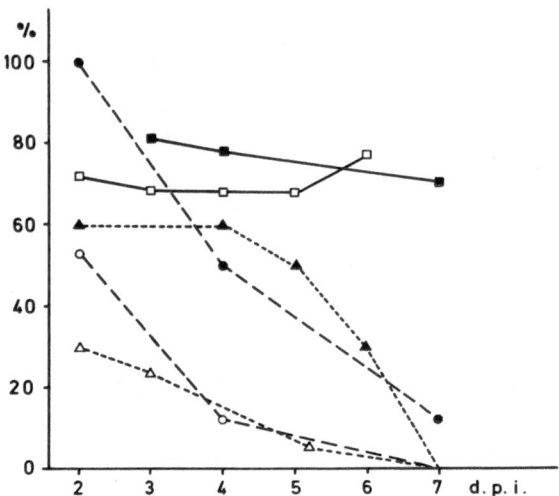

Fig. 4   Percentage of positive swabs after vaginal infection of NMRI mice with wild virus strains of HSV-1 ——— and HSV-2 ——— , syn mutant strains of HSV-1 o----o and HSV-2 o----o, and TK⁻ strains of HSV-1 .... and HSV-2 .... .

TABLE 6   Vaginal infection with wild and mutant strains of HSV. *Tested in C57 Bl mice for reasons mentioned above.

	HSV-1 wild-type*	HSV-1+2 syn	HSV-1+2 TK⁻
Titer in the vagina, 2 d.p.i.	$10^{3,5}$	$10^{2,4}$	$10^{1,4}$
Latency established	$\frac{47}{67}$ (70 %)	$\frac{4}{18}$ (22 %)	$\frac{0}{26}$ (0 %)
Lethality	$\frac{34}{108}$ (31 %)	$\frac{0}{31}$ (0 %)	$\frac{0}{27}$ (0 %)

CONCLUSION

It is known that the capacity of establishing latency is controlled by viral genes and, under special conditions, independent of virus replication (Lofgren et al., 1977). Taking

the non-injured mucous membranes as inoculation site, however,
adequate virus production in the epithelium seems to be
required for the invasion of the virus into the nervous system.
In the ganglia the acute productive infection is changed to
latent infection, and infected cells are eliminated to some
extent (Walz et al., 1976). The effectiveness of this change
and elimination determines the spread of virus in the ganglia
and the possible invasion into the central nervous system.
Depending upon the mode of immunization, immune factors
influenced both the peripheral and ganglionic infection. The
natural resistance of the host, however, manifested itself
predominantly in ganglionic infection, and the virulence of
viral strains, predominantly in epithelial infection. In the
case of TK⁻ strains, there may be another mechanism, which
inhibits the reactivation of latent virus (Price and Khan,
1981).

REFERENCES

Dubbs, D.R. and Kit, S. 1964. Mutant strains of herpes
    simplex deficient in thymidine kinase-inducing activity.
    Virology, 22, 493-502.
Hilfenhaus, J., Christ, H., Köhler, R., Moser, H., Kirchner,
    H., Levy, H.B. 1981. Protectivity of herpes simplex
    virus antigens: Studies in mice on the adjuvant effect
    of PICLC and on the dependence of protection on T cell
    competence. Med. Microbiol. Immunol., 169, 225-235.
Kaerner, H.C., Baumgartl, D., Zeller, H., Schatten, R.,
    Ott-Hartmann, A. 1981. Peripheral pathogenicity in mice
    acquired by an originally non-pathogenic strain of
    herpes simplex virus after serial passages in mouse
    brain. Int. Workshop on Herpesviruses Bologna, Italy,
    July 27-31, 1981, page 151.
Lofgren, K.W., Stevens, J.G., Marsden, H.S., Subak-Sharpe, J.
    H. 1977. Temperature-sensitive mutants of herpes simplex
    virus differ in the capacity to establish latent infec-
    tions in mice. Virology, 76, 440-443.
Lopez, C. 1975. Genetics of natural resistance to Herpesvirus
    infections in mice. Nature, 258, 152-153.
Munk, K. and Donner, D. 1963. Cytopathischer Effekt und
    Plaque-Morphologie verschiedener Herpes-Simplex-Virus-
    Stämme. Arch. ges. Virusforsch., 13, 529-540.
Price, R.W. and Khan, A. 1981. Resistance of peripheral auto-
    nomic neurons to in vivo productive infection by herpes
    simplex virus mutants deficient in thymidine kinase
    activity. Inf. Immun., 34, 571-580.
Schneweis, K.E., Sommerhäuser, H., Huber, D. 1972. Biologic
    and immunologic comparison of two plaque variants of

herpes simplex virus type 1. Arch. ges. Virusforsch.,
38, 338346.

Schneweis, K.E., Gruber, J., Hilfenhaus, J., Möslein, A.,
Kayser, M., Wolff, M.H. 1981. The influence of different
modes of immunization on the experimental genital herpes
simplex virus infection of mice. Med. Microbiol.
Immunol., 169, 269279.

Schneweis, K.E., Olbrich, M., Saftig, V., Scholz, R. 1982.
Effects of genetic resistance against herpes simplex
virus in vaginally infected mice. Manuscript submitted
to Med. Microbiol. Immunol.

Sturn, B. and Schneweis, K.E. 1978. Protective effect of an
oral infection with herpes simplex virus type 1 against
subsequent genital infection with herpes simplex virus
type 2. Med. Microbiol. Immunol., 165, 119127.

Thouless, M.E. 1972. Serological properties of thymidine kinase produced in cells infected with type 1 or type 2 herpesvirus. J. gen. Virol., 17, 307315.

Walz, M.A., Yamamoto, H., Notkins, A.L. 1976. Immunological
response restricts number of cells in sensory ganglia
infected with herpes simplex virus. Nature, 264, 554556.

Supported by Deutsche Forschungsgemeinschaft Nr. SCHN 174/6-1

DIFFERENCES OF HSV2 STRAINS IN THEIR EFFICIENCY OF ESTABLISHING LATENT INFECTIONS IN GANGLIA OF GUINEA PIGS

M. Scriba

Sandoz Forschungsinstitut, Brunnerstr. 59,
A-1235 Wien, Austria

ABSTRACT
    Pathogenesis of HSV2 infections in guinea pigs after s.c. or i.d. inoculation is described as characterized by primary lesions, continuous virus persistence in ganglia and skin and spontaneously developing recurrent herpes. In contrast to 9 HSV2 strains assayed previously in this model which were all found to behave similarly, three more HSV2 strains studied were found to have reduced pathogenicity. They induced less primary lesions, rare or no recurrent herpes and had reduced capacity to establish latent ganglionic infection. They persisted, however, in peripheral tissues to the same extent as the virulent strains. One of these three strains was a thymidine kinase negative mutant. In the case of the other two strains the molecular basis for the lack of pathogenicity and failure to establish latency in ganglia is not clear.

Infections of guinea pigs with herpes simplex virus type 2 (HSV2) either subcutaneously (s.c.) or intradermally (i.d.) into the footpad lead to development of primary herpes at the site of inoculation, characterized by inflammation and vesiculation. These lesions usually resolve spontaneously within 2 to 3 weeks. A life-long clinically asymptomatic infection is established thereafter during which the virus persists in a latent state in the sensory ganglia subserving the initially inoculated foot. Unlike in experimentally infected mice or rabbits or naturally infected humans, however, in guinea pigs the virus persists in addition to and independently from ganglionic infection, in the initially inoculated site of the skin. After s.c. inoculation virus is found even more regularly to persist locally than in ganglia (Table 1). In both sites virus is not dectable by any direct assay but only after cultivation of the explanted tissue in vitro (Scriba and Tatzber, 1981). Yet the virus persists probably in different states in ganglia and skin: in ganglia virus is most likely to reside in a latent, i.e. non-replicative, state, whereas some indirect evidence was obtained that virus in the skin is maintained as a low-grade productive infection (Scriba, 1981). The asymptomatic infection may often be interrupted by phases of virus reactivation and subsequent appearance of recurrent herpes at the site of initial inoculation. The recurrent herpes develops spontaneously and so far no mechanism triggering these exacerbations could be identified. The majority of these recrudescences are apparently induced by virus reactivated in latently infected ganglia. The role of virus persisting in the peripheral tissue for the pathogenesis of the infection is still unclear. We have assayed the pathogenicity of 9 different strains of HSV2 in this model, including old laboratory strains as well as a number of recent clinical isolates (Scriba and Tatzber, 1981). All 9 strains tested were found to induce primary and recurrent herpes to a similar extent suggesting that all these strains do not also differ in their ability to establish latent infections in ganglia.

In continuation of these studies we assayed a number of laboratory strains in this model and found so far 3 strains to be non-pathogenic for guinea pigs, namely C5a, HG52 and N9 (Table 2). C5a is a thymidine kinase negative (tk) mutant of the pathogenic strain 72, the strain with which most of our animal experiments have been performed; HG52 was obtained from Dr. Subak-Sharpe's laboratory in Glasgow; N9 is a derivative of strain MS, adapted to growth at $25^{o}C$ by Dr. H.F. Maassab, Ann Arbor (Maassab and McFarland, 1973). Clone N9 was isolated by 3 cycles of plaque-purification from his stock of this so called "cold variant".

After s.c. inoculation with these 3 strains the incidence of primary herpes was markedly lower than after infection with strain 72; this difference was most pronounced after infection with strain HG52 (18% versus 75% in 72-infected controls). After i.d. infection only the HG52 infected animals showed a reduced proportion of primary herpes; all 3 strains induced, however, less severe symptoms than strain 72. More interesting is the considerably reduced proportion of animals developing recurrent herpes after infection with these attenuated strains, most pronounced again in the HG52-infected animals, where none

TABLE 1   Recovery of HSV2, strain 72 from explants of footpad skin and dorsal root ganglia after s.c. or i.d. footpad infection

Day after infection	Subcutaneous		Intradermal	
	Footpad	Ganglia	Footpad	Ganglia
20 – 100	37/37 (100)[+]	45/75 (60)	14/17 (82)	18/21 (86)
100 – 400	78/83 (94)	37/79 (47)		17/32 (53)

[+] Number of animals positive/number tested (percent)

TABLE 2 Clinical observations and persistent infections after s.c. or i.d. inoculation with HSV strains

Inoculation	Strain	Clinical observations		Recovery of virus from	
		Primary lesions	Recurrent lesions	Footpad	Ganglia
s.c.	72	24/32*	21/31	28/28	11/24
	C5a	8/25	2/25	22/22	0/21
	HG52	3/17	0/17	34/34[+]	2/32
	N9	5/16	3/16	11/11	0/11
i.d.	72	12/12	6/12	8/12	10/11
	C5a	5/6	1/6	5/6	0/6
	HG52	11/17	0/17	4/17	3/17
	N9	6/6	1/6	1/5	1/5

* Number of animals positive/number tested

+ Virus isolation ratios of HG52 infected animals are the summary of 2 separate experiments. In the first experiment no clinical observation had been performed

TABLE 3   In vitro characteristics of HSV 2 strains

Strain	Virus yield[a] in		TK activity[d] induced in		Virus yield at 38.5°/34°C in	
	GPF[b]	Vero[c]	Vero	GPF	Vero	GPF
72	1.2×10^4	7.1×10^4	83.2	42.9	0.39	7.10
C5a	1.8×10^4	6.4×10^4	0.6	0.6	0.11	5.26
HG52	1.2×10^4	6.0×10^4	68.8	51.6	0.03	3.29
N9	5.8×10^3	8.2×10^4	75.5	n.t.[f]	0.01	4.23
Mock			0.4	0.6		

a PFU/0.2 ml

b moi 0.03, 72 h incubation 36°C

c moi 0.003, 48 h incubation 36°C

d cpm x 10^{-3} of [^{125}I] deoxycytidine phosphorylated in a 20 min assay (performed as described by Fong and Scriba 1980)

e PFU obtained after 72 h incubation at 38.5°C/PFU obtained after 72 h at 34°C

f not tested

of 34 animals developed recurrent lesions.

Animals were then assayed for virus persisting in dorsal root ganglia and footpad skin by cocultivation of these tissues on primary rabbit kidney cells. All s.c. infected animals were shown to harbor virus in their inoculated footpad, demonstrating that successful infection had occurred in all animals with all 4 strains of virus. In none of the C5a or N9 infected animals and in only 6% of HG52 infected animals was virus detectable in ganglia, whereas strain 72 was recovered from ganglia of 46% of the guinea pigs. After i.d. inoculation HSV2 persists less regularly in the footpad skin but more frequently in the ganglia than after s.c. infection. After this route of infection C5a was shown to remain in the skin only, the proportion of positive animals being even higher than in the 72-infected group. HG52 and N9 on the other hand were found in both sites, skin and ganglia, at reduced ratios.

The reduced incidence of latent ganglionic infections established by these 3 strains could be the consequence of reduced replication in peripheral tissue and accordingly of less virus reaching the ganglia. To test this possibility we measured virus replication in the footpad skin after s.c. infection. Figure 1 demonstrates that after infection with the virulent virus 72 infectious virus was detectable in all animals assayed at 24 h post infection (p.i.), the percentage of positive animals decreasing thereafter until day 11, by which time virus was undetectable in tissue homogenates. Also highest titers of virus were usually observed around 24 - 48 h p.i. (Figure 2). Virus titers in the skin were, therefore, determined at 24 and 48 h after infection with the various virus strains (Figure 3). Another virulent strain, K979, was included in this experiment in additon to strain 72. Virus titers varied considerably among animals of the same group. Since only 3 animals were assayed per virus and time point these data have to be viewed with caution. There is no evidence, however, that strains N9 and HG52 would replicate less well in the skin than the virulent strains. Only C5a reached lower titers than strain 72 at 24 h p.i., a difference which was no longer observed at 48 h. Thus, an impaired

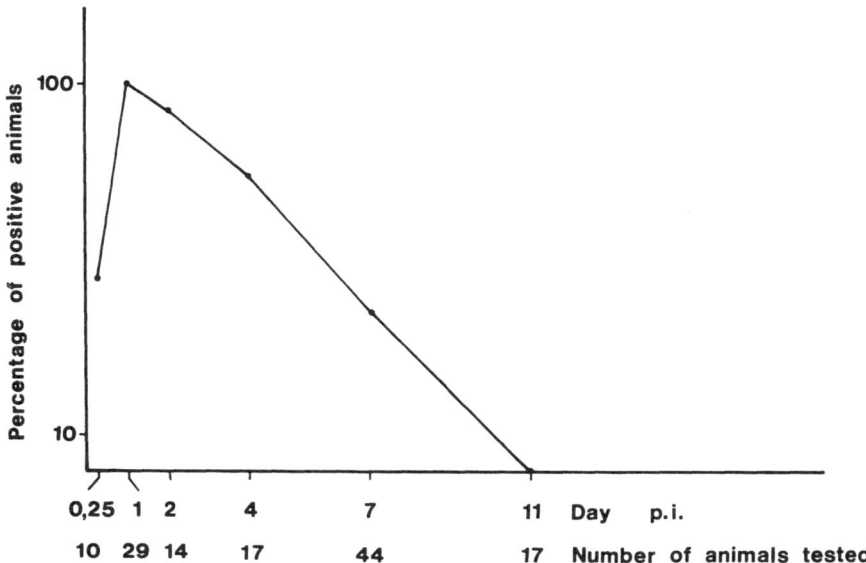

<u>Figure 1</u> Percentage of animals in which virus was detectable in homogenized footpad skin after s.c. infection with 10^4 PFU of HSV 2 strain 72.

capacity to replicate in the skin is probably not the explanation for the failure of these strains to effectively induce latent infections in ganglia.

Inability to induce latent infections in the nervous system has so far been reported for two types of mutants of HSV1: temperature-sensitive (ts) and tk mutants. Thus Lofgren and coworkers (1977) have shown that some but not all ts mutants of HSV1 were unable to establish latency in the dorsal root ganglia or the brain of mice. No specific mutation could however be associated with the latency negative strains. A specific mutation namely the lack of tk could on the other hand be related to a failure to establish latency in ganglia of mice and guinea pigs (Tenser and Dunstan, 1979; Tenser, Miller and Rapp, 1979). Such mutants cannot replicate in neurons, which are non-dividing cells and, therefore, probably lack any enzymes needed for thymidylate synthesis, be it by de-novo or by salvage pathways. Tk viruses can, however, grow in peripheral tissue, i.e. in potentially dividing cells.

58

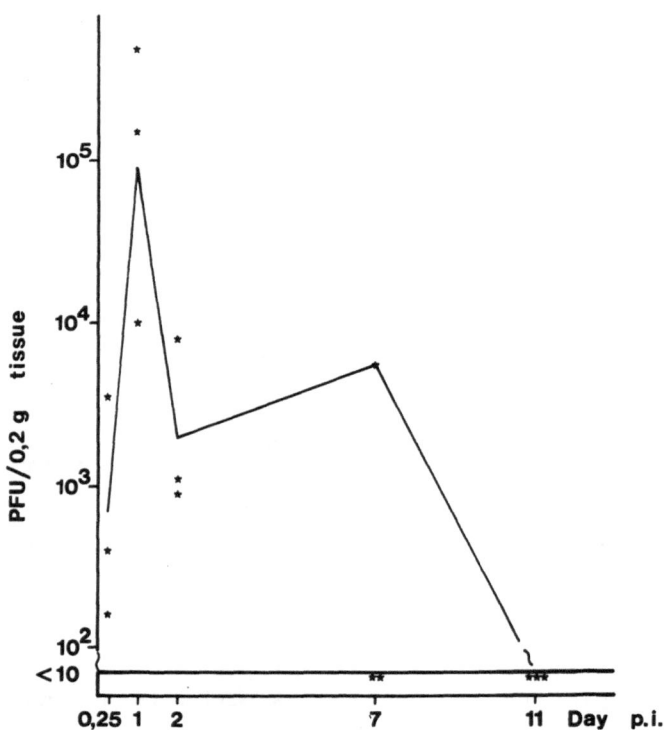

Figure 2 Virus titers in homogenized footpad skin after
s.c. infection with strain 72. Three animals were assayed
per time point. Stars indicate individual titers, the line
shows geometric means.

It was, therefore, not unexpected, that our tk⁻ mutant of
HSV2 would not induce latent infections in ganglia. The fact
that it gave rise to a few recurrent exacerbations can probably
be interpreted as evidence that occasionally also the virus
resident in the skin can be activated to induce recurrent
lesions. The basis for the reduced ratios of latency and of
subsequent recurrent infections induced by the other two
strains, HG52 and N9, is not clear. Particularly striking is
the total inability of HG52 to induce recurrent infections
although it was at least occasionally detectable in ganglia.
    The strains were tested for their growth capacity in
guinea pig cells in vitro, for tk induction and for growth at

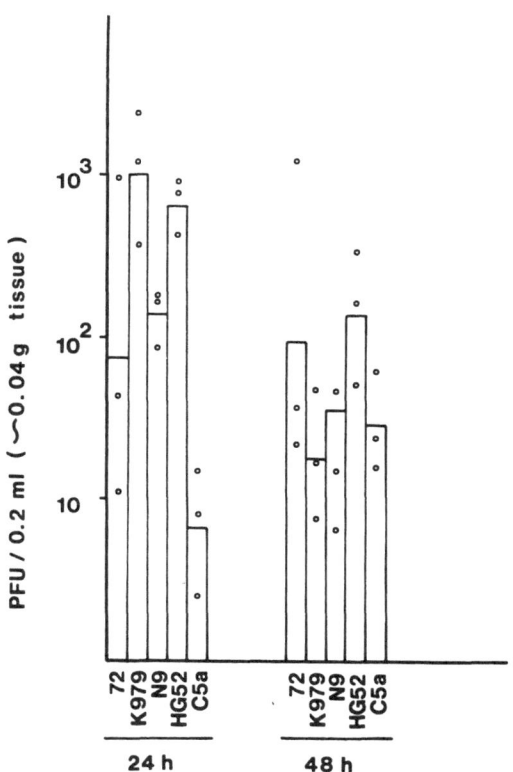

Figure 3 Virus titers in footpad skin 24 and 48 h after s.c. infection with 10^4 PFU of five different strains. Circles indicate individual titers, columns represent the geometric mean of three animals tested.

elevated temperatures (Table 3). N9 and HG52 induced tk activity similar to strain 72 in Vero cells as well as in guinea pig fibroblasts (GPF). Also, virus yields were essentially similar in both types of cells, although highest titers were obtained later in GPF than in Vero (72 h in GPF inoculated at a moi of 0.03, 48 h in Vero cells inoculated at a moi of 0.003). However, this was true for all four virus strains tested. To assay for ts markers, virus growth at $34^{\circ}C$ was compared to that at $38.5^{\circ}C$. Strains 72 and C5a were only slightly reduced at $38.5^{\circ}C$ in Vero cells, whereas both strain N9 and HG52 showed more than one log reduction. This did not, however, hold in GPF, where all four strains exhibited better growth at $38.5^{\circ}C$ than at $34^{\circ}C$.

Thus, for both strains HG52 and N9 lack of tk, temperature sensitivity or host range mutation was not the explanation for their inability to efficiently induce latent ganglionic infections in guinea pigs. We have so far not studied whether these strains can replicate in neurons. The question also remains open for all three strains studied here, whether the failure to recover virus from ganglia was really due to the inability of these strains to establish latent infections or rather due to the inability to be reactivated. Failure to replicate in neurons, which has at least been demonstrated for tk⁻ strains of HSV1, might well prevent reactivation in vivo as well as in vitro. Accordingly other techniques should be applied than cocultivation to search for latent virus, before differences in the efficiency with which virus strains establish latency can be proved.

I would like to speculate in this context, that differences among virus strains in going latent or even more in being reactivated from a latent state in neurons are an explanation for the different courses of herpes infections observed in the natural human infection. Inherent differences of the herpes strains may be the reason why a large proportion of humans who have antibodies against the virus and, therefore, most likely carry a latent infection, never develop overt recurrent disease, whereas in others frequent recurrences develop. It would, therefore, be very interesting to compare the pathogenicity of virus strains recovered from ganglia of individuals without history of recurrent herpes with the pathogenicity of isolates obtained from recurrent lesions.

REFERENCES

Fong, B.S. and Scriba, M. 1980. Use of (^{125}I)deoxycytidine to detect herpes simplex virus-specific thymidine kinase in tissues of latently infected guinea pigs. J. Virol., 34, 644-649.
Lofgren, K.W., Stevens, J.G., Marsden, H.S. and Subak-Sharpe, J.H. 1977. Temperature-sensitive mutants of herpes simplex virus differ in the capacity to establish latent infections in mice. Virology, 76, 440-443.

Maassab, H.F. and McFarland, C.R. 1973. Characterization of herpes simplex virus types 1 and 2 adapted to growth at 25°C. J. gen. Virol., 19, 151-153.

Scriba, M. 1981. Persistence of herpes simplex virus infection in ganglia and peripheral tissues of guinea pigs. Med. Microbiol. Immunol., 169, 91-96.

Scriba, M. and Tatzber, F. 1981. Pathogenesis of herpes simplex virus infections in guinea pigs. Infect. Immun., 34, 655-661.

Tenser, R.B. and Dunstan, M. 1979. Herpes simplex virus thymidine kinase expression in infection of the trigeminal ganglion. Virology, 99, 417-422.

Tenser, R.B., Miller, R.L. and Rapp, F. 1979. Trigeminal ganglion infection by thymidine kinase-negative mutants of herpes simplex virus. Science, 205, 915-917.

HERPES SIMPLEX VIRUS TYPES 1 AND 2 GENES AFFECTING LATENCY IN MOUSE FOOTPAD AND SENSORY GANGLIA

J.H. Subak-Sharpe, S.A. Al-Saadi*, G.B. Clements

Institute of Virology, University of Glasgow,
Church Street, Glasgow, G11 5JR, England
*University of Baghdad

Following a primary infection in man, Herpes Simplex Virus (HSV) usually persists in the latent state and remains there lifelong. However periodically it may become spontaneously reactivated and infectious virus is produced - which can result in overt clinical disease (Wildy et al., 1982). The latent HSV genome persists in sensory ganglia both in man and in some laboratory animals, and can be experimentally reactivated by explantation of ganglia and culture in vitro (Stevens and Cook, 1971; Bastian et al., 1972; Stevens, 1975; Barringer, 1975).

The viral genome appears to be latent within the sensory neuroses of dorsal root ganglia (McLennan and Darby, 1980), but recovery from central nervous tissue, autonomic ganglia and the adrenal gland have also been reported (Nesburn et al., 1972; Knotts et al., 1973; Price et al., 1975; Cook and Stevens, 1976; Warren et al., 1978). Skin explants from the sites in man at which HSV recurrences had been observed have not yielded virus (Rustigan et al., 1976). However, recurrent HSV has been observed in patients with 'blow-out' fractures which had severed the nerve supply to the area of skin involved (Hoyt and Billson, 1976).

HSV-1 and HSV-2 have been isolated from the site of isolation (footpad and vagina) of latently infected guinea pigs (Scriba, 1976, 1977; Donnenberg et al., 1980). HSV-1 has been isolated also from the ear skin (the site of inoculation) in 8% of latently infected mice in the absence of overt clinical lesions (Hill et al., 1980). In the course of experiments aimed to study the viral genes influencing the ability of HSV to induce latency in mice, we have made new observations highly relevant to the above problem and have to date recovered HSV-1 and HSV-2 from the mouse footpad as well as dorsal root ganglia three months or more after inoculation.

HSV-1 strain 17 <u>wt</u>, HSV-2 strain HG52 <u>wt</u> and derived temperature sensitive <u>(ts)</u> mutants (Timbury, 1971; Brown et al., 1973; Halliburton and Timbury, 1973, 1976; Marsden et al., 1976) were used to inoculate Biozii (high antibody responder) strain mice via the rear footpad. The mouse core body temperature (38.5°C) is nonpermissive for the <u>ts</u> mutants used. Though the footpads may be somewhat below the core temperature when the mice are active, while they are close packed asleep in the nest the footpads will be at or near the core temperature. The mice were kept minimally for three months after infection and then tested by explanting the dorsal root ganglia (DRG) and footpad skin (FP) into culture and incubating at 31°C with daily screening for production of infectious virus. Following infection with HSV-1 <u>wt</u> at doses between 10^5-10^6 pfu/mouse, the Biozzi mice showed some initial footpad swelling and reddening of the skin, but none became permanently paralysed and all survived (Clements and Subak-Sharpe, 1983). None of the mice infected with HSV-1 <u>ts</u> mutants or with HSV-2 <u>wt</u> or <u>ts</u> mutant virus showed any evidence of illness and none died (Al-Saadi et al., 1983). The Biozzi strain thus is a member of the resistant group of mouse strains like the C57 Bl/6 strain described by Lopez (1975) and Kirchner et al. (1977).

Virus was never detected in the supernatant from explanted DRG earlier than the sixth day after explantation. The majority of BHS reactivations from explanted ganglia first appeared between days 7 and 14 and the latest time at which virus was first detected was 24 days after DRG explantation. To our initial surprise we reproducibly obtained virus reactivation also from footpad explants in mice infected with 10^5/10^6 pfu of HSV-1 and HSV-2 wt. No virus was recovered from the footpad of the 19 mice inoculated with less than 10^5 pfu of HSV-1 wt, though their DRG explants were positive in 14 cases (Table 1). The footpad

cultures never shed virus before the tenth day after
explantation and on one occasion not until the 42nd day. We
have never detected virus in tissue homogenates made
immediately after explantation, which is in accord with other
reports (Cook and Stevens, 1976; Hill and Blyth, 1976). At
the doses of HSV used in the present study virus was never
recovered from the left DRG or the left footpad,
contralateral to the site of inoculation. The virus which
reactivated from mice initially infected with a ts mutant in
every case (except for two mice inoculated with tsI) proved
to have retained the ts phenotype. Using the restriction
enzymes BamHI, BglII, HindIII, KpnI and EcoRI (Lonsdale et
al., 1979; Lonsdale, 1979), the DNA fragment profiles of
reactivated viruses were compared with the profiles of the
virus used for initial infection and in very case shown to be
unchanged.

As can be seen from Table 1, HSV-2 wt virus was
recovered with high efficiency from the DRG but much less
frequently from the footpad. As far as the HSV-2 ts mutants
are concerned, ts 5 and ts 10 have not been recovered either
from DRG or from the footpad; mutants ts 3, ts 9 and ts 12
have only been recovered from explanted footpad; mutants ts
11 and ts 13 have been recovered from DRG only; the remaining
six HSV-2 mutants were all recoverable both from DRG and
footpad; but whilst ts 1, ts 6 and ts 7 were obtained from
either site with approximately equal frequency, ts 2, ts 4
and ts 8 reactivated much more frequently from the DRG. HSV-1
wt virus, after initial inoculation with >10^5 pfu, was
readily recovered from DRG or footpad. There is efficient
recovery from DRG of latent HSV-1 sw (these mice were
initially inoculated with 10^3 or more pfu) and the HSV-1
mutants D syn, tsI syn and tsF syn; ts G syn and ts K syn
have not been recovered so far from the DRG of Biozzi strain
mice; ts K syn is the only HSV-1 ts mutant so far tested to
have been recovered from the footpad. The pattern of recovery
of these HSV-1 ts mutants from the latent state in mice
differs in some respects (eg tsI) from that previously

TABLE 1   Recovery of HSV (wt) and (ts) mutants following
           explantation of dorsal root ganglia and footpad
           from latently infected mice (three months after
           initial inoculation into the footpad of the right
           hind limb)

Virus inoculated	pfu/mouse inoculated	DNA phenotype	DRG positive/ total (%)		Footpad positive/ total (%)	
HSV-1						
wt 17 syn$^+$	10^6-10^7	+	Yes$^+$		7/7	(100)
wt 17 syn$^+$	10^5-10^6	+	Yes$^+$		7/9	(78)
wt 17 syn$^+$	10^4-10^5	+	11/15	(73)	0/15	(0)
wt 17 syn$^+$	10^3-10^4	+	3/4	(75)	0/4	(0)
ts D syn	6×10^5	–	3/5	(60)	0/5	(0)
ts I syn	1×10^6	+	10/10	(100)	0/9	(0)
ts F syn	1×10^7	+	8/12	(67)	0/12	(0)
ts G syn*	3.7×10^6	+	0/15	(0)	0/14	(0)
ts K syn	1×10^5	–	0/10	(0)	2/10	(20)
HSV-2						
wt HG52	1×10^6	+	6/6	(100)	2/6	(33)
wt HG52	1×10^5	+	11/13	(85)	1/14	(7)
ts 1	1×10^5	–	4/11	(36)	2/10	(20)
ts 2	1.7×10^6	–	8/17	(47)	1/16	(6)
ts 3	1.2×10^5	+	0/16	(0)	5/15	(33)
ts 4	5×10^6	+	12/14	(86)	1/14	(7)
ts 5	1.7×10^6	+	0/12	(0)	0/12	(0)
ts 6	1×10^6	–	1/16	(6)	1/16	(6)
ts 7	8×10^5	–	2/14	(14)	1/11	(9)
ts 8	2.5×10^5	–	5/14	(35)	1/9	(11)
ts 9	7.5×10^5	–	0/11	(0)	1/11	(18)
ts 10	2.5×10^5	–	0/13	(0)	0/9	(0)
ts 11	4.2×10^5	–	1/12	(8)	0/12	(0)
ts 12	5×10^5	+	0/14	(0)	1/14	(7)
ts 13	6×10^5	+	2/14	(14)	0/14	(7)

+   Assayed after dissociation of ganglia pooled from
     several mice thus no data available on individual mice.
*   Thymidine kinase negative at both the permissive and
     non-permissive temperatures.

Legend to Table 1:

Three to four week old Biozzi (high antibody responder) mice were injected subcutaneously into the right rear footpad with 10^4-10^6 pfu/mouse of HSV-1 wt, HSV-2 wt or one of five HSV-1 or thirteen HSV-2 ts mutants. At least three months after primary infection (when the mice were totally asymptomatic), the mice were killed using chloroform. Nine ipsilateral (one sacral, six lumber, two thoracic) and two contralateral dorsal root ganglia (DRG) were dissected out and explanted under aseptic conditions. In addition, footpad tissue from both the left and the right sides was also explanted from each mouse and cultured as organ culture in vitro at 31°C. In 18 cases out of the total of 286, the explanted footpad became contaminated during culture and had to be discarded. Explant cultures of individual ganglia and footpad tissue were maintained in Eagle's minimum essential medium (Glasgow modified) supplemented 50% foetal calf serum, penicillin 100/units/ml, streptomycin 100 ug/ml, gentamicin 25 ug/ml and nystatin 25 units/ml. Released virus was detected by screening the supernatant on semi-confluent BHK cells grown in microtitre plates. The screening procedure was carried out daily for the explanted footpad cultures and twice weekly for DRG. Recovered viruses were screened for growth on C13 cells both at 31°C and 38.5°C (the permissive and non-permissive temperatures). A mouse in which either the footpad or any ganglion released infectious virus was scored as positive. The first screening always took place within 24 hours after explantation.

reported (Lofgren et al., 1977; Watson et al., 1980), but major differences distinguish the two experimental systems used: notably the route of inoculation, the mouse strain and the method of screening, though the same virus mutants were used in both studies.

The distribution of ganglia from which HSV-2 was recovered differed between the latency positive mutants; wt, ts 1, ts 2 and ts 4 were recovered from a number of ganglia, while the other mutants were shed from only one or two ganglia innervating the footpad (Table 2).

Our results suggest the following tentative conclusions:

1. Non-recovery of HSV-1 ts G syn and HSV-2 ts 5 and ts 10 from either site may indicate that these three mutants are deficient in functions necessary to establish or maintain latency in Biozzi mice or for successful reactivation following explantation.

2. The recovery of HSV-2 mutants (ts 3, ts 9 and ts 12) and of HSV-1 mutant ts K syn only from explanted footpads suggests that HSV can go latent in mouse tissues other than, and apparently independent of, the DRG.

3. Recovery only from DRG of the HSV-1 mutants ts D syn, ts I syn, and ts F syn and HSV-2 mutants ts 11 and ts 13 further supports the notion of independent states of latency in footpad and DRG.

4. Only a minority of mice produced virus both from the footpad and from DRG following explantation, one infected with HSV-2 wt and one each with ts 4, ts 7 and ts 8. (In the case of HSV-1 wt, the ganglia from several mice were pooled and it is not possible to correlate release of virus from the DRG and footpads). This further supports the hypothesis that HSV-2 can produce latent infection independently at the two sites.

5. The observed differences in recoverability of HSV-1 and HSV-2 ts mutants suggest that the genetic control of the ability of HSV to produce latent infection is not simple and involves several virus gene functions. It is relevant that some DNA positive and some DNA negative

TABLE 2   Anatomical distribution of DRG* from which HSV-2 was successfully reactivated in latently infected Biozzi mice **

Virus***	Dose (pfu/mouse)	No.mice dissected	No.mice +ve	Right Sacral	Right Lumbar						Right Thoracic	
				1	6	5	4	3	2	1	13	12
wt	1×10^5	13	11	1	1	5	6	2	1	0	0	0
wt	1×10^6	6	6	0	3	5	3	0	0	0	0	0
ts 1	1×10^5	11	4	0	1	2	1	0	0	0	0	0
ts 2	1.7×10^6	17	8	2	4	3	2	0	0	0	0	0
ts 4	5×10^6	14	12	2	5	6	4	0	0	0	0	0
ts 6	1×10^6	16	1	0	0	0	1	0	0	0	0	0
ts 7	8×10^5	14	2	0	0	2	2	0	0	0	0	0
ts 8	2.5×10^5	14	5	0	3	2	0	0	0	0	0	0
ts 11	4.2×10^5	12	1	0	1	0	0	0	0	0	0	0
ts 13	6×10^5	14	2	0	2	1	0	0	0	0	0	0
Total		197	52	5	20	26	19	2	1	0	0	0

*   No virus was ever recovered from left sided DRG.

**   The figures under each column indicate the numbers of mice positive with regard to virus recovery from that DRG.

***   ts 3 (18 mice), ts 5 (12), ts 9 (11), ts 10 (15) and ts 12 (14) have not been recovered from DRG.

mutants were shown to induce latent infection while others failed to do so (Table 1).

With the exception of two isolates from mice inoculated with ts I, all the reactivants retained the ts phenotype which excludes reversion to wt as an explanation for their successful recovery from latency. We cannot rule out the possibility that some leakiness allowing replication may have occurred, particularly in the footpad which may not always have been at the mouse core temperature. Any leak-through would allow the mutant genes parial function and therefore could favour the establishment of latency. Thus some ts mutants with latency relevant function may have escaped detection. But the non-recovery of mutants ts G, ts 5 and ts 10 strongly suggests that their functions are essential for the establishment of or reactivation from latency.

We have recovered virus from the footpads of 16 HSV-1 inoculated and 17 HSV-2 inoculated Biozzi mice which had been asymptomatic for at least three months. In the case of HSV-1 mutant ts K and HSV-2 mutants ts 3, ts 9 and ts 12 virus has only been recovered from the footpad and not from the DRG. Scriba (1981) has reported the recovery of HSV-2 from footpad skin, but not the dorsal root ganglia of guinea-pigs infected with virus into the footpad 10 days after surgical denervation. Recovery of virus from the peripheral regions may be due either to reactivation of virus latent within nervous tissue which subsequently travels via a nerve to the peripheral site, or to the presence of virus over a long period in some cells at peripheral sites: although these two possibilities are not mutually exclusive. We think it most unlikely that the input virus could have persisted either as such or in a slowly replicating form during the three months or more between inoculation and dissection. Moreover we have never recovered virus directly from homogenates of the footpad immediately after such explantation. This includes four cases when we cut a footpad lengthwise in half and homogenised one half while explanting the other with subsequent sucessful reactivation. We are forced to conclude that the virus is capable of establishing a latent infection in the footpad and, as neural cell bodies have never been described as located in the footpad, it follows that HSV can become latent in cells of the mouse other than neurones. The difference in timing of reactivation from the footpad and dorsal root ganglia may be a reflection of this. However, at present we cannot exclude the possibility that mechanical trapping after reactivation but before release of virus from the footpad tissue contribute to the difference in timing. It does not seem very likely that trapping alone could lead to the large and consistent difference observed.

Our overall conclusions are: 1) that HSV wt and HSV-2 and some ts mutants can be recovered from the footpad of latently infected totally asymptomatic Biozzi mice. 2) Recovery of virus from the footpad is apparently dose-dependent as suggested by the results using HSV-1 wt (Table 1). 3) Both HSV-1 and HSV-2 can be recovered from the dorsal root ganglia. 4) HSV can establish latent infection in dorsal root ganglia and footpad independently and 5) the ability to go latent at these sites is affected by ts mutations in several different HSV genes.

We wish to thank Miss M. Braidwood for her excellent technical assistance with this study.

REFERENCES
Al-Saadi, S.A., Clements, G.B. and Subak-Sharpe, J.H. 1983. J. gen. Virol. In press.
Barringer, J.R. 1975. Progress in Medical Virology, 20, 1-26.
Bastian, F.O., Rabson, A.S., Yee, C.L. and Tralka, T.S. 1972. Science, 178, 306-307.
Brown, S.M., Ritchie, D.A. and Subak-Sharpe, J.H. 1973. J. gen. Virol., 18, 329-346.
Clements, G.B. and Subak-Sharpe, J.H. "Progress in Brain Research". (P.O. Behan and V. Ter. Meulen, Eds.). In press. Elsevier, Holland.
Cook, M.L. and Stevens, J.G. 1976. J. gen. Virol., 31, 75-80.
Donnenberg, A.D., Chaikof, E. and Aurelian, L. 1980. Infect. and Immun., 30, 99-109.
Halliburton, I.W. and Timbury, M. 1973. Virology, 54, 60-68.
Halliburton, I.W. and Bimbury, M. 1976. J. gen. Virol., 30, 207-220.
Hill, T.J. and Blyth, W.A. 1976. Lancet (i), 397-399.

Hill, T.J., Harbour, D.A. and Blyth, W.A. 1980. J. gen.
    Virol., 47, 206-207.
Hoyt, C.S. and Billson, F.A. 1976. Lancet (ii), 1346-1365.
Kirchner, H., Hirt, H.M., Kochen, N. and Munk, K. 1978.
    Zschr. Immunitätsf. exp. Therapie, 154, 147-154.
Knotts, F.B., Cook, M.L. and Stevens, J.G. 1973. J. exp.
    Med., 138, 740-744.
Lofgren, K.W., Stevens, J.G., Marsden, H.S. and Subak-Sharpe,
    J.H. 1977. Virology, 76, 440-443.
Lonsdale, D.M., Brown, S.M., Subak-Sharpe, J.H., Warren, K.G.
    and Koprowski, H. 1979. J. gen. Virol., 43, 151-171.
Lonsdale, D.M. 1979. Lancet (i), 849-852.
Lopez, C. (1975). Nature (London), 258, 152-153.
Marsden, H.S., Crombie, I.R. and Subak-Sharpe, J.H. 1976. J.
    gen. Virol., 31, 347-372.
McLennan, J.L. and Darby, G. 1980. J. gen. Virol., 51,
    233-243.
Nesburn, A.B., Cook, M.L. and Stevens, J.G. 1972. Arch.
    Ophthalmology, 88, 411-418.
Price, R.W., Katz, B.J. and Notkins, A.L. 1975. Nature
    (London) 257, 686-688.
Rustigan, R., Smulow, J.B., Tye, M., Gibson, W.A. and
    Shindell, E. 1966. J. Investigative Dermatology, 47,
    218-221.
Scriba, M. 1976. Med. Microbiol. Immunol., 162, 201-208.
Scriba, M. 1977. Nature (London), 267, 529-531.
Scriba, M. 1981. Med. Microbiol. Immunol., 169, 91-96.
Stevens, J.G. 1975. Curr. Topics Microbiol. Immunol., 70,
    31-50.
Stevens, J.G. and Cook, M.L. 1971. Science, 173, 843-845.
Timbury, M.C. 1971. J. gen. Virol., 13, 373-376.
Warren, K.H., Brown, S.M., Wroblewska, Z., Gilden, D.,
    Koprowski, H. and Subak-Sharpe, J.H. 1978. New Engl. J.
    Med., 298, 1o68-1069.
Watson, K., Stevens, J.G., Cook, M.L. and Subak-Sharpe, J.H.
    1980. J. gen. Virol., 49, 149-159.
Wildy, P., Field, H.J. and Nash, A.A. 1982. In "Virus
    Persistence" SGM Symposium 33 (B.W.J. Mahy, A.C. Minson
    and G.K. Darby, Eds.), pp. 133-167. Cambridge University
    Press.

SESSION I

HUMAN, SIMIAN AND MURINE HERPESVIRUSES

Part 2

Chairman: J.H. Subak-Sharpe
Co-chairman: J.B. Hudson

NEW RESULTS ON THE BIOLOGY OF EPSTEIN-BARR-VIRUS

H. Wolf, G.J. Bayliss, R. Seibl

Max von Pettenkofer-Institut für Hygiene und
Medizinische Mikrobiologie, University of Munich, FRG

ABSTRACT

Epstein-Barr virus has been linked to infectious
mononucleosis and to the neoplastic diseases nasopharyngeal
carcinoma and Burkitt's lymphoma. The initial evidence for
these relationships was derived from seroepidemiological
studies. Since then other techniques such as nucleic acid
hybridization with tumor material have confirmed these
conclusions. Many studies from various groups have
contributed data. Some of these do not seem to fit into a
unifying concept - for example, EBV is a lymphotropic virus,
but the NPC tumor cells, which carry EBV, are epithelial.
From published data and experimental results obtained in our
laboratory a hypothetical model for the interaction of EBV
with its host - man - is developed.

INTRODUCTION

Epstein-Barr virus (EBV) is a human lymphotropic (human
herpesvirus 4). Its natural target cells are B-lymphocytes,
and receptors for EBV have been demonstrated only on this
cell type. The virus is the causative agent of infectious
mononucleosis and is associated with African Burkitt's
lymphoma, lymphoepithelial carcinoma of the nasopharynx, one
of the most frequent tumors of man in certain areas of
Southeast Asia, and fatal lymphoproliferative disorders in
immunologically compromised individuals (for recent reviews
see Henle and Henle, 1979; Wolf, H., 1981; Purtilo and Klein,
1981). The virus has been shown to be oncogenic for marmosets
(Miller et al., 1972) and is capable of transforming B-cells
from humans and other primates in vitro (Diehl et al., 1969;
Gerber et al., 1969). After primary infection the virus
remains latent in B-lymphocytes of the peripheral blood for
the remainder of the patient's life (Nilsson et al., 1971).
Each of the disease states associated with EBV has a
particular serological pattern (these are shown in Table 1;
data are taken from Henle and Henle, 1979).

EBV can be isolated from throat washings of apparently
healthy persons who have had a previous EBV infection (Gerber

TABLE 1   Antibodies to EBV antigen.

Disease	VCA: IgG	IgM	IgA	EA	EBNA
Normal adults	+	−	−	−	+
Acute infection (early)	++	+	−	+	−
Chronic infection	+	+	−	+	+
Reactivation	+	+	−	+	+
NPC	++	−	+	+(D)	+
BL	++	−	−	+(R)	+

et al., 1972). As shown in Table 1, these individuals have antibodies to EBV virus capsid antigen (VCA) and to the nuclear antigen (EBNA) but not to EBV early antigen (EA). These observations raise a number of questions which must be answered before we can understand the relationship between the virus and its host.

1) What is the source of virus in the throat washings of apparently healthy persons and why do apparently normal individuals who shed virus have antibodies only to VCA and EBNA?

2) How does the virus infect epithelial cells which apparently lack receptors for the virus?

3) How does the virus persist in cells lifelong and what are the molecular mechanisms underlying the regulated expression of EBV?

4) Can we develop a model including all observations described so far which could explain the uneven risk for NPC by taking into account additional parameters?

RESULTS

1) It might have been predicted that the EBV carrying lymphocytes in the oropharynx which escaped host control mechanisms would have been the source of the virus which can be obtained from healthy individuals. Studies of others (Morgan et al., 1979) indicated that EBV could be isolated from saliva collected from Stenson's duct.

Studies by us on parotid salivary gland tissue (Wolf et
al., 1981a,b) have suggested that the cells which
surround or are present in the lumen of the ducts of
this gland are capable of supporting a productive cycle
of EBV replication (Fig.1a,b). Production of EBV in
salivary duct cells could also explain the absence of
certain EBV specific serum antibodies in normal adults
(see also discussion). Searches of other tissues of the
oropharynx (e.g. tonsils from healthy individuals
Fig.1c) proved negative as no productively infected cell
could be found using in situ hybridization techniques.
In situ hybridization studies using tonsillar carcinoma

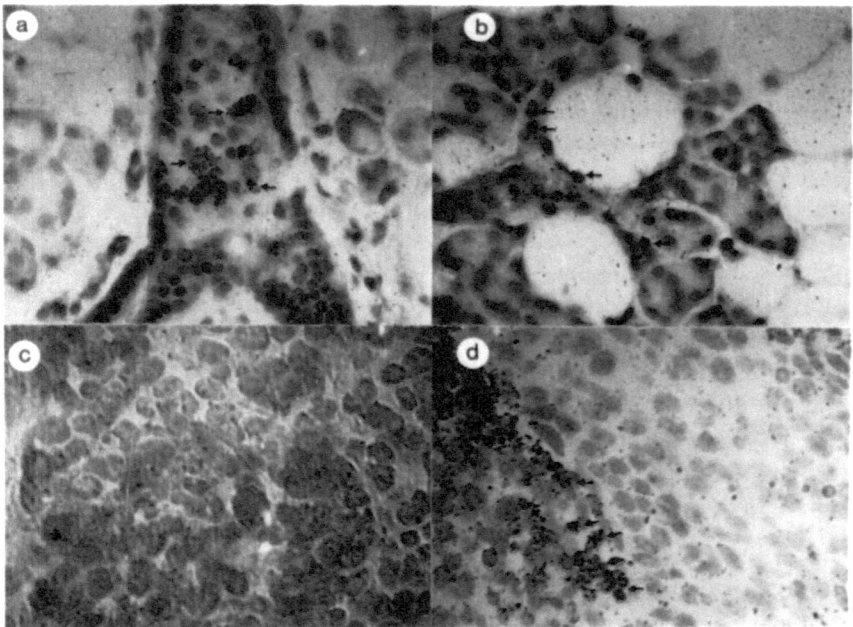

Fig. 1   In situ DNA-DNA hybridization of cryosections
of a,b) normal parotid gland, c) normal tonsil, d)
non-keratinizing tonsillar carcinoma. Cloned EBV DNA
which was labelled in vitro with ^{32}P-orthophosphate by
nick translation was used as a probe (see Wolf et al.,
1981b for methodology). Note that the producing cells
(arrow) in the parotis surround, or are present in, the
ducts (a+b), that the normal tonsil is EBV genome free
(c) and that the tonsillar carcinoma contains EBV
carrying cells (arrow) (d).

(T.C.) tissue, however, showed that 25% of the specimens
so far tested carried EBV in the epithelial cells
(Fig.1d). This situation resembles somewhat that seen
with Marek's disease virus, where the transformed cells
are T-cells but the lytic expression of the virus occurs
in the germinative epithelium of the feather follicle
(Calnek and Hitchner, 1969).

2) To date receptors for EBV have been demonstrated only on
B lymphocytes (Jondal and Klein, 1973; Wolf,H.,
unpublished observations) and no other normal
nonmalignant cell type. How then does the virus enter
such cells and persist within them? Initially
microinjection of EBV DNA into a wide variety of
receptor negative cells (Graesmann et al., 1980) and
later transfection with EBV DNA using the calcium
phosphate co-precipitation technique (Stoerker et al.,
1981; Miller et al., 1981) and the implantation of
receptor into the membranes of receptor negative cells
(Volsky et al., 1981) have been used to demonstrate that
once EBV overcomes the barrier to penetration, normal
expression of the virus can occur although synthesis of
EBNA was not observed when only lytic expression was
induced. It was proposed some time ago that syncitium
inducing viruses such as paramyxovirus might induce
fusion between lymphocytes and epithelial cells, thus
allowing the virus to gain access to such cells. Since
then we have demonstrated that EBV itself can induce
fusion. When densely packed monolayers of lymphoblastoid
cells (Bayliss and Wolf, 1981a) were infected with EBV
derived from the EBV producing cell line P3HR1, we
observed the formation of polykaryocytes. Further
studies in which we prepared mixed monolayers containing
both receptor positive (Raji) cells and receptor
negative cells (human fibroblasts, epithelioid cells or
T-lymphoblastoid cells) showed that an infected, EBV
expressing B-lymphoblastoid cell was capable of fusing
with a non-infected receptor negative cell. The

involvement of the receptor negative cell line in the
fusion event was clearly demonstrated when human
T-lymphoblasts were used in the mixed cultures, since we
could show the presence of T-cell specific antigens on
the surface of the polykaryocytes (Bayliss and Wolf,
1980). A close cell to cell contact as it occurs in
monolayers is necessary for the development of
polykaryocytes. The viral nature of the fusion event and
the mechanisms involved have been studied in detail
using chemical activation of latent genomes and various
metabolic inhibitors. It was shown that an early viral
protein was responsible for the fusion event (Bayliss
and Wolf, 1981b). More recent experiments (Fig.2) have
further substantiated the viral origin of the fusion
inducing protein(s). Purified EBV DNA was transfected
into unrelated cells (NIH 3T3 cells). In addition to the
synthesis of EBV EA, fusion of the transfected cells was
also observed. Further studies with this technique using
cloned fragments of the EBV genome should permit the
mapping of gene(s) encoding the fusion protein(s) on the
EBV genome.

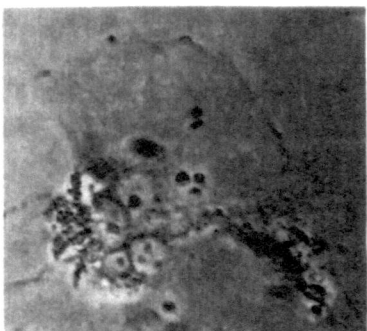

Fig. 2   The formation of polykaryocytes in NIH 3T3
cells transfected with EBV DNA. EBV DNA was purified
from virions isolated from cultures of P3HR1 cells. 10
µg EBV DNA was mixed with 10 µg of NIH 3T3 cell DNA as
carrier and co-precipitated with calcium phosphate
(according to Graham and van der Ebb, 1973). The
precipitate was added to the indicator cells and after
4 h at 37°C the cultures were washed and refed. 24 h
later the cultures were photographed using a phase
contrast photomicroscope. Note the presence of many
nuclei in the polykaryocyte.

3) Very little is known at the molecular level of the
    mechanisms which regulate the response of the cell to
    infection with EBV. As far as we know, all EBV carrying
    cell lines express a single viral antigen - EBNA. This
    protein could be a repressor protein which prevents

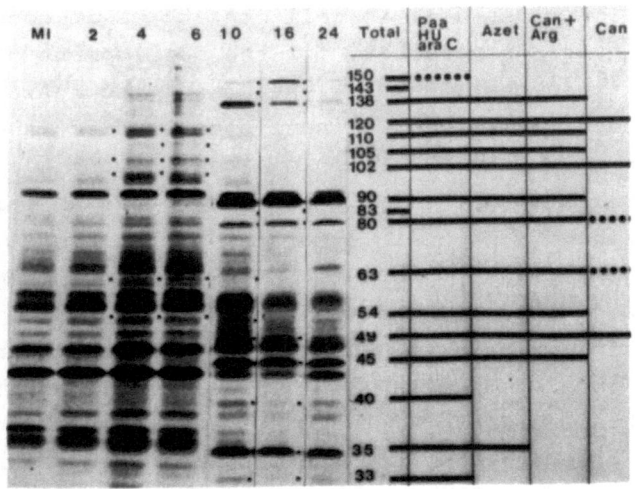

Fig. 3   A summary of the published data on control of
EBV protein synthesis (taken from Bayliss and Wolf,
1981c; Bayliss and Wolf,1982). Synthesis of proteins in
EBV-super-infected Raji cells. Raji cells were
superinfected with EBV derived from P3HR1 cultures and
pulse labelled with ^{35}S-methionine at various times
after infection (the starting times in h for the 30-min
pulses are given above the tracks; approximate molecular
masses are given in kilodaltons at the side of the gel)
In a series of similar experiments various metabolic
inhibitors were added at the time of infection and the
cells were labelled at 12-16 h after infection. Solid
lines on the right indicate protein synthesis in the
presence of the inhibitor named in the column heading.
PAA, phosphonoacetic acid at 200 ug/ml; HU, hydroxyurea
at 4 mg/ml; ara C, cytosine arabinonucleoside at 50
ug/ml; Azet, azetidine at 500 ug/ml; Can + Arg,
canavanine at 500 ug/ml in normal arginine-containing
medium; and Ca, canavanine at 500 ug/ml in arginine-free
medium. The clumn headed "Total" indicates the spectrum
of proteins seen in uninhibited infected Raji cells. The
150-kilodalton protein is synthesized in cultures
treated with phosphonoacetic acid or hydroxyurea but not
in cultures treated with cytosine arabinonucleoside; the
80- and 63-kilodalton proteins can be identified in
extracts of canavanine-treated cells only after
immunoprecipitation because they are relatively poorly
synthesized under these conditions.

lytic expression. If EBV-carrying cell lines are
infected with a sufficiently high multiplicity, a lytic
cycle will occur (Bayliss and Wolf, 1981c) with the
synthesis of at least 30 virus induced or specific
proteins. These proteins can be divided into 3 groups
according to their kinetics of synthesis, response to
inhibition of DNA synthesis, and requirement for
virus-specified factors. These data are summarized in
Fig.3. Do these observations have ony relevance to
regulated expression of EBV during the stepwise
induction of a lytic cycle by the virus in the absence
of inhibitors? The experiment shown in Fig. 4 indicates
that this is the case. If Raji cells are infected with
decreasing amounts of virus, then the intermediate and
late proteins are no longer synthesized at a certain cut
off value.

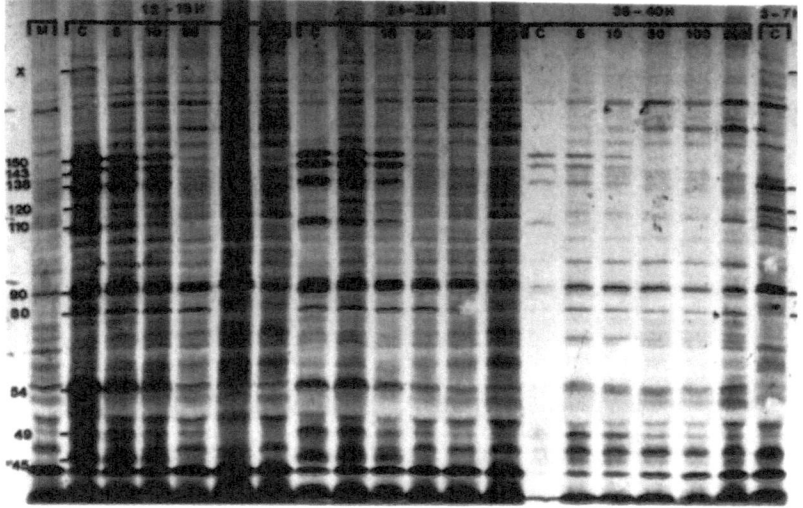

Fig. 4   Raji cells were superinfected with various
dilutions of a stock of P3HR1 EBV; 12, 24 and 36 h post
infection the infected cells were labelled for 4 h with
^{35}S-methionine, extracts of the cells were subjected to
immune precipitation and the precipitates analyzed on
SDS-polyacrylamide gels (for methodology see Bayliss and
Wolf, 1981c). At dilutions of 1:5 or 1:10 the same
spectrum of viral proteins is induced as with the
concentrated (c) virus stock. At dilutions of 1:50 or
lower a very limited spectrum of proteins can be
identified.

However, a certain subset of the early antigen complex
is made and it is the same subset as that obtained by
chemically induced Raji cells. Similar observations have
been made using an EBV genome negative cell line (BJA).
Immunoprecipitation of EBV proteins allows further
characterization and a linkage to serological data.
These data (Fig. 5) show also that proteins of the EA
complex are synthesized in considerable amounts during
the replication of EBV; yet normal adults do not have
antibodies against these proteins even if they shed
virus.

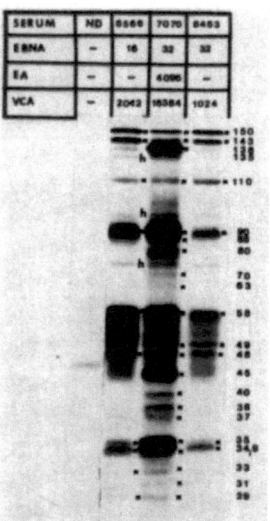

Fig. 5   An analysis of EBV specified polypeptides by
immunoprecipitation using sera having different
reactivities to EBV specified antigens. ND is a serum
free of EBV antibodies. 6966 and 84 63 have high titers
against VCA but not EA, serum 7070 has high titers
against both VCA and EA. Proteins 138, 88, 45, 40, 38,
37 are only pecitpitated by the EA positive sera. These
results are representative for a much larger panel of
sera which we have tested.

In an attempt to further substantiate the viral nature
of the polypeptides and to map the genes on the viral
genome which is essential for detailed studies on the
molecular basis for the regulation of viral gene
expression we selected mRNA from

a producer cell line (P3/HR1) by hybridization to cloned
EBV DNA fragments. This mRNA was then translated in
vitro using a rabbit reticulocyte translation system
(NEN). With this technique we were able to identify 22
proteins as EBV specific and have mapped their positions
on the EBV genome. These data are summarized in Fig. 6.

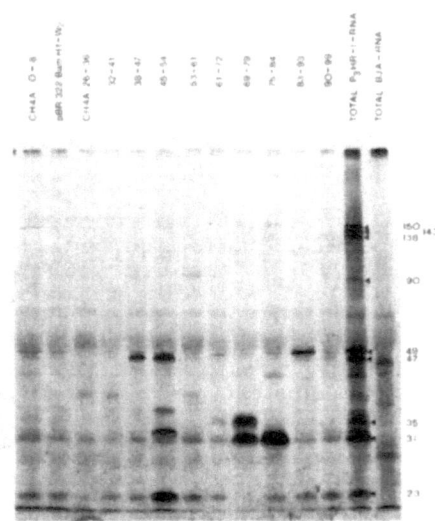

Fig. 6   A) In vitro translation of EBV specific mRNA.
EBV DNA fragments cloned in Charon 4a (Buell et al.,
1981) or pBR322 (a gift from D.Hayward) were used to
select virus specified mRNA from virus producing cells
(P3HR1) by hybridization. The selected mRNAs were
translated in vitro using the rabbit reticulocyte
system. After translation the synthesized proteins were
analyzed by immune precipitation and SDS gel analysis.

One interesting observation which awaits
explanation is that if mRNA from EBV genome negative
cells (BJA-B) is selected using EBV DNA, a mRNA is
obtained which hybridizes to the region spanning 61-72
map units of the EBV genome. This RNA can be translated
in vitro to yield a polypeptide of 85,000 mol.wt. This
region of the EBV genome is known to hybridize to
cellular DNA under stringent conditions and may
represent cellular sequences which have been
incorporated into the viral genome during the course of
evolution.

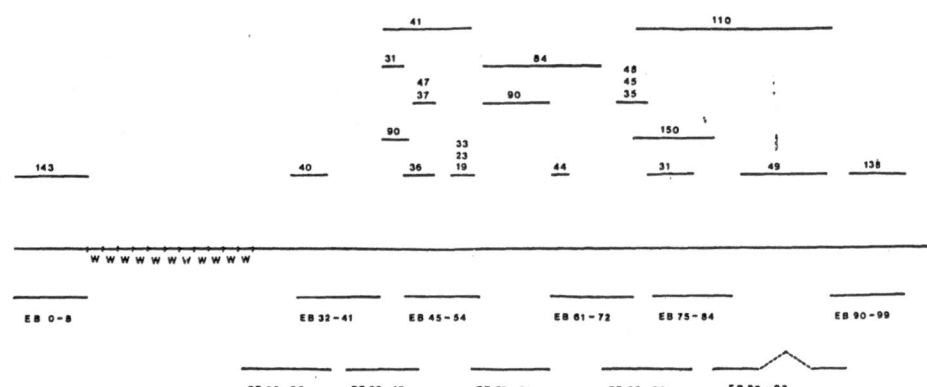

Fig. 6   B) A schematic representation of the data presented in panel A and additional data obtained by using cloned Bam Hl-fragments of EBV (Skare and Strominger, 1980). The coding regions for the 22 polypeptides (labelled with their molecular weights in kilodaltons) are illustrated. As pp 143, 41, 84, 90, 150, 110, 138 were only characterized by Charon clones, their map positions were not as precisely defined.

4)   A model has been developed which attempts to include the available data and should be useful to predict certain events or measurable parameters and to design further experiments, thus allowing the hypothesis to be further tested. For explanation of the model see legend Fig. 7 and discussion.

DISCUSSION

As suggested in Fig. 7, EBV will infect B lymphocytes during acute or primary infection, and due to the lack of immune response the cells will enter into the lytic cycle and produce a full set of viral antigens (Fig. 6). It seems probable that not all B-lymphocytes are capable of supporting a fully lytic infection due to a cellular factor which prevents expression of EBV (block 1) and these will be selected for and go on to become the cells which carry EBV specified antigens, antibodies will be developed against EA, VCA and EBNA (Table 1). As the immune defense mechanisms of the body remove the lytically infected cells from the circulation (block 2), the antibody levels will start to fall

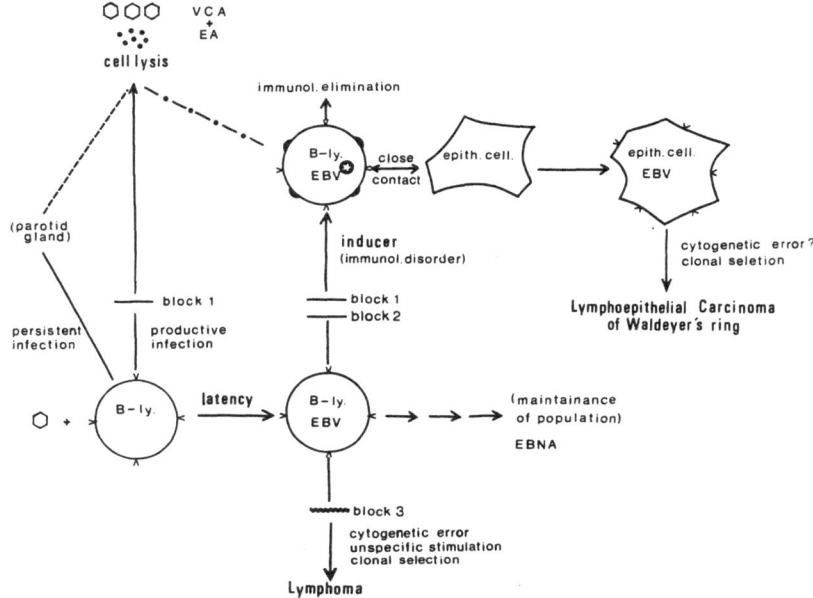

Fig. 7   The scheme summarizes the suggested biological
effects of EBV described in the text. Block 1 and 2
inhibit the lytic expression of EBV, block 3 suppresses
the proliferation of EBV genome containing lymphoid
cells in the periphery. Block 1: Block at cellular level
(endogenous block). Evidence: only a certain percentage
of cells from cloned cell lines produces virus. This
block is responsible for poor production of virus. Block
2: Block from the outside (exogenous block,
immunological control?). Evidence: in peripheral blood
from patients with infectious mononucleosis, in fresh BL
or NPC biopsies no viral particles can be found. After
explantation into tissue culture a few cells start to
produce virus. EBV   :activated EBV genes;   EBV
receptors;   virus specific membrane changes.

during the convalescent phase. After a certain period
antibodies to the early antigens disappear. However, as
mentioned above, EBV is produced in the parotid gland. The
viral particles and intracellular virus associated antigens
including EA will be shed into the saliva and reach the
oropharynx. Here the viral particles (but not EA) could bind
to the B-lymphocytes and be presented to the body as
antigens, thus maintaining the antibody titers to VCA; EA,
however, cannot bind to the lymphocytes and will be degraded

by proteases and not be available to the body as antigens. On the other hand, the circulating lymphocytes which carry EBV latently contain EBNA and as far as we know no other EBV specified protein. These lymphocytes will be subject to the normal turnover processes, and as they die, EBNA will be released into the blood stream and thus antibodies to this antigen will persist. Thus normal convalescent sera will have low level IgG anti-VCA and anti-EBNA antibodies (Table 1). If immunosuppresion occurs, either because of other disease (e.g. Hodgkins's disease) or due to immunosuppressive therapy, some of the circulating peripheral blood lymphocytes (PBLs) will escape the normally tight control mechanism and enter into a cycle of virus replication, causing a secondary increase in the titers to EA, VCA and EBNA. The very strong block 3 (see Fig. 7) may, under rare circumstances, be ineffective and allow the clonal selection of a cell which differs in its antigenic makeup. This may be true of the factors which lead to the development of Burkitt's lymphoma. Environmental mutagens (Birnboim, 1982) and unspecific "mitogens" (Malaria) (Burkitt, 1969) which facilitate clonal selection through proliferation may favour this event. Specific karyotypes in the selected clones (Manolova et al., 1979) may correlate to the altered antigenic makeup of these cells. A different view of the steps involved in the development of Burkitt's lymphoma has been published by Klein (1979).

Specific genetic constellations (XLP) or acquired conditions (immunesuppressed transplant recipients) determine a reduced efficiency of block 3 (cellular response to proliferating cells). Therefore the selective pressure on peripheral B-lymphocytes (which already have a potential for unlimited growth by virtue of the resident EBV genomes) may be weaker. Under less stringent selective pressure more cells may favour initial proliferation and facilitate the selection of cell clones. A specific cytogenetic error (Purtilo, 1980) may occur under therapy and may induce a change from polyclonality to monoclonality.

A close contact between epithelial cells and
B-lymphocytes, which may carry EBV genome, has been descirbed
for the lymphoepithelial ring of the throat (Waldeyer's
ring). This unique tissue may provide the necessary
conditions for EBV-induced fusion between the two cell types,
thus unabling the EBV genome to enter the epithelial cell. If
this hypothesis is true, the EBV should be associated with
other tumors which arise within this tissue. Studies of
patients with non-keratinizing carcinomas arising in
Waldeyer's ring show in several cases a serological picture
similar to that seen in NPC (Table 2). This prompted us to
look for the presence of EBV genomes in such tumors by in
situ hybridization with cloned EBV DNA. So far we have
detected EBV DNA in two poorly differentiated tonsillar
carcinomas (T.C.) (see Fig. 1d). The major difference between
T.C. and NPC is that only 25% of the limited number of T.Cs
so far tested were serologically related to EBV, whereas 100%
of the NPCs are EBV genome positive; at the moment we cannot
explain these findings. This proposal would be in good
agreement with the proffered model.

Table 2   EBV antibodies in patients with carcinomas located in Waldeyer's Ring

Tonsillar carcinoma

Name	Date of birth	IgA(VCA)	IgG(VCA)	IgA(EA)	EBNA	histologic type
W.M.	02.02.02	1:32	1:1024	neg.	1:16	lymphoepithelial Ca
M.M.	06.09.16	1:256	1:4000	neg.	1:32	lymphoepithelial Ca
B.M.	11.06.39	1:16			1:128	poorly differen-tiated cell Ca
P.D.	19.12.25	1:160	1:512	neg.	unsp.	undifferentiated Ca
H.M.	21.08.32	1:32	1:64	neg.	1:4	lymphoepithelial Ca

Carcinomas of the tongue

W.M.	08.01.34	1:32	1:1024	neg.	1:64	undifferentiated Ca
G.H.	02.11.09	1:16	1:128	neg.	1:8	lymphoepithelial Ca
S.J.	29.03.25	1:64	1:2048	neg.	1:128	undifferentiated Ca

Carcinomas of the gum

O.M.	31.98.21	1:16	1:1024	1:4	1:16	lymphoepithelial Ca

Ito observed that certain plant extracts could induce latent EBV and somehow increase the risk for NPC (Ito et al., 1981). Croton oil was one of the first suspected medicaments. However, it is highly irritant and is used only under close medical supervision and is therefore unlikely to be a NPC related risk factor. More recently both Ito and Zeng Yi (personal communication) have tested altogether over 500 different extracts from 100 plant families and found that 20 of them were capable of activating latent EBV. Some of the extracts were active in the aqueous form and thus open the possbility that traditional Chinese herbal medicines, often applied as teas, may contain EBV-inducing principles. One difference in the EBV serology of the populations with low and high risk for NPC development is that in high risk areas the level of antibody to EBV antigens remains high throughout life when compared to low risk populations (Zeng Yi, personal communication). Thus EBV activating substances could continually stimulate the latently infected B-cells to enter into a lytic cycle (explaining the consistently high antibody titers). If follow-up studies could demonstrate a match between the areas with high risk for NPC and the use of the discussed plant extracts, a multifactorial causation of NPC would be further substantiated.

REFERENCES
Bayliss, G.J. and Wolf, H. 1980. Epstein-Barr virus induced cell fusion. Nature (London), 287, 164-165.
Bayliss, G.J. and Wolf, H. 1981a. The spontaneous and induced synthesis of Epstein-Barr virus antigens in Raji cells immobilized on surfaces coated with antilymphocyte globulin. J. Gen. Virol., 54, 397-401.
Bayliss, G.J. and Wolf, H. 1981b. An Epstein-Barr virus early protein induces cell fusion. Proc. Natl. Acad. Sci. USA, 78, 7162-7165.
Bayliss, G.J. and Wolf, H. 1981c. The regulated expression of Epstein-Barr virus. III. Proteins specified by EBV during the lytic cycle. J. Gen. Virol., 56, 105-118.
Bayliss, G.J. and Wolf, H. 1982. Effect of the arginine analogue canavanine on the synthesis of Epstein-Barr virus-induced proteins in superinfected Raji cells. J. Virol., 41, 1109-1111.
Birnboim, H.C. 1982. DNA strand breakage in human leukocytes exposed to a tumor promotor phorbol myristate acetate. Science, 215, 1247-1249.

Buell, G.N., Reisman, D., Kintner, C., Crouse, G. and Sugden, B. 1981. Cloning overlapping DNA fragments from the B95-8 strain of Epstein-Barr virus reveals a site of homology to the internal repetition. J. Virol., 40, 977-982.

Burkitt, D.P. 1969. Etiology of Burkitt's lymphoma - an alternative hypothesis to a vectored virus. J. Natl. Cancer Inst., 42, 19-28.

Calnek, B.W. and Hitchner, G.B. 1969. Localization of viral antigen in chickens infected with Marek's disease herpes virus. J. Natl. Cancer Inst., 43, 935-949.

Diehl, V., Henle, G., Henle, W. and Kohn, G. 1969. Effect of a herpes group virus (EBV) on growth of peripheral leukocyte cultures. In Vitro, 4, 92-99.

Gerber, P., Nonoyama, M., Lucas, S., Perlin, E. and Goldstein, L.I. 1972. Oral excretion of Epstein-Barr virus by healthy subjects and patients with infectious mononucleosis. Lancet II, 988-989.

Gerber, P., Whang Peng, J. and Monroe, J.H. 1969. Transformation and chromosome changes induced by Epstein-Barr virus in normal human leukocyte cultures. Proc. Natl. Acad. Sci. (USA), 63, 740-747.

Graessmann, A., Wolf, H. and Bornkamm, G.W. 1980. Expression of Epstein-Barr virus genes in different cell types after microinjection of viral DNA. Proc. Natl. Acad. Sci. (USA), 77, 433-436.

Graham, F.O. and van der Ebb, A.J. 1973. A new technique for the assay of infectivity of human adenovirus 5 DNA. Virology, 52, 456-467.

Henle, W. and Henle, G. 1979. Seroepidemiology of the virus. In "The Epstein-Barr virus" (Ed. M.A. Epstein and B.G. Achong). (Springer, New York). pp. 62-78.

Ito, Y., Kishishita, M., Yanase, S. and Harayama, T. 1981. Epstein-Barr virus-activating principles in medicinal plants. In "Herpesvirus. Clinical, pharmacological and basic aspects". Proceedings of an International Symposium. (Ed. H. Shiota, Y.-C. Cheng and W.H. Prusoff). (Excerpta Medica, Amsterdam).

Jondal, M. and Klein, G. 1973. Surface markers on human B and T lymphocytes II. Presence of Epstein-Barr virus receptors on B lymphocytes. J. Exp. Med., 138, 1365-1378.

Klein, G. 1979. Lymphoma development in mice and humans: Diversity of initiation is followed by convergent cytogenetic evolution. Proc. Natl. Acad. Sci. USA, 76, 2442-2446.

Manolova, Y., Mandov, G., Keiler, J., Levan, A. and Klein, G. 1979. Genesis of the 14q+ marker in Burkitt's lymphoma. Hereditas, 90, 5-10.

Miller, G., Grogan, E., Heston, L., Robinson, I., Smith, D. 1981. Epstein-Barr viral DNA: infectivity for human placental cells. Science, 212, 452-455.

Morgan, D.G., Miller, G., Niedermann, J.C., Smith, H.W. and Dowalby, J.M. 1979. Site of Epstein-Barr virus replication in the oropharynx. Lancet I, 1154-1155.

Nilsson, K., Klein, G., Henle, W. and Henle, G. 1971. The
    establishment of lymphoblastoid lines from adult and
    fetal lymphoid tissue and its dependence on EBV. Int. J.
    Cancer, 8, 443-450.
Purtilo, D.T. 1980. Epstein-Barr virus-induced oncogenesis in
    immune deficient individuals. Lancet I, 300-303.
Purtilo, D.T. and Klein, G. 1981. Introduction to
    Epstein-Barr virus and lymphoproliferative diseases in
    immunodeficient individuals. Vsmvrt Trd-. 41, 4209-4210.
Purtilo, D.T. 1981. Immune deficiency predisposing to
    Epstein-Barr virus-induced lymphoproliferative disease:
    the X-linked lymphoproliferative syndrome as a model. In
    "Advances in Cancer Research ". (Ed. G. Klein and S.
    Weinhouse). (Academic Press, New York). pp. 279-312.
Skare, J. and Strominger, J.L. 1980. Cloning and mapping of
    Bam H1 endonuclease fragments of DNA from the
    transforming B95-8 strain of Epstein-Barr virus. Proc.
    Natl. Acad. Sci. USA, 77, 3860-3864.
Stoerker, J., Parris, D., Yajima, Y. and Glaser, R. 1981.
    Pleiotropic expression of Epstein-Barr virus DNA in
    human epithelial cells. Proc. Natl. Acad. Sci. USA, 78,
    5852-5855.
Volksky, K.J., Klein, G., Volsky, B. and Shapiro, I.M. 1981.
    Production of infectious Epstein-Barr virus in mouse
    lymphocytes. Nature (London), 293, 399-401.
Wolf, H. 1981. The use of nucleic acid hybridization
    exemplified with Epstein-Barr virus-associated diseases.
    Verh. Dtsch. Ges. Path., 65, 47-57.
Wolf, H., Wilmes, E. and Bayliss, G.J. 1981a. Epstein-Barr
    virus: its site of persistence and its role in the
    development of carcinomas. Haematology and Blood
    transfusion, 26, 191-196.
Wolf, H., Bayliss, G.J. and Wilmes, E. 1981b. Biological
    properties of Epstein-Barr virus. In "Cancer Campaign,
    Vol.5, Nasopharyngeal Carcinoma". (Ed. E. Grundmann).
    (Gustav Fischer Verlag, Stuttgart). pp. 101-109.

TREE SHREW HERPESVIRUS: PATHOGENICITY AND LATENCY

G. Darai, H.-G. Koch

Institut für Medizinische Virologie der Universität Heidelberg,
Im Neuenheimer Feld 324, 6900 Heidelberg, F.R.G.

ABSTRACT
    The study of the pathogenicity of different isolates of
Tupaia herpesvirus in its indigenous host, marmosets, and rodents, revealed that intravenous administration of this virus
led to the death of infected juvenile Tupaias only. The
clinical picture was manifested by a generalized virus
infection predominantly inflammatory, hemorrhagic, and with
necrosis of the lungs. In contrast, the majority of the
intraperitoneally inoculated tree shrews survived the
infection. The state of latency of differnt Tupaia herpesvirus
isolates was investigated in vivo using rodents, Tupaias and
marmosets. It was found that Tupaia herpesviruses persist only
in the spleens of Tupaia and New Zealand rabbits infected
previously with different Tupaia herpesvirus isolates. The
identification of the viruses recovered from the spleens of
Tupaia and rabbits by genomic analysis of DNAs revealed no
alteration as compared to the original inoculum.

INTRODUCTION

    Tupaia (the tree shrew), a member of the family Tupaiidae,
is regarded as one of the most primitive prosimians bridging
the gap between insectivores and primates. The first discovery
of herpesvirus-like particles in tree shrews (THV isolate no.1)
was reported in 1970 by Mirkovic et al. from Melnick's
laboratory; this was isolated from a degenerating lung tissue
culture from an apparently healthy animal. Our laboratory has
been intensively involved in investigating the virological
aspects of tree shrews and has succeeded in isolating five
further isolates (THV no. 2 to 6) from different individual
animals. The transmissibility and pathway mechanisms for the
persistence of latent virus in tree shrews is of special
importance since THV-1 to 4 were isolated from imported animals
and THV-5 and 6, which are similar, or identical, to THV-4,
were isolated from animals bred in captivity (F2 and F8
generation). These studies are subject of this review.

History of tree shrew herpesvirus

    The data on the isolation of the different strains of

Tupaia herpesvirus are summarized in Table 1.

TABLE 1 History of different Tupaia herpesvirus isolates

Isolate/ strain	Age of animal	Source
isolate 1 strain: 1	?*	degenerating lung tissue culture from an apparently healthy tree shrew; Mirkovic et al. (1970).
isolate 2 strain: 2	8 years*	degenerating cell culture from a malignant lymphoma of a moribund tree shrew; Darai et al. (1979).
isolate 3 strain: 3	9 years*	degenerating cell culture from a Hodgkin's sarcoma of a moribund tree shrew; Darai et al. (1979 and 1980).
isolate 4 strain: 4	11 years*	degenerating cell culture from spleen of a moribund tree shrew; Darai et al. (1981 and 1982).
isolate 5 strain: 4	7 years**	degenerating cell culture from spleen of a healthy tree shrew; Darai et al. (1983).
isolate 6 strain: 4	4 years***	degenerating cell culture from spleen of a healthy tree shrew; Darai (1981, unpublished).

*   imported animals
**   second breeding generation (F2) in captivity
***   eighth breeding generation (F8) in captivity

Biological properties of tree shrew herpesvirus
     The morphology of the different Tupaia herpesvirus isolates was investigated using the electron microscope (McCombs et al., 1971; Darai et al., 1979, 1980, 1982). The

intra- and/or extracellular herpesvirus structure was observed in infected cells. Naked virus capsids of about 100 nm diameter were measured. Some of the envelope particles contained several virus capsids in agreement with the first description of THV-1 by McCombs et al. in 1971. The diameter of the envelope ranged between 200 and 350 nm.

For determination of host range and virus growth a variety of cell cultures from different species were screened for their susceptibility to different THV isolates. It was found that the cells of choice for the propagation and plaque assay of THV isolates are Tupaia embryonic and/or baby fibroblasts. The maximum infectivity (1×10^7 to 5×10^7 p.f.u. $\times$ ml^{-1}) was reached 5 days after infection as described previously (Darai et al., 1979, 1982). In contrast, all other cell cultures, except primary rabbit kidney cells (5×10^5 p.f.u. $\times$ ml^{-1}), human embryonic fibroblasts (2.5×10^3 p.f.u. $\times$ ml^{-1}), and marmoset skin fibroblasts (2×10^2 p.f.u. $\times$ ml^{-1}), showed no cytopathic effect (c.p.e.) during a six-week observation period. The non-susceptible cell cultures tested were as follows: primary monkey kidney cells (Cercopithecus aethiops), African green monkey kidney cells (Vero, CV-1), dog kidney cells (NBL-2), dog thymus cells (Fcf2th), rat embryonic fibroblasts, hamster embryonic fibroblasts, mouse embryonic fibroblasts, and chicken embryonic fibroblasts.

Physical properties of Tupaia herpesvirus DNA

A precise determination of the buoyant density of THV-DNA by analytical ultracentrifugation gave a value of = 1.724 g $\times$ ml^{-1} corresponding to a G0C content of 65.4%. The other value was determined from the ultraviolet absorbance-temperature profile of the DNA. The viral DNAs were cleaved with different restriction endonucleases, and the cleavage sites of different restriction enzymes on THV DNA of strains 1 to 6 were determined. The DNA cleavage pattern of THV strains 1 to 6 after digestion with the restriction enzyme Hind III (A/AGCTT) are given in Figure 1 and with Eco RI (G/AATTC) in Figure 2; the data for THV strains 1 to 4 after digestion with the

94

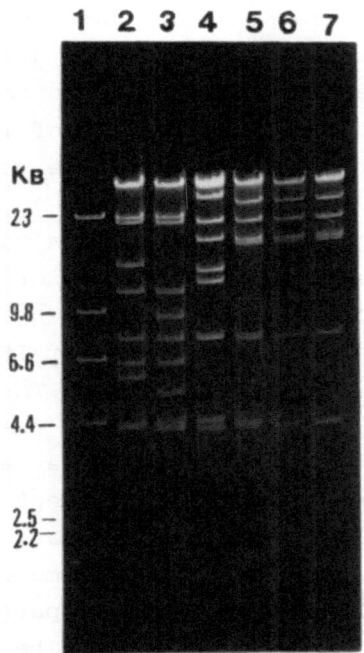

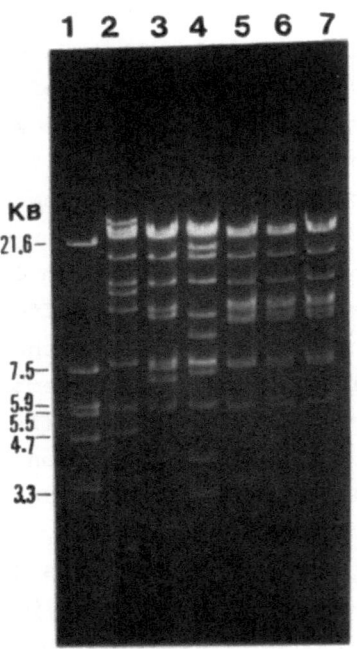

Fig.1   Hind III cleavage
pattern of DNAs of Tupaia
herpesviruses 1 to 6;
lanes: 1 = lambda DNA
cleaved with Hind III
and served as internal
marker, 2 = THV-1, 3 =
THV-2, 4 = THV-3, 5 =
THV-4, 6 = THV-5, and
7 = THV-6. Agarose slab
gel electorphoresis
(0.5% agarose).

Fig.2   Eco RI cleavage
pattern of DNAs of
Tupaia herpesviruses
1 to 6; lanes: 1 =
lambda NDA cleaved
with Eco RI and served
as internal marker, 2 =
THV-1, 3 = THV-2, 4 =
THV-3, 5 = THV-4, 6 =
THV-5, and 7 = THV-6.
Agarose slab gel
electrophoresis (0.5%
agarose).

restriction enzyme Bam HI (G/GATCC) are shown in Figure 3.
These analyses demonstrate clearly that THV-1 to 4 can be
distinguished from each other. The cleavage patterns of THV-4
and 5 show only minor differences, for example the Hind III
fragment H of THV-4 is not present in the cleavage pattern of
the THV-5 isolate with the same enzyme. This indicates that
THV-4 and 5 must be similar, and the subtile differences are
due to strain variations between both isolates (Darai et al.,
1983). The physical map of HSV-2 was constructed using Hind III
and Eco RI restriction endonucleases.

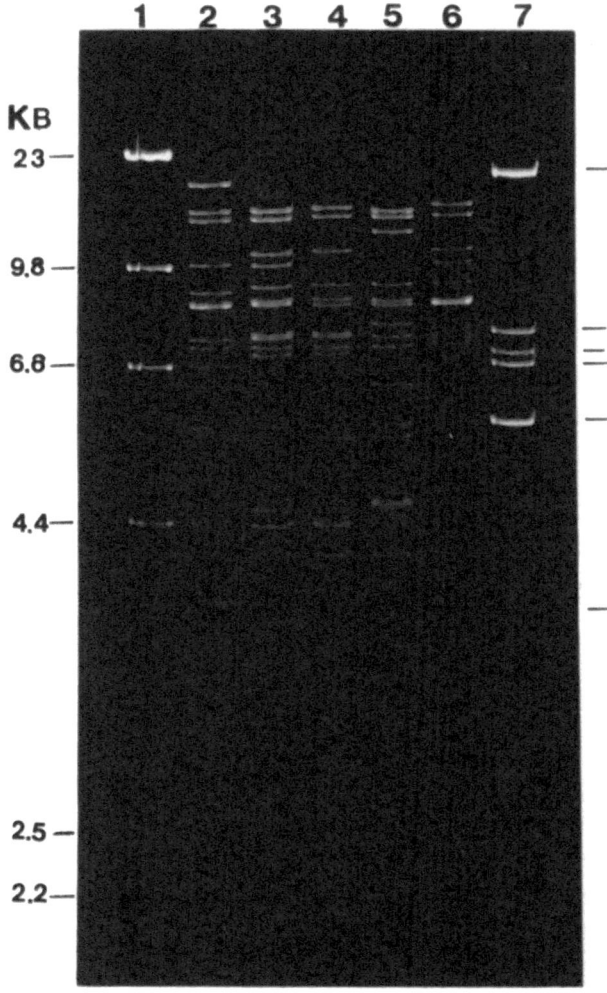

Fig. 3 Bam HI cleavage pattern of DNAs of Tupaia herpesviruses 1 to 4 and a recombinant no. R26 of two different isolates (THV-2/THV-3) which was generated in vitro as described previously (Darai et al., 1981a); lanes: 1 = lambda DNA cleaved with Hind III and lane 7 = with Bam HI served as marker, 2 = THV-1, 3 = THV-2, 4 = R26 generated in vitro between THV-2/THV-3, 5 = THV-3 and 6 = THV-4. Agarose slab gel electrophoresis (0.8% agarose).

The molecular weights of the THV DNAs were determined by electron-microscopic measurement of the contour length, which resulted in a value of about 130 Megadaltons for THV-1 to 4

(Darai et al., 1981). Single-stranded THV DNA was prepared for electron-microscopy by heating the viral DNA in formamide and isolating the single-strands from agarose gel (Koller et al., 1978). It was found that single-stranded THV DNA does not display any extended stem-loop structures. Thus the structure of THV genomes seems to be unique when compared to the DNAs of other known herpesviruses from other species.

Sequence homologies of the DNAs of THV-1 to 4 were determined using blot hybridization experiments between DNAs of THV-1 to 4.

Virion polypeptides of tree shrew herpesvirus

The virion polypeptides of the different isolates of the Tupaia herpesvirus were analysed by SDS-polyacrylamide slab gel electrophoresis and by isoelectric focusing. The viral proteins from either non-radioactive or ^{35}S-methionine-labeled virions formed distinct patterns of at least 35 polypeptides ranging in molecular weight from 12.000 to 230.000. Whilst the majority of the analogous polypeptides of these viruses were of indistinguishable electrophoretic mobility, some (e.g. polypeptides of 82 to 84 K) showed small differences in apparent molecular weight which were characteristic of the virus strain (Faissner et al., 1982). The two-dimensional electropherograms revealed at least 47 discernible protein spots some of which were specific for a given THV isolate and which were detectable even in lysates of THV-infected cells. In addition five glycoproteins were found in purified THV virions (Faissner et al., 1982; Flügel et al., 1983).

A protein kinase activity was found to be associated with tree shrew (Tupaia) herpesvirus. The protein kinase was characterized with respect to its requirements for enzymatic activity (Flügel and Darai, 1982).

A new thymidine kinase activity is present in Tupaia baby fibroblast cells infected with the tree shrew herpesvirus (THV, isolate 2) (Flügel and Darai, 1982a).

Pathogenicity of tree shrew herpesvirus

The pathogenicity of different Tupaia herpesvirus isolates was investigated in vivo using rodents, Tupaias, and marmosets. Clinical disease did not develop in rats, mice, hamsters, and marmosets. In contrast it was found that the different THV isolates (THV-1 to 4) are highly pathogenic for juvenile tree shrews when the animals were inoculated intravenously. However, the majority of intraperitoneally inoculated animals survived the infection. The clinical picture was manifested as inflammatory haemmorhagic necrosis of the lungs and generalized herpes infection as described previously (Darai et al., 1982, 1983). Death occurred on the 4th to 8th day after inoculation. The tissues and whole blood of these animals were titrated for the determination of the virus yield in different organs using a plaque assay (Darai et al., 1979, 1982). The results indicate that the main organs for the propagation of the Tupaia herpesviruses are lung, spleen, and liver.

In addition it was found that isolate 2 induced malignant lymphoma in its indigenous host. The first tumour developed three and a half years after administration. Infectious virus was recovered after culturing the tumour cells in tissue culture. The examination of the genome structure of the recovered virus which was performed using restriction enzyme analysis of the virion DNA resulted in the same cleavage pattern as the DNA of the THV, which had been inoculated three and a half years earlier (Darai et al., 1983, 1983a). Parallel to this observation it was found that THV-2 and 3 are capable of inducing hyperplasia of the thymus in rabbits, and when newborn animals were inoculated with THV-2 and 3, they developed malignant thymoma in a few (8%) cases (Darai et al., 1980, 1983, 1983a).

The state of viral latency

Latency of different isolates of tree shrew herpesvirus was studied in a variety of laboratory animals and in its indigenous host. It was found that those juvenile tree shrews which survived the THV infection (administered intraperitoneally) are carriers of persisting virus. Infectious viruses were recovered from the cultured spleens of these animals only. For this study previously infected animals were sacrificed and/or splenectomized between 1 and 3 days after inoculation.

Similar results were obtained using New Zealand rabbits which were inoculated with THV isolates 1 to 4. Infectious viruses were recovered only from the spleen of those animals which were sacrificed several months and/or years post infection. The cultured spleen cells of these animals developed cytopathic lesions and released infectious viruses which led to total cell lysis of the spleen cell cultures (Darai et al., 1981b, 1982, 1983). The identification of such recovered viruses from the spleens of Tupaias and rabbits by genomic analysis of the DNA of reisolated viruses was performed using restriction enzyme analysis of the viral DNA. Alterations were not detectable when the cleavage pattern of the viral DNA of the recovered viruses was compared to its original inoculum. In cotrast, latent infectious viruses were not recovered from infected mice, rats, hamsters, and marmosets which were sacrificed months after the administration of THV-1 to 4, although a variety of specimens including blood, kidney, thymus, and spleen were tested.

CONCLUSION

Four strains of Tupaia herpesvirus have been classified from six isolates of different individual animals. With the exception of isolate no. 1 (strain 1) (Mirkovic et al., 1970) all other isolates were obtained from lymphatic tissues of tree shrews. Isolate no. 2 (strain 2) and isolate no. 3 (strain 3) were isolated from spontaneously developed lymphatic tumours of tree shrew (Darai et al., 1979, 1980, 1982a; Hofmann et al., 1981). Isolates no. 4, 5, and 6 (strain 4) were obtained from cultured spleen cells of three different tree shrews (Table 1). The history, and the origin of the detection of all these isolates indicate that the tree shrew herpesviruses (strain 1 to 4) persist as latent viruses in tree shrews. This state of

TABLE 2 Properties of Tupaia herpesvirus

| | THV strains | | | |
	1	2	3	4
Number of isolates	1	1	1	3
Host range	Tupaia embryonic fibroblasts (max.titer 2.0×10^7 PFUxml^{-1}) Tupaia embryonic kidney cells (max.titer 5.0×10^7 PFUxml^{-1}) Primary rabbit kidney cells (max.titer 7.0×10^5 PFUxml^{-1}) Human foreskin fibroblasts (max.titer 3.0×10^4 PFUxml^{-1}) Marmoset skin fibroblasts (max.titer 2.0×10^2 PFUxml^{-1}) Tupaia, rabbit, and human leukocytes (max.titer 5.0×10^5 PFUxml^{-1})			
Reproductive cycle	Maximal infectivity was reached 4 to 6 days p.i. on Tupaia embryonic fibroblasts, which were infected at an M.O.I. of 0.01 PFU/cell			
Cytopathic effect	Enlargement of infected cells, inclusion bodies in nucleus and cytoplasma			
Properties of DNA: G+C content %			65-66 81	
T$_m$ °C (0.1 SSC)				
Buoyant density in CsCl (gxml^{-1})			1.724	
Molecular weight by contour length measurement	129±3	133±2	130±2	132±3
Number of isomeric arrangements	1	1	1	1
Arrangement of reiterated sequences	not present			

TABLE 2 Properties of Tupaia herpesvirus (continued)

	THV strains			
	1	2	3	4
Number of polypeptides of virions:	35	37	36	37
Glycoproteins in purified THV virions		at least five		
Enzyme associated with Tupaia herpesvirus:		Protein kinase and specific phosphate acceptor proteins		
Thymidine kinase activity	ND	+	ND	ND
Pathogenicity in indigenous host	Lethal for juvenile and young adult Tupaia by i.v. infection (100%) and (25%) by i.p. application			
Latency	Infectious virus recovered several months (over 2 years) from cultured spleens of infected Tupaias, which survived the acute infection. Tupaia herpesvirus persists as latent virus in the spleen of New Zealand rabbits and can be recovered several months after administration from the cultured spleen of the animals.			
Oncogenicity	Induced hyperplasia of thymus (8% malignant thymoma) in New Zealand rabbits. THV-2 induces malignant lymphoma in tree shrew.			

ND = not done

viral latency can also be established experimentally in tree shrews using these four virus strains.

A number of herpesviruses have been isolated from different animal species including primates, and according to their biological properties they have been classified into three subfamilies, namely Alpha, Beta, and Gammaherpesvirinae (Roizman et al., 1981). Classification of herpesviridae using the properties of their genomes resulted in the grouping of different well investigated herpesviruses into groups A, B, C, D, and E (Roizman et al., 1981). The detailed analysis of Tupaia herpesvirus strains 1 to 4 as described above and summarized in Table 2 does not allow the assignment of the Tupaia herpesviruses to any one of the three known herpesvirus subfamilies, or to the groups A to E. At this stage of investigation it seems appropriate to emphasize that Tupaia herpesviruses constitute the first members of a new herpesvirus subgroup.

ACKNOWLEDGMENT

We extend our thanks to Dr. D.M. Taylor, University of Heidelberg, for critical reading of this manuscript.

REFERENCES

Darai, G., Matz, B., Schröder, C.H., Flügel, R.M., Berger, U., Munk, K. and Gelderblom, H. 1979. Characterization of a tree shrew herpesvirus isolated from a lymphosarcoma. J. Gen. Virol., 43, 541-551.

Darai, G., Zöller, L., Matz, B., Flügel, R.M., Hofmann, W. and Gelderblom, H. 1980. Herpesvirus Tupaia: Isolation, Characterization and Oncogenicity. In "Advances in Comparative Leukemia Research 1979" (Ed. B.A. Lapin, D.S. Yohn). (USSR Acad. Med. Sci. / IEP&T-Moscow). pp. 141-148.

Darai, G., Flügel, R.M., Matz, B. and Delius, H. 1981. DNA of Tupaia herpesviruses. In "Herpesvirus DNA" (Ed. Y. Becker). (M. Nijhoff Publishers, The Hague). pp. 345-362.

Darai, G., Zöller, G., Matz, B., Flügel, R.M., Möller, P., Hofmann, W., Gelderblom, H. and Delius, H. 1982. Tupaia herpesviruses: Characterization and biological properties. Microbiologica, 5, 285-298.

Darai, G., Koch, H.-G. and Flügel, R.M. 1981a. Recombinants between Tupaia herpesviruses. Analysis of their genome structure and biological properties. In "International Workshop on Herpesviruses" (Ed. A.S. Kaplan et al.). (Esculapio Publ. Co., Bologna, Italy). p. 28.

102

Darai, G. and Zöller, L. 1981b. Latent state of Tupaia herpesviruses in the New Zealand Rabbit. In "The Human Herpesviruses" (Ed. A. Nahmias et al.). (Elsevier, New York).
pp. 622-623.

Darai, G., Koch, H.-G., Flügel, R.M. and Gelderblom, H. 1983
(in press). Tree shrew (Tupaia) herpesviruses. In
"Herpesvirus of Man and Animal, Developments in Biological
Standardization" (Karger, Basel).

Darai, G., Koch, H.-G., Möller, P., Hofmann, W., Gelderblom, H.
and Flügel, R.M. 1983a (in press). Is the tree shrew a
model system for the investigation of Hodgin's Disease? In
"Proceedings of the Symposium on the Use of Nonhuman
Primates in Exotic Viral and Immunologic Diseases" (Ed.
S.S. Kalter).

Darai, G., Zöller, L., Hofmann, W., Möller, P., Schwaier, A.
and Flügel, R.M. 1982a. Spontaneous malignomas in Tupaia
(tree shrew). Am. J. Primatol., 2, 177-189.

Faissner, A., Darai, G. and Flügel, R.M. 1982. Analysis of
polypeptides of the tree shrew (Tupaia) herpesvirus by gel
electrophoresis. J. Gen. Virol., 58, 139-148.

Flügel, R.M., Faissner, A., Koch, H.-G. and Darai, G. 1983. (in
press). Analysis of viral proteins and glycoproteins of
Tupaia herpesviruses. In "Herpes Virus of Man and Animal,
Developments in Biological Standardization" (Karger,
Basel).

Flügel, R.M. and Darai, G. 1982. Protein kinase and specific
phosphate acceptor proteins associated with Tupaia
herpesviruses. J. Virol., 43, 410-415.

Flügel, R.M. and Darai, G. 1982a. Thymidine kinase induced by
Tupaia herpesvirus. In "Herpesvirus Workshop, Abstracts of
papers presented at the sixth Cold Spring Harbor meeting
on Herpesviruses, August 31 - September 5, 1982". p. 126.

Hofmann, W., Möller, P., Schwaier, A., Flügel, R.M., Zöller, L.
and Darai, G. 1981. Malignant tumours in Tupaia (tree
shrew). J. med. Primatol., 10, 155-163.

Mirkovic, R., Voss, W.R. and Benyesh-Melnick, M. 1970.
Characterization of a new herpes-type virus indigenous for
tree shrews. In "Proceedings of the 10th International
Congress of Microbiology" (Mexico City). pp. 181-189.

McCombs, R.M., Brunschwig, J.P., Mirkovic, R. and Benyesh-
Melnick, M. 1971. Electron microscopic characterization of
a herpes-like virus isolated from tree shrews. Virol., 45,
816-820.

Koller, B., Delius, H., Bünemann, H. and Müller, W. 1978. The
isolation of DNA from agarose gels by electrophoretic
elution onto malachite green-polyacrylamide columns. Gene,
4, 227-239.

Roizman, B., Carmichael, L.E., Deinhardt, F., de-The, G.,
Nahmias, A.J., Plowright, W., Rapp, F., Sheldrick, P.,
Takahashi, M. and Wolf, K.: The Herpesvirus Study Group,
The International Committee on Taxonomy of Viruses. 1981.
Herpesviridae: definition, provisional nomenclature, and
taxonomy. Intervirol., 16, 201-217.

ONCOGENIC HERPESVIRUSES OF NON-HUMAN PRIMATES - PERSISTENCE OF VIRAL DNA IN TRANSFORMED LYMPHOID CELLS

B. Fleckenstein, Sabine Schirm, Christine Kaschka-Dierich

Institut für Klinische Virologie, University of Erlangen-Nürnberg, Federal Republic of Germany

ABSTRACT

Herpesvirus (H.) saimiri and H.ateles are highly oncogenic in various non-human primates and in rabbits, causing rapidly progressing malignant T-cell lymphomas upon experimental infection. Cell lines derived from virus-induced tumors and in vitro transformed lymphoid cells contain non-integrated circular viral DNA in high multiplicity. Persisting viral DNA molecules of cell lines that do not produce infectious virus are highly methylated in the unique L-DNA and repetitive (H) DNA sequences. Partial denaturation mapping has shown that some DNA circles contain duplications of L-DNA segments; however all non-producer cell lines investigated so far have L-DNA segments that are considerably shorter than the L-DNA region of virion DNA (110 kbp). The deletions in the circular molecules of H.saimiri transformed cells were mapped by hybridizations with cloned probes of virion L-DNA. In the circular DNA of two cell lines derived from virus induced marmoset lymphomas (1670, 70N2), a 20 kbp segment of L-DNA is missing which corresponds to the virion L-DNA between map coordinates 0,52 and 0,70. The rabbit tumor cell line 7710 bears an L-DNA deletion of about 30 kbp (L-DNA map units 0.23 to 0.50). Two sublines of the in vitro immortalized H1591 cells were investigated. The circular DNA of one line is missing about 42 kbp of virion DNA; in the circles of the other H1591 subline at least 47% of the viral genetic information was found to be absent. The L-DNA missing in the circular viral genomes could not be found in the linear fraction of each cellular DNA at the sensitivity level where 0.5 single copy gene/cell would have been clearly detected. Apparently, an internal L-DNA stretch of at least 63 kbp, representing 56% of the total viral genetic information, does not code for viral gene functions that would be consistently required to guarantee continuous extrachromosomal persistence or to maintain the state of growth transformation in lymphoid cells. The high amount of persisting viral DNA stands in remarkable contrast to low concentration of viral RNA and virus-coded proteins. The Herpesvirus ateles-associated nuclear antigen (HATNA) was detected in transformed lymphoid cells with very high genome copy number; but no trace of viral protein synthesis was found in other non-producer cell lines.

CHARACTERIZATION OF HERPESVIRUS SAIMIRI AND HERPESVIRUS ATELES INDUCED PROTEINS

S. Modrow, H. Wolf

Max von Pettenkofer-Institut für Hygiene and Medizinische
Mikrobiologie, University of Munich, West-Germany

ABSTRACT

Herpesvirus saimiri-induced cell proteins and structural
proteins labelled with ^{35}S-methionine, ^{32}P-orthophosphate and
^{14}C-Glucosamine respectively were analysed after
electrophoresis in SDS-polyacrylamide gels. Early proteins
were accumulated by the use of amino acid analogues.
Thirty-one virus-induced polypeptides were identified, 7 of
these were found to be glyco- and six to be phosphoproteins.
Twenty-one of the H.saimiri-induced cellular proteins were
localized on the virion. By surface iodination, five of these
were located at the envelope and four at the capsid.
Immunoprecipitation with various sera from natural and
experimental hosts revealed antibodies to a specific subset
of viral proteins in tumor-developing animals. Other antibody
species were identical to those found in the natural host,
whereas a further subset was characteristic only for the
natural host with its characteristic subclinical infection.
Using labelled proteins from Herpesvirus saimiri 11
(H.saimiri 11) and the attenuated strain H.saimiri 11 att
respectively, a diference was shown after precipitation with
a serum raised against infected cell proteins of H.saimiri
11.

INTRODUCTION

Herpesvirus saimiri, an endogenous virus of squirrel

monkey (Saimiri sciureus) populations (Meléndez et al., 1968,

1969) is highly tumorigenic in a variety of experimental

hosts, especially in marmosets of the genus Saguinus

(S.oedipus, S.nigricollis, S.fuscicollis) (Deinhardt et al.,

1974), owl monkeys (Aotus trivirgatus) (Hunt et al., 1970,

Meléndez et al., 1971) and New Zealand white rabbits (Daniel

et al., 1974, 1975; Rangan et al., 1976). All these animals

develop a fatal, rapidly proliferating neoplastic disease

with lymphoma in the local and systemic lymph nodes with or

without peripheral lymphoblastic leukemia. Especially the

organs of the reticuloendothelial system show massive

infiltrations with lymphoid cells following virus infection.

In contrast to marmoset monkeys, where the incidence of

neoplastic disease is 100%, the appearance of tumors in owl

monkeys is often delayed and about 20% of the animals do not develop tumors. H.saimiri infected New Zealand white rabbits show a disease pattern similar to that of primates; the incidence of tumors after infection varies between 20 and 75% in different studies.

Squirrel monkeys, the natural hosts, are lifelong virus carriers following inapparent infection early in life. Virus can be isolated from lymphocytes after cocultivation with susceptible cells; there is no evidence that virus is produced in peripheral lymphocytes, suggesting a biological behaviour similar to that in Marek's disease virus (Calnek et al., 1970) and EBV (Deinhardt and Deinhardt, 1979; Wolf and Bayliss, 1979; Wolf et al., 1981; Wolf et al., this volume).

Both viruses are lymphotropic and tumorigenic and have specialized target cells within the body of the host, permitting a steady virus production. The suppression of viral replication in carrier cells and in tumor cells therefore seems to be an established fact.

To study the regulation of gene expression of H.saimiri, we characterized the virus-specific proteins synthesized during the lytic cycle. The time-ordered appearance of proteins during lytic infection might suggest their possible regulatory functions. Blocking experiments with translation inhibitors and especially the use of amino acid analogues (Honess and Roizman, 1974; Fenwick and Walker, 1978; Bayliss and Wolf, 1981, 1982) have proved particularly helpful for further characterization of early proteins which control the synthesis of polypeptides produced late in the cycle. A further characterization of the structural proteins and their localization in the virion by surfac iodination studies led to a detailed analysis of viral structural proteins. Based on our protein data, we were able to study the different gene expression in natural and experimental tumor-bearing hosts. We immunoprecipitated polypeptides obtained from lytically infected cells with sera from squirrel monkeys, owl monkeys, marmosets and New Zealand white rabbits.

In all experiments an attenuated mutant (H.saimiri 11

att, Schaffer et al., 1975) of the oncogenic H.saimiri 11 was
included. This virus strain is not oncogenic in marmosets
(Wright et al., 1977, 1980) and induces a latent or
persistent infection, similar to that of the oncogenic strain
in squirrel monkeys.

MATERIAL AND METHODS

1. Virus-induced cell proteins

Owl monkey kidney cells (OMK-cells) were cultured in 32
ounce glass prescription bottles or plastic Petri plates
using Minimal Essential Medium (MEM Earl's salts, Gibco)
supplemented with 10% heat-inactivated fetal calf serum
(Seromed). Cells were infected with H.saimiri 11 or H.saimiri
att at 1-2 PFU/cell and treated as described (Modrow and
Wolf, 1983a). At the times indicated in the experiments,
cells were labelled with 10 µCi/ml ^{35}S-methionine (NEN) in
methionine-free medium, 7.5 µCi/ml ^{32}P-phosphate (NEN) in
phosphate-free medium or 0.75 µCi/ml ^{14}C-glucosamine (NEN) in
glucose-free medium containing 1.1 mg/ml fructose. At the end
of the labelling period cells were rinsed three times with
cold phosphate buffered saline (PBS) to stop amino acid
incorporation, solubilized in solubilization buffer (0.05 M
Tris-HCl, pH 7.0, 2% SDS, 5% mercaptoethanol, 3% sucrose,
bromephenolblue), sonicated for 15 sec with a Branson
sonifier (microtip at its maximum output), heated 5 min at
100°C and stored at -20°C.

Amino acid analogues - 500 µg/ml canavanine (Sigma) in
arginine-free MEM or 500 µg/ml azetidine (Sigma) were added
in a part of the experiments after the adsorption period.

Aliquots of 5 µl of the labelled cell extracts were
spotted on Whatman 3 MM filter paper discs, air dried, washed
twice in cold 5% trichloracetic acid (TCA) for 10 minutes and
twice in 95% ethanol. After drying at room temperature,
filters were placed in vials with aquasol 2 (NEN) and
counted.

20000 cpm per slot for ^{35}S-methionine, 10000 cpm for
^{32}P-phosphate and 2000 cpm for ^{14}C-glucosamine labelled

samples were submitted to electrophoresis in 10%
SDS-polyacrylamide gels (Modrow and Wolf, 1983a).

For in vitro labelling of glycosylated proteins,
unlabelled infected cell extracts were separated in 10%
SDS-polyacrylamide gels and electroblotted onto
nitrocellulose paper sheets (Schleicher and Schuell, BA85,
pore size 0.45 μm) using two carbon plates as electrodes
(25cm x 25cm x 2cm; grade CC, Deutsche Carbone, Frankfurt).
These were covered with 2 sheets of conductive sponge,
available from electronic supply shops. Blotting was
basically done according to the methods of Renart et al.,
(1979) and Towbin et al. (1979) using buffer containing 192
mM glycine, 25 mM Tris-HCl, pH 7.5, 10% methanol with a
constant current of 3 mA/cm² for 2 hours. After the transfer,
sheets were incubated for one hour in 3% BSA, 154 mM NaCl, 10
mM Tris-HCl, pH 7.4 at 40°C before ^{125}I-Concanavalin A
(Medac, iodinated with lactoperoxidase iodination system,
NEN) in 154 mM NaCl, 10 mM Tris-HCl, pH 7.4, 5 mM EDTA, 0.05%
NP40, 3% BSA was added. The filter membranes were incubated
overnight at room temperature, washed in 154 mM NaCl, 10 mM
Tris-HCl, pH 7.4, 5 mM EDTA, 0.05% NP40 and exposed to Kodak
XOMatS film with intensifying screens (Lightning Plus,
DuPont) at -70°C.

2.   Structural proteins

OMK-cells were infected with H.saimiri 11, H.saimiri 11
att, H.ateles 73 or H.ateles 810 and labelled as described
above. Virions were purified from the supernatant over two
combined isopycnic Percoll (Pharmacia) and sucrose gradients
(Modrow and Wolf, 1983b). The labelled proteins were analysed
in 10% SDS-polyacrylamide gels. Capsids were prepared by
incubation in 0.5% NP40 at 4°C for 15 min and pelleted. The
surface proteins of purified intact virions and capsids were
iodinated using the carrier coupled NEN-lactoperoxidase
iodination system, the labelled proteins were
immunoprecipitated with a serum directed against structural
proteins of H.saimiri 11 and separated in 10%
SDS-polyacrylamide gels.

3. Immunoprecipitation

OMK-cells were infected with H.saimiri 11 or H.saimiri 1 att and labelled with ^{35}S-methionine as described above. At the end of the labelling period, cells were rinsed three times in cold PBS and solubilized in 0.5 ml per 1x10 infected cells immunoprecipitation buffer (IP-buffer, 1% Triton X-100, 0.1% SDS, 0.137 M NaCl, 1 mM $CaCl_2$, 1 mM $MgCl_2$, 10% glycerol, 20 mM Tris-HCl, pH 9.0, 0.01% NaN_3, 1 µg/ml phenylmethylsulphonylfluoride) and disrupted by sonification. The extracts were clarified by centrifugation at 100 000 g for 30 min at 4°C and stored at -20°C.

In order to remove antibodies directed against cellular proteins, 10 µl of each serum were incubated with 0.5 ml of an extract of uninfected unlabelled OMK-cells (1x10^7 cells/ml) overnight at 4°C. 3 mg protein A sepharose-beads (Pharmacia) preswollen in 100 µl IP-buffer, were added and the reaction incubated at 4°C for another 2 hours. 0.5 ml of the labelled protein extracts was added and the immune complexes were allowed to form during a 3 hours incubation period at room temperature. The beads were washed with IP-buffer until supernatants contained no detectable radioactivity. The washed beads were resuspended in solubilization buffer and heated 5 min at 100°C to dissociate the immune complexes and analysed in 10% SDS-polyacrylamide gels.

4. Sera

The sera of squirrel monkeys (Ss1, Ss2, Ss3) and owl monkeys (At1, At2, At3) were a gift of L.Falk, New England Primate Research Center, Southborough, Mass. The Saguinus nigricollis serum (Sn1) was obtained from a monkey which died of a neoplastic disease 7 weeks after inoculation i.m. with 1x10^6 PFU H.saimiri 11. The Saguinus fuscicollis (Sf1) was infected with H.saimiri 11 att and developed a lifelong virus carrier status without showing any signs of disease. The serum was obtained 7 years after inoculation. The New Zealand

white rabbit (NZWR1) was inoculated intravenously with $1x10^6$
PFU H.saimiri 11 and died 3 weeks after inoculation. A serum
against viral structural proteins was obtained from a rabbit
(R1) inoculated intracutaneously with multiple doses of
H.saimiri 11 in the presence of complete Freund's adjuvans. A
serum against virus-induced infected cell proteins was
obtained from a goat inoculated with multiple doses of
H.saimiri 11 infected cells (gift of F. Deinhardt, Munich).

RESULTS

1.   <u>Time ordered synthesis of viral proteins</u>

a)   labelling with ^{35}S-methionine

To study the course of protein synthesis during the
lytic cycle of virus replication, infected cell cultures were
labelled at various times after infection (Fig. 1).
Twenty-one polypeptides were synthesized starting 9 to 10
hours post infection (Fig. 1, lane L-P) and are most likely
late proteins, since their synthesis increased further and
they could also be identified in purified virions (Fig. 4a).
Early proteins could be detected in trace amounts only.

The use of amino acid analogues proved to be helpful to
enrich these early polypeptides and facilitated their
detection and distinction from late proteins. Eleven
virus-induced proteins were synthesized in the presence of
canavanine (Fig. 1, lane B-F); addition of azetidine allowed
six polypeptides to be produced (Fig. 1, lane G-K). Three of
the proteins synthesized in the presence of amino acid
analogues were also found in the virion (gp 88, pp 57, p 28).
When canavanine and azetidine were added to the cultures
simultaneously, the protein pattern appeared
indistinguishable from the one obtained with canavanine alone
(not shown). All protein data are summarized in Table 1.

b)   Labelling with ^{32}P-phosphate

Labelling with ^{32}P-orthophosphate showed, that five
viral polypeptides became phosphorylated during the course of
infection (Fig. 2): pp 57, pp 46, pp 28 were found to be late

viral polypeptides, pp 163, pp 57, pp 41, pp 28 were
synthesized in the presence of canavanine, pp 163, pp 57 and
pp 41 with azetidine added to the cultures.

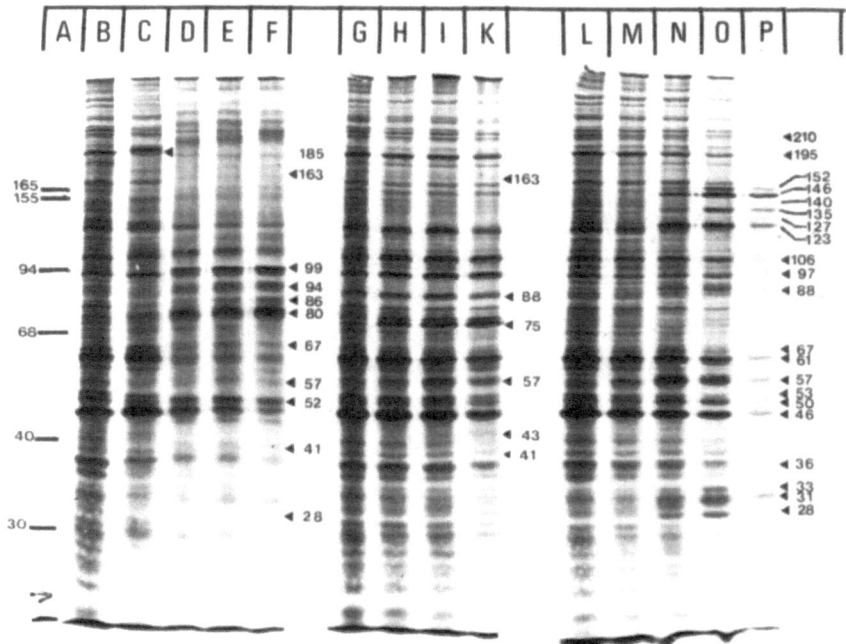

Fig. 1   Protein profiles from H.saimiri 11-infected
cells labelled at various times after infection with
^{35}S-methionine. Samples of 20000 cpm were applied per
slot. A: molecular weight marker proteins; B:
mock-infected cells, labelled 24-26 hours after mock
infection; virus-infected cells, treated with canavanine
and labelled from 0-4 (C), 4-9 (D), 9-15 (E) and 15-24
(F) hours after infection; virus-infected cells treated
with azetidine and labelled from 0-4 (G), 4-9 (H), 9-15
(I), 15-24 (K) hours after infection; virus-infected
cells labelled without analogues 0-4 (L), 4-9 (M), 9-15
(N), 15-24 (O), 24-26 (P) hours after infection.

c)   Labelling with ^{14}C-glucosamine

In vivo labelling of viral proteins with (Fig. 3, A-F)
or without subsequent immunoprecipitation (Fig. 3, N-S)
identified seven glycosylated viral polypeptides: gp 152, gp
140, gp 127, gp 88, gp 67, gp 53, gp 50. In the presence of
canavanine, no viral glycoproteins could be identified after

immunoprecipitation, in the presence of azetidine, gp 127, gp 88, gp 67, gp 53, gp 50 were synthesized in trace amounts.

d)   in vitro labelling of glycoproteins

By electroblotting of virus-infeced proteins and detection of glycosylated proteins with ^{125}I-Con A, which binds specifically to glucose and mannose residues (Goldstein et al., 1965), the same polypeptides could be identified as glycoproteins as by in vivo labelling with ^{14}C-glucosamine (Fig. 3, T-Y).

2.   Structural proteins

The protein profiles of the various H.saimiri and H.ateles strains are shown in Fig. 4a. Twenty-one structural polypeptides could be identified for the H.saimiri strains by labelling with ^{35}S-methionine; two of these proteins (pp 135, pp 57) were found to be phosphorylated. A comparison of the protein pattern of H.saimiri 11 and H.saimiri 11 att showed no differences in the molecular weight of the single protein bands.

For H.ateles 73 and H.ateles 810, twenty different virion proteins could be identified by ^{35}S-methionine labelling. Three of these were found to be phosphorylated (pp 136, pp 57, pp 56). The molecular weights of H.ateles 810 polypeptides differed slightly from H.ateles 73 proteins and were distinguishable from the protein patterns observed with H.saimiri isolates.

By surface iodination of purified H.saimiri 11 and H.saimiri 11 att virions and capsids (Fig. 4b), 5 viral polypeptides (gp 88, gp 67, pp 57, p 46, p 28) could be identified as parts of the virus envelope and four polypeptides as capsid proteins (gp 152, p 146, gp 140, pp 135). No difference was found between the two strains of H.saimiri.

3.   Immunoprecipitation

a)   Precipitation with sera from Saimiri sciureus

H.saimiri infected cell proteins were labelled early (6-8 hours p.i.) middle (15-17 hours p.i.), late (24-26 hours

p.i.) and in the presence of azetidine with ^{35}S-methionine.
The labelled polypeptides were precipitated with three
different sera from squirrel monkeys (Ss1, Ss2, Ss3). In
azetidine-treated cells and at early times after infection
only a few viral proteins were precipitated: gp 152, gp 53,
gp 50, pp 28 in azetidine treated cells and gp 152, p 97, gp
53, p 46 in early labelled cells. A subset of viral proteins,
which are mostly viral structure proteins was identified when
cells were labelled at intermediate and late times p.i. (Fig.
5): p 195, gp 152, p 146, pp 135, gp 127, p 123, p 106, p 97,
gp 88, gp 67, p 61, gp 53, gp 50, pp 28. A serum against
virion proteins produced in rabbits (R1) was used as positive
control. All sera were tested with mock infected cells to
exclude unspecific binding (not shown).

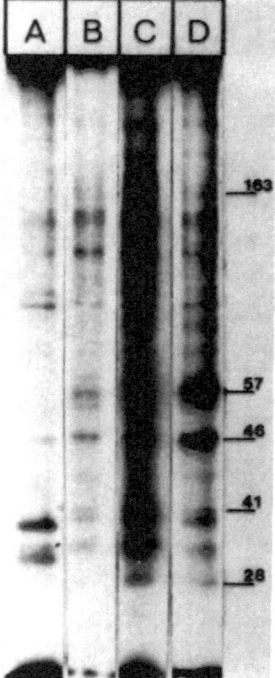

Fig. 2   Protein profiles from H.saimiri 11 infected
cells labelled with ^{32}P-orthophosphate. Samples of 10000
cpm were applied per slot; cells were labelled 24-26
hours after infection. A: mock-infected cells, B:
infected cells, treated with canavanine, C: infected
cells, treated with azetidine, D: infected cells without
analogues.

b)   Precipitation with sera of experimental hosts

^{35}S-methionine labelled proteins were precipitated with sera from three different owl monkeys (At1, At2, At3), one Saguinus nigricollis (Sn1), and one New Zealand white rabbit (NZWR1). All these animals were dying of neoplastic disease after infection with H.saimiri. Sera from the experimental hosts precipitated at middle and late (Fig. 5) times after infections a limited number of viral proteins: gp 152, gp 127, p 115, p 80, p 55-57 (p 55 for Aotus trivirgatus, p 57 for S.nigricollis and NZWR), gp 53, gp 50, pp 28. p 146 and pp 135 were only precipitated with some owl monkey sera in very small quantities, p 195, p 123, p 106, p 97, gp 88, gp 67, p 61 were never seen. Three proteins, however, were not found to be precipitated with the sera of the natural hosts: p 115, p 80, p 55-57. p 115 and p 55-57 are synthesized already at an early stage after infection, p 115 was not found in the presence of azetidine.

H.saimiri infected cell proteins were precipitated with a serum of a Saguinus fuscicollis (Sf1) which was persistently infected with H.saimiri 11 att. The protein profiles obtained after precipitation were very similar to those obtained with sera of Saimiri sciureus, most of the proteins being structural polypeptides (Fig. 5).

c)   Comparison of H.saimiri 11 and H.saimiri 11 att infected
      cell proteins

All sera from the natural and experimental hosts showed no differences in the protein profiles of H.saimiri 11 and H.saimiri 11 att infected cell proteins. By immunoprecipitation with a serum against H.saimiri 11 infected cell proteins in a goat, one polypeptide in H.saimiri 11 infected cells was precipitated which was not found in H.saimiri 11 att infected cells (Fig. 6); the protein had a molecular weight of about 55.000 D.

DISCUSSION

The repression of the lytic cycle is essential for the manifestation of the oncogenic potential of a virus of the

herpes group, since replication invariably causes the death
of the host cells. It seems reasonable to conclude from
observations with other herpesviruses, that the expression of
viral genes follows a regulated pattern. It would be of great
interest to know where this cascade of regulated expression
is interrupted in the tumor cell (Wolf and Bayliss, 1979) and
eventually to understand the mechanisms responsible for this
regulation. Whereas the highly lytic Herpes simplex virus
allowed detailed analysis of the lytic cycle (Honess and
Roizman, 1974, 1975; Morse et al., 1978; Wolf and Roizman,
1978), it is extremely difficult to obtain results for
Epstein-Barr virus, where an efficient lytic system is not
known (Wolf and Bayliss, 1979; Kallin et al., 1979; Feighny
et al., 1981; Bayliss and Wolf, 1981, 1982). In order to
study the regulation of gene expression, we examined the
course of protein synthesis in cells lytically infected with
H.saimiri.

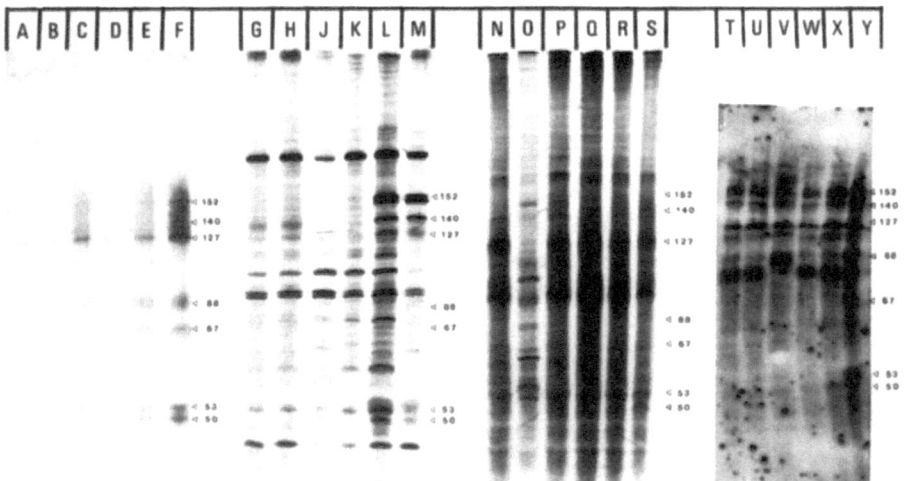

Fig. 3   Glycosylation of H.saimiri-induced proteins.
A-F: cells labelled with ^{14}C-glucosamine and
immunoprecipitated, G-M: cells labelled with
^{35}S-methionine and immunoprecipitated, N-S: cells
labelled with ^{14}C-glucosamine, T-Y: cells
electroblotted, labelled with ^{125}I-Con A.
A, G, N, T: mock-infected cells, labelled 24-26 hours
after mock-infection; B, H, O, V: cells infected with
H.saimiri 11 treated with canavanine, labelled 24-26
hours after infection; C, I, P, U: cells infected with
H.saimiri 11, treated with azetidine, labelled 24-26

hours after infection. D, K, Q, W: cells infected with
H.saimiri 11, labelled 6-8 hours after infection. E, L,
R, X: cells infected with H.saimiri 11, labelled 15-17
hours after infection. F, M, S, Y: cells infected with
H.saimiri 11, labelled 24-26 hours after infection.

Analysis of electrophoretically separated polypeptides
revealed at least 31 virus-induced proteins synthesized
during the course of infection. The polypeptides could be
characterized and classified according to their molecular
weights, their modification and their kinetic appearance in
the lytic cycle. All these data are summarized in Table 1.

As for other members of the herpesvirus group, the
function of early proteins is essential for the synthesis of
polypeptides produced later in the lytic cycle. The amino
acid analogues canavanine (for arginine) and azetidine (for
proline) are incorporated into the polypeptide chains in
place of the corresponding amino acids. By this they affect
the function of the proteins whithout detectably changing
their molecular weights. In the presence of azetidine six
different viral proteins were synthesized (Fig. 1): pp 163,
gp 88, pp 57, p 43, pp 41. In the presence of canavanine 11
polypeptides were produced: p 185, pp 163, p 99, p 94, p 86,
p 80, gp 67, pp 57, p 53, pp 41, pp 28, three of these being
identical with those synthesized in the presence of
azetidine: p 52, pp 41, pp 28. This suggests that two groups
of proteins may belong to a first class of early proteins.
According to the content of arginine and proline and their
participitation in active groups in the polypeptide chains,
their function may be inhibited by the incorporation of
either of the amino acid analogues. The synthesis of a second
class of proteins does not follow. Some of the proteins
synthesized in the presence of analogues were not found in
untreated infected cells. An explanation for this effect may
be that the enrichment in cells with the analogues is
essential for their detection. Alternatively, an altered
posttranslational modification could be responsible for these
proteins.

Twenty-one polypeptides could be identified as late proteins (Fig. 1), the synthesis of which started about 9 to 10 hours post infection (p 210, p 195, gp 152, p 146, gp 140, pp 135, gp 127, p 123, p 106, p 97, gp 88, gp 67, p 61, pp 57, gp 53, gp 50, pp 46, p 36, p 33, p 31, pp 28). The synthesis of these polypeptides was dependant on prior DNA-replication; when inhibitors of the viral DNA-synthesis were added during infection, only a subset of early proteins was produced (Modrow and Wolf, 1983a). Some of these late proteins are also synthesized in the presence of amino acid analogues (gp 88, pp 57, pp 28) and possibly are polypeptides whose synthesis is required during the whole cycle. By labelling with ^{32}P-phosphate (Fig. 2), five phosphoproteins were identified during the course of infection: pp 163, pp 57, pp 46, pp 41, pp 28. pp 135 was found to be phosphorylated in the virions. This process of phosphorylation might occur during or be essential for the assembly of the virion.

The viral glycoproteins were identified by two different methods: (I) by in vivo glycosylation with ^{14}C-glucosamine and (II) by in vitro labelling with ^{125}I-Concanavalin A. Both methods gave similar results - seven viral proteins were found to be glycosylated: gp 152, gp 140, gp 127, gp 88, gp 67, gp 53, gp 50. These were all late viral proteins as they were not synthesized at early times after infection or in the presence of canavanine. When ^{14}C-glucosamine labelled proteins were separated without prior immunoprecipitation, all late viral glycoproteins could be identified beside a number of host glycoproteins (Fig. 3, N-s). In canavanine-treated cells (Fig. 3, O) some additional proteins were detected, which were not seen in immunoprecipitation experiments. These bands may represent a subset of early viral proteins which are not recognized by the serum used here. Alternatively, they may be artefacts due to the presence of the analogue.

In the in vitro labelling experiments with ^{125}I-Con A, all glycoproteins with glucose and mannose or derivatives of

118

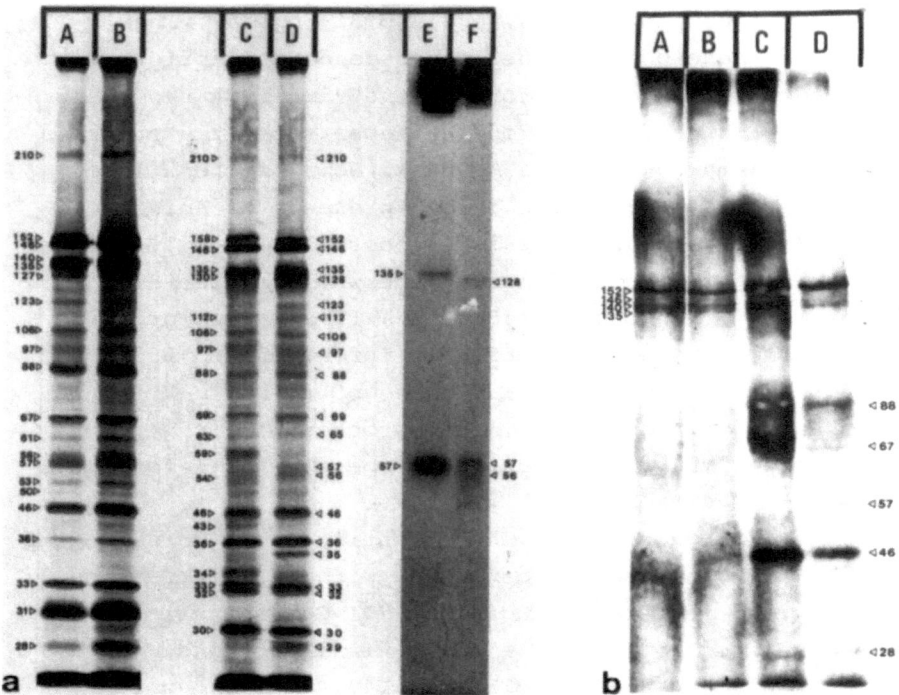

Fig. 4   a) Structural proteins of H.saimiri and
H.ateles. A-D: labelled with ^{35}S-methionine, E-F:
labelled with ^{32}P-orthophosphate. A: H.saimiri 11; B:
H.saimiri 11 att, C: H.ateles 810, D: H.ateles 73, E:
H.saimiri 11, F: H.ateles 73. b) ^{125}I-labelled surface
proteins. A: H.saimiri 11 att capsids, B: H.saimiri 11
capsids, C: saimiri 11 att virions, D: H.saimiri 11
virions.

these sugars are identified by their binding capacity for
^{125}I-Con A, regardless whether they are of cellular or viral
origin. Due to the experimental procedure no host shut-down
can be observed and viral proteins can be observed as
additional bands only.

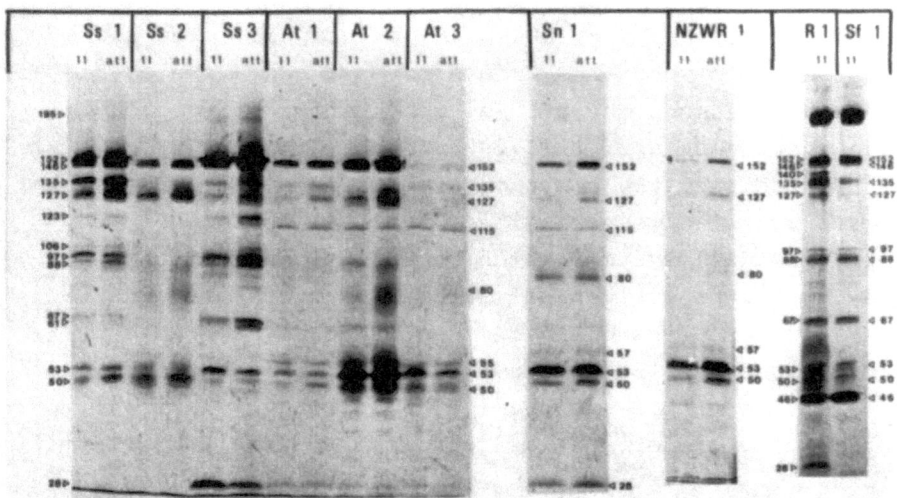

Fig. 5   H.saimiri-infected cells, labelled with
³⁵S-methionine from 24-26 hours after infection and
immunoprecipitated with the sera indicated.
11: H.saimiri 11 infected cells; att: H.saimiri 11 att
infected cells. Ss1, Ss2, Ss3: sera of Saimiri sciureus,
infected with H.saimiri 11; At1, At2, At3: sera of Aotus
trivirgatus, infected with H.saimiri 11; Sn1: serum of
S.nigricollis, infected with H.saimiri 11; Sf1: serum of
S.fuscicollis, infected with H.saimiri 11 att. NZW1:
serum of a New Zealand white rabbit, infected with
H.saimiri 11; R1: rabbit serum against structural
proteins of H.saimiri.

The analysis of purified virions of H.saimiri 11 and
H.saimiri 11 att revealed 21 polypeptides as viral structural
proteins (Fig. 4a). All these proteins were also identified
as late viral polypeptides being produced late during the
lytic cycle. Two of these proteins located in the virion were
found to be phosphorylated. For H.ateles 73 and H.ateles 810,
20 different proteins could be identified, three of these
were phosphorylated (pp 136, pp 57, pp 56). The molecular
weights of H.ateles 73 proteins differed slightly from
H.ateles 810 polypeptides and were distinguishable from the
protein pattern observed with H.saimiri isolates. The overall
pattern of the protein profiles of the various H.saimiri and
H.ateles strains, however, was fairly similar, 8 proteins

being conserved according to their molecular weights (p 210, gp 146, p 106, p 97, gp 88, p 46, p 36, p 33). The close relationship of proteins from H.saimiri and H.ateles reflects the relatedness of their DNAs, which show 35% homology (Fleckenstein et al., 1978).

To identify the components of virions and capsids, the surface proteins were labelled with ^{125}I using the lactoperoxidase system, which is a very gentle method, allowing the selective iodination of surface proteins. By this, four proteins could be identified as capsid polypeptides (gp 152, p 146, gp 140, pp 135) and five as parts of the viral envelope (gp 88, gp 67, pp 57, p 46, p 28; Fig. 4b). No difference was found between the two H.saimiri strains.

To study the gene expression in the various natural and experimental hosts, H.saimiri-induced cell proteins were immunoprecipitated with sera from these animals. In the natural hosts (Saimiri sciureus) most antibodies are directed against late viral polypeptides, which are mostly structural components of the H.saimiri virion (Fig. 4). A very similar picture was obtained with a serum from a Saguinus fuscicollis (Sf 1), which was infected with H.saimiri 11 att (Schaffer et al., 1975). This virus strain is reported to be non-oncogenic in different marmoset species, and induces a latent or persistent infection (Falk et al., 1976; Wright et al., 1977, 1980). Thus the etiological behaviour of H.saimiri 11 att in marmosets is very similar to that of H.saimiri 11 in squirrel monkeys. This fact could be demonstrated by immunoprecipitation experiments: the sera of squirrel monkeys infected with the oncogenic wild type showed the same antibody pattern as that obtained from a marmoset infected with H.saimiri 11 att.

Sera from experimental hosts infected with H.saimiri which had died from a neoplastic disease showed by immunoprecipitation, that their antibody specificity was different from that obtained from the natural host, but very similar amongst the different species (owl monkey, marmoset,

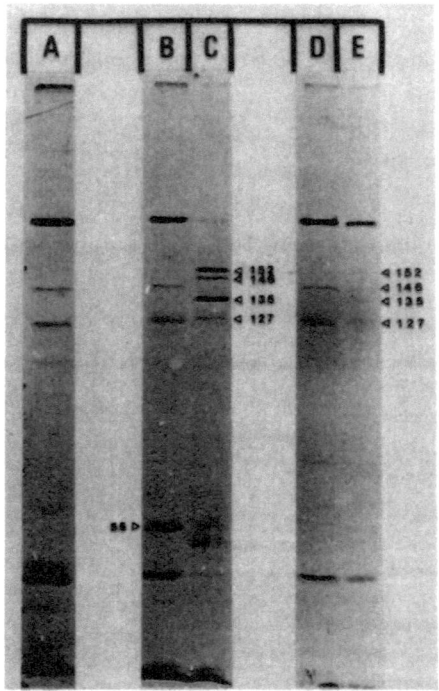

Fig. 6   Cells infected with H.saimiri, labelled with
^{35}S-methionine and immunoprecipitated with a goat serum
directed against H.saimiri 11 infected cell protein. A:
mock-infected cells labelled 24-26 hours after
mock-infection; B: H.saimiri 11 infected cells, labelled
8-10 hours after infection; C: H.saimiri 11 infected
cells, labelled 24-26 hours after infection; D:
H.saimiri 11 att infected cells, labelled 8-10 hours
after infection; E: H.saimiri 11 att infected cells,
labelled 24-26 hours after infection.

New Zealand white rabbit). With the sera of all these hosts,
three proteins were precipitated, which were never
precipitated with sera from squirrel monkeys: p 115, p 80, p
55 in owl monkeys and p 57 in S.nigricollis and NZWR
respectively. The slight difference in the molecular weight
(p 55 - p 57) may be due to a different modification in the
various hosts with the antibodies directed against the
modification. p 115 and p 55-57 may be due to a different
modification in the various hosts with the antibodies
directed against the modification. p 115 and p 55 - 57 were

synthesized already at an early stage after infection; the synthesis of p 115, however, was inhibited by the treatment of azetidine and thus may belong to a second regulatory group of early proteins.

Since all animals developing H.saimiri-induced neoplastic disease are reported to have high anti-EA titers (Klein et al., 1973; Pearson et al., 1973, 1974), which increase with the development of malignant tumors, one might

TABLE 1

Mol.wt x10⁻³	Time after synthesis with H.saimiri 11 (0 2 4 6 8 10 12 14 16 18 20 22 24)	synthesis with canavanine	synthesis with azetidine	phospho-rylation	glyco-sylation	structural proteins
210						•
195						•
185		•				
163		•	•	•		
152					•	•
146						•
140					•	•
135						•
127					•	•
123						•
106						•
99		•				
97						•
94		•				
88			•		•	•
86		•				
80		•				
75			•			
67		•			•	•
61						•
57		•	•	•		•
53					•	•
52		•				
50					•	•
46				•		•
43			•			
41		•	•	•		
36						•
33						•
31						•
28		•		•		•

conclude, that the three proteins p 115, p 80, p 55 - 57 are components of the EA-complex. In natural hosts the anti-EA titers were found to decline some weeks after the primary infection.

Between the protein profiles obtained from H.saimiri 11 and H.saimiri 11 att infected cell proteins precipitated with squirrel monkey, owl monkey, marmoset and NZWR sera respectively, no differences could be detected. However, one protein could be identified in H.saimiri infected cells when the extracts were precipitated with a serum raised in a goat against H.saimiri 11 infected cells. The molecular weight of the protein was found to be 55000 D. This protein may either be a viral protein which is deleted in H.saimiri 11 att, or a cellular protein, whose synthesis is not induced during infection with H.saimiri 11 att. As a third possibility, the differences in the protein patterns may be due to a different protein modification of H.saimiri 11 and H.saimiri 11 att induced polypeptides.

The characterization of the polypeptides which present, themselves in the various experimental and natural hosts as antigens may be a step towards a better understanding of the regulatory mechanisms involved in the development of the H.saimiri induced malignant disease. At least our experiments show that tests for antibodies directed against specific antigens could be useful to discriminate between tumor bearing and non-tumor bearing hosts and that antibodies reacting with other antigens may be used for a nondiscriminating diagnosis of the immune status. Although this may be of interest for hosts infected with H.saimiri, similar work may prove important for the diagnosis of infections or neoplastic disease caused by Epstein-Barr virus and other herpesviruses in man.

REFERENCES

Bayliss, G.J. and Wolf, H. 1981. The regulated expression of Epstein-Barr virus III. Proteins specified by EBV during the lytic cycle. J. Gen. Virol., 56, 105-118.

Bayliss, G.J. and Wolf, H. 1982. Effect of the analogue canavanine on the synthesis of Epstein-Barr virus-induced proteins in superinfected Raji cells. J. Virol., 41, 1109-1111.

Calnek, B.W., Adldinger, H.K. and Kohn, D.E. 1970. Feather follicle epithelium. A source of enveloped and infectious cell-free herpesvirus from Mark's disease. Avian Disease, 14, 219-233.

Daniel, M.D., Hunt, R.D., DuBoise, P., Silva, D. and Melendez, L.V. 1975. Induction of Herpesvirus saimiri lymphoma in New Zealand white rabbits inoculated intravenously. In "Oncogenesis and Herpesviruses II", Part 2 (Ed. G. de Thé, M. Epstein and H.zurHausen). (IARC, Lyon). pp. 205-208.

Daniel, M.D., Melendez, L.V., Hunt, R.D., King, N.W., Anver, M., Fraser, C.E.O., Barahona, H.H. and Baggs, R.B. 1974. Herpesvirus saimiri VII. Induction of malignant lymphoma in New Zealand white rabbits. J. Natl. Cancer Inst., 53, 1803-1807.

Deinhardt, F. and Deinhardt, J. 1979. Comparative aspects in oncogenic animal herpesviruses. In "The Epstein-Barr Virus" (Ed. M.A. Epstein and B.G. Achong). (Springer Verlag, Heidelberg). pp. 374-415.

Deinhardt, F., Falk, L.A. and Wolfe, L.G. 1974. Simian herpesviruses and neoplasia. Adv. Cancer Res., 19, 169-205.

Falk, L.A., Wright, J., Deinhardt, F., Wolfe, L.G., Schaffer, P.A. and Benyish-Melnick, M. 1976. Experimental infection of squirrel and marmoset monkeys with attenuated Herpesvirus saimiri. Cancer Res., 36, 707-710.

Feighny, R.J., Henry II, B.E. and Pagano, J.S. 1981. Epstein-Barr virus polypeptides: Effect of inhibition of viral DNA replication on their synthesis. J. Virol., 37, 61-71.

Fenwick, M.L. and Walker, M.J. 1978. Suppression of the synthesis of cellular macromolecules by Herpes simplex virus. J. Gen. Virol., 41, 37-51.

Fleckenstein, B., Bornkamm, G.W., Mulder, C., Werner, F.-J., Daniel, M.D., Falk, L.A., Delius, H. 1978. Herpesvirus ateles DNA and its homology with Herpesvirus saimiri nucleic acid. J. Virol., 25, 361-373.

Goldstein, I.J., Hollerman, C.E. and Smith, E.E. 1965. Protein-carbohydrate-interaction. II. Inhibition studies on the interaction of concanavalin A with polysaccharides. Biochemistry, 4, 876-883.

Honess, R.W. and Roizman, B. 1974. Regulation of Herpesvirus macromolecular synthesis I: Cascade regulation of the synthesis of three groups of viral proteins. J. Virol., 14, 8-19.

Hunt, R.D., Meléndez, L.V., King, N.W., Gilmore, C.E., Daniel, M.D., Williamson, M.G. and Jones, T.C. 1970. Morphology of disease with features of malignant lymphoma in marmosets and owl monkeys inoculated with Herpesvirus saimiri. J. Natl. Cancer Inst., 44, 447-465.

Kallin, B., Luke, J. and Klein, G. 1979. Immunochemical

characterization of Epstein-Barr virus-associated early and late antigens in N-butyrate-treated P3HR1 cells. J. Virol., <u>32</u>, 710-716.

Klein, G., Pearson, G.R., Rabson, A., Ablashi, D.V., Falk, L., Wolfe, L., Deinhardt, F. and Rabin, H. 1973. Antibody reactions to Herpesvirus saimiri (HVS)-induced early and late antigens (EA and LA) in HVS-infected squirrel monkeys, marmosets and owl monkeys. Int. J. Cancer., <u>12</u>, 270-289.

Meléndez, L.V., Daniel, M.D., Hunt, R.D. and Garcia, F.G. 1968. An apparently new herpesvirus from primary kidney cultures of the squirrel monkey (Saimiri sciureus). Lab. Anim. Care, <u>18</u>, 374-381.

Meléndez, L.V., Hunt, R.D., Daniel, M.D., Blake, J.B. and Garcia, F.G. 1971.Acute lymphocytic leukemia on owl monkeys inoculated with Herpesvirus saimiri. Science, <u>171</u>, 1161-1163.

Meléndez, L.V., Hunt, R.D., Daniel, M.D., Garcia, F.G. and Fraser, C.E.O. 1969. Herpesvirus saimiri II. Experimentally induced malignant lymphoma in primates. Lab. Anim. Care, <u>19</u>, 378-386.

Modrow, S. and Wolf, H. 1983a, Herpesvirus saimiri-induced proteins in lytically infected cells. I. Time ordered synthesis. J. Gen. Virol.

Modrow, S. and Wolf, H. 1983b, Characterization of Herpesvirus saimiri and Herpesvirus ateles structural proteins. Virology.

Morse, L.S., Pereira, L., Roizman, B. and Schaffer, P. 1978. Anatomy of Herpes Simplex Virus (HSV) DNA X: Mapping of viral genes by analysis of polypeptides. J. Virol., <u>26</u>, 389-410.

Pearson, G.R., Orr, T., Rabin, H., Cicmanec, I., Ablashi, D. and Armstrong, G. 1973. Antibody pattern of Herpesvirus saimiri (HVS) induced antigens in owl monkeys infected with HVS. J. Natl. Cancer Inst., <u>51</u>, 1939-1943.

Pearson, G.R., Rabin, H., Wallen, W.C., Neubauer, R.H., Orr, T.W. and Cicmanec, I.L. 1974. Immunological and virological investigations on owl monkeys infected with Herpesvirus saimiri. J. Med. Primatology, <u>3</u>, 54-67.

Rangan, S.R.S., Martin, L.N., Enright, F.M. and Allen, W. 1976. Herpesvirus saimiri-induced malignant lymphoma in rabbits. J. Natl. Cancer Inst., <u>57</u>, 151-156.

Renart, I., Reiser, I. and Stark, G.R. 1979. Transfer of proteins from gels to diazobenzylomethyl-paper and detection with antisera: a method for studying antibody specificity and antigen structure. Proc. Natl. Acad. Sci. USA, <u>76</u>, 3116-3120.

Schaffer, P.A., Falk, L.A. and Deinhardt, F. 1975. Attenuation of Herpesvirus saimiri for marmosets after successive passage in cell culture at 39°C. J. Natl. Cancer Inst., <u>55</u>, 1243-1246.

Towbin, H., Staehelin, T. and Gordon, J. 1979. Electro-phoretic transfer of proteins from polyacrylamide gels to nitrocellulose sheets: procedure and some applications. Proc. Natl. Acad. Sci. USA, <u>76</u>, 4350-4354.

Wolf, H. and Bayliss, G.J. 1979. The role of host-virus
    interaction for the development of herpesvirus induced
    malignancies of New World primates. In "Antiviral
    mechanisms in the control of neoplasia". (Ed.
    P.Chandra). (Plenum Publ. Corp.). pp. 315-329.
Wolf, H., Bayliss, G.J. and Wilmes, E. 1981. Biological
    properties of Epstein-Barr virus. In "Cancer Campaign,
    Vol.5, Nasopharyngeal Carcinoma". (Ed. Grundmann,
    Ablashi, Krüger). (Gustav Fischer Verlag, Stuttgart).
    pp. 101-109.
Wolf, H. and Roizman, B. 1978. The regulation of γ
    (structural) polypeptide synthesis in herpes simplex
    virus types 1 and 2 infected cells. In "Oncogenesis and
    Herpesviruses III, Part 1". (Ed. G. de Thé, W. Henle and
    F. Rapp). (IARC, Lyon). pp. 327-336.
Wright, J., Falk, L.A., Wolfe, L.G. and Deinhardt, F. 1980.
    Herpesvirus saimiri: protective effect of attenuated
    strain against lymphoma induction. Int. J. Cancer, 26,
    477-482.
Wright, J., Falk, L.A., Wolfe, L.G., Ogden, J. and Deinhardt,
    F. 1977. Susceptibility of common marmosets (Callithrix
    jacchus) to oncogenic and attenuated strains of
    Herpesvirus saimiri. J. Natl. Cancer Inst., 59,
    1475-1478.

FACTORS INVOLVED IN PERSISTENT MURINE CYTOMEGALOVIRUS
INFECTIONS - A REVIEW

J.B. HUDSON

Division of Medical Microbiology, Faculty of Medicine,
University of British Columbia, Vancouver, Canada V6J 1W5

ABSTRACT
    This presentation will review what is known about the
factors involved in persistent murine cytomegalovirus (MCMV)
infections, by considering studies on infected mice and cell
lines infected in vitro. In mice of various strains, MCMV
establishes a productive infection in numerous tissues,
although specific cell types within a tissue may be spared.
Dissemination of the virus may be facilitated by a temporary
and generalized immunosuppression. Eventually a variety of
anti-viral responses help to terminate the acute phase of
infection, which is then replaced by a chronic type of
infection in certain tissues, and a true latent infection in
others. Some of the factors which are important in determining
the severity of the acute infection and the establishment and
duration of the chronic phase are: the strain and precise
history of the virus itself; age and strain of mice; the
presence of physical barriers to virus or immune cells (eg.
basement membranes in acini of submaxillary glands);
macrophages, which may control virus dissemination or promote
persistence; and the immune status of the mouse.
    The virus has frequently been reactivated from several
tissues of persistently infected mice. The two methods which
have proven successful in reactivation are: immunosuppressive
therapy of the animals; and explantation of tissues, usually
in the presence of embryonic fibroblast cultures. These
studies implicate the presence of virus-controlling factors in
persistently infected animals.
    Infections in vitro have been done on numerous cell lines
of murine and non-murine origin. Different responses have been
observed, ranging from efficient production of virus to
limited viral gene expression with no production of virus.
These in vitro studies have indicated the relevance of cell
cycle parameters, and other host cell factors, in determining
the extent of viral gene expression and persistence.

INTRODUCTION

    Murine Cytomegalovirus (MCMV) is a herpes virus which is
capable of infecting and persisting in various wild and
laboratory strains of mice. Most of the biochemical and
biological features of the virus have been discussed in two
recent reviews (Hudson, 1979; Osborn, 1982). This presentation
considers only those aspects which are thought to be relevant
to persistent MCMV infections, and hence relevant to

persistent herpes infections in general.[1]

The term 'persistent infection' is used, because in many instances it is not clear whether experimental mice have been chronically infected (producing low levels of infectious virus) or latently infected (no detectable infectious virus). The mouse can have both types of infection concurrently. Thus the virus may be in a true latent state in one type of tissue or group of cells, while another tissue is continuously shedding small amounts of virus. Even the designation of 'latent infection' as applied may be misleading, since insufficient amounts of the tissue may have been sampled for virus assay. This point will be raised again in a later section.

The old term 'salivary gland virus' reflects the fact that infected mice commonly shed small quantities of virus in their saliva for long periods of time. This probably represents the normal mode of transmission of MCMV. As a consequence the mouse probably reinfects itself periodically.

Therefore the problem requiring investigation may not be simply: 'What factors determine whether or not the virus replicates', but rather: 'What determines the level of virus production in a specific tissue'. In this respect CMV's may differ fundamentally from herpes simplex type viruses.

FACTORS AFFECTING MCMV INFECTIONS IN THE MOUSE

Figure 1 summarizes the kinetics of virus growth in selected tissues and the accompanying host responses. The graph is somewhat idealised in that all of these parameters have not been compared within a specific mouse strain, although there are enough data to indicate that several different strains follow a similar pattern of events, at least qualitatively. The basic model used in our laboratory is the SWR/J mouse, which responds to an intraperitoneal infection of

---

[1] In the following text only selected references are given. A more comprehensive bibliography is found in the reviews mentioned above.

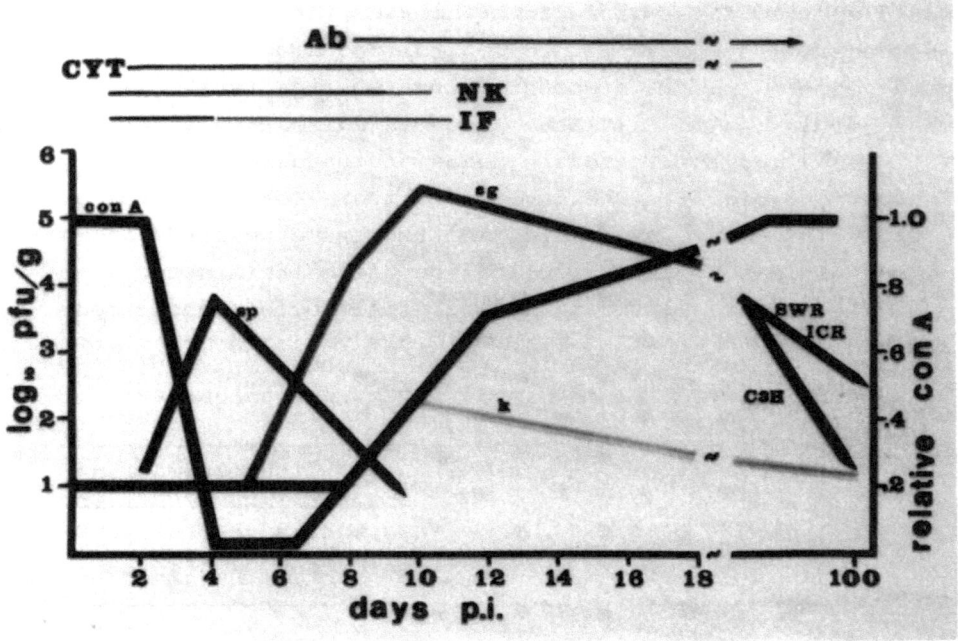

Fig. 1   Kinetics of virus growth and host responses.
Data for infectious virus (pfu per g. of tissue)   and
concanavalin A response of spleen cells are taken from
our studies with SWR/J mice (sg = submaxillary gland; sp
= spleen; k = kidney). Corresponding data for circulating
anti-MCMV antibody (Ab); cytotoxic T-cells (CYT); natural
killer cell activity (NK), and serum interferon (IF),
have been compiled from various published studies
utilizing various strains of mouse. In the upper part of
the diagram the solid lines represent the times of
maximal function, and the broken lines represent times of
uncertainty or disagreement in connection with a
function.

MCMV by replicating the virus transiently in visceral tissues
(as exemplified by the spleen in Fig. 1) and more extensively
in submaxillary glands and kidney. A dramatic but temporary
immunosuppression is observed after three days. This is
illustrated by the abrogation of the concanavalin A response
by spleen cells. The immunosuppression appears to be general,
and may allow the virus to disseminate throughout the body.
However, interferon and natural killer cell activity have been
detected shortly after infection, and eventually circulating
antibody and cytotoxic T-cells are found in abundance. It is

not clear how these different responses interrelate, although
in concert they do appear to control the amount of virus
produced, and may be responsible for terminating the acute
phase of infection in tissues such as spleen and liver.

The virus then enters a phase of gradually decreasing
production (Fig. 1). The duration of this 'chronic' phase is
clearly influenced by some of the factors enumerated in Table
1, but ultimately virus replication can be terminated.

The factors listed in Table 1 will now be considered
individually.

TABLE 1   Factors involved in MCMV pathogenesis

Factor	Involvement in	
	Acute Infection	Persistent Infection
Virus:		
strain (genotype)	+	?
history (virulent; attenuated)	+	+
Host:		
age	+	+
strain (H-2 genes)	+	+
physical barriers	?	+
macrophages	+	+
cell differentiation	+	?
cell cycle	+	±
immune status (NK cells; cortisone)	+	+

(i)   Strain of Virus

There exist at least two, and probably many more,
genetically distinguishable strains of MCMV, viz: the so-
called Smith strain, the one deposited in the American Type
Culture collection many years ago, which itself has probably
diverged considerably in different laboratories; and the
'virulent' K181 strain selected by Osborn. These two strains

differ in their restriction endonuclease patterns and in virus protein composition (Misra and Hudson, 1980; Dimmock and Hudson, unpublished data). Although they differ markedly in virulence, i.e. with respect to the acute infection, they do not appear to have been compared in regard to persistent infection.

(ii) History of the Virus

Murine CMV obtained from infected mice rapidly attenuates upon passage in cell culture (Osborn and Walker, 1971). The resultant attenuated virus retains the capacity to replicate in submaxillary glands (whereupon it reverts to virulence), but not in visceral tissues such as spleen and liver. The attenuation is accompanied by changes in virus protein composition (Dimmock and Hudson, unpublished data). The submaxillary-passaged virus tends to persist longer in the mouse than does virus repeatedly passaged in fibroblast cultures (Misra, 1977). It is not known if these differences are caused by cultivation of the virus in different cell types, i.e. acinar epithelial cells in the submaxillary gland compared with fibroblasts in vitro, or by some other feature of cultivation in vivo compared with in vitro (Selgrade et al, 1981).

(iii) Age of Mouse

In common with numerous other viruses, MCMV is much more virulent towards young immature mice than older mature mice. In addition we have found that infected immature SWR/J mice give rise to a more prolonged chronic phase than do infected adults (unpublished data). This may be explained by a quantitatively greater dissemination of the virus during the earlier stages of infection, when the immune system is not properly developed, with the results that tissues are seeded with more virus.

(iv) Strain of Mouse

A notable host contribution to MCMV pathogenesis is the

histocompatibility gene status, which has been studied
extensively by Chalmer (Chalmer et al, 1977; Chalmer, 1979).
Table 2 presents a few examples of the relative effect of H-2
genes on mortality in MCMV-infected adults. In general the b
and d haplotypes confer sensitivity to the virus, sensitivity
being dominant in crosses. Other non-H2 genes also contribute
however, and Chalmer has argued for the involvement of at
least four genetic loci (two H-2 linked, two non H-2 linked),
some of which correlate with specific histopathological
effects in certain tissues (Chalmer, 1979).

TABLE 2   Influence of host strain.

Strain	H2 haplotype	Relative LD_{50}[a]	Influence in persistent infection
DBA/1	q	<0.4	?
Balb/c	d	1.0	?
C57/BL	b	1.8	?
C3H/HeJ	k	>8.2	+
CBA	k	>8.2	?
SWR/J	q	>10[b]	+

[a]These data are examples taken from Chalmer (1979) and
represent LD_{50} values for young adults.

[b]Data from our laboratory under conditions approximating
those of Chalmer.

The host strain also influences the duration of the
chronic infection. This is illustrated in Fig. 1, from which
it can be seen that the chronic phase is more prolonged, at
least in submaxillary glands, in ICR and SWR mice than in C3H.

(v)   Physical Barriers

Conceivably the presence of 'barriers' such as basement
membranes could render a tissue or group of cells relatively
inaccessible to virus, and to immune responses once infection
were established. This could explain why salivary glands
require a long time to become infected in the first place, and
why the infection is then prolonged after this. Henson's group
has shown that the duration of the chronic phase in
submaxillary glands is inversely related to the efficacy of

the inflammatory response. Ultimately the attack on the acini
is successful and leads to destruction of infected and
adjacent uninfected cells. This process can be alleviated by
cortisone, with the result that virus continues to be produced
and shed (Henson and Neapolitan, 1970).

(vi) Macrophages

Studies from Mims' laboratory and from ours' have
focussed on the roles played by these cells in MCMV
infections. Mims and Gould (1978) have shown that peritoneal
macrophages and Kupffer cells can restrict the spread of MCMV,
although this restriction was relatively ineffective for
salivary gland passaged virus compared with cell-culture
passaged virus. This is an important distinction since wild
mice presumably are exposed to salivary gland virus.
Furthermore, in view of the invariable finding that
blood-borne virus is cell associated rather than free virus,
then perhaps the importance of the macrophage as a 'guardian'
against entry of virus into tissues has been exaggerated. In
fact the few macrophages which do become infected in vivo may
serve as reservoirs for later reinfection. In support of this
concept is the evidence that MCMV can persist in, and can be
reactivated from, spleen and peritoneal macrophages following
infection in vitro or in vivo (Hudson et al., 1978; Brautigam
et al., 1979; and unpublished data).

Thus the macrophage may well be an important factor in
persistent MCMV infections, but for reasons different from
those usually considered relevant to viruses.

(vii) Cell Differenciation

Probably few people would deny the likelihood that MCMV
gene expression is influenced by the state of differentiation
of the host cell, although very little evidence supports this
hypothesis.

Recently Dutko and Oldstone (1981) showed that modulation
of gene expression in teratocarcinoma cell lines could affect
MCMV transcription and replication, the more 'differentiated'

state favoring replication. Although this behaviour is quite different from other viruses tested in the same cell lines, it is evident that MCMV is subject to intracellular host control. This is also relevant to persistent infections since a cell carrying a latent MCMV genome may lose this control if host gene expression is modulated through differentiation or extracellular factors.

(viii) Cell Cycle

Studies in our laboratory (Muller and Hudson, 1977) indicated that MCMV can only replicate in fibroblasts if they are traversing the cell cycle. Specifically a cellular event associated with early S-phase seems to be required. Further discussion of this phenomenon appears below. Other cell types may show a similar requirement. The relevance to persistent infection stems from the hypothesis that, if a G_o-phase fibroblast carried a latent MCMV genome, then any event which forced that fibroblast into the cell cycle would also permit virus replication.

(ix) Immune Status

Several workers have shown that MCMV infection enhances NK cell activity. The importance of this response in the control of infection has been inferred from experiments with beige mutants, which lack significant NK activity and which are especially susceptible to the virus (Bancroft et al., 1981). It is generally assumed that the other immune responses depicted in Fig. 1 are also important in limiting the acute infection, although they do not prevent the establishment of persistent infection. Nevertheless, evidence for a continuing role of the immune system in controlling the virus has been adduced from the many experiments in which immunosuppressive treatments have led to the emergence of infectious virus (see Table 2 and next section).

REACTIVATION OF MCMV

Table 3 summarizes the successful attempts to reactivate

TABLE 3   Reactivation of MCMV

Experimental Material	Reactivation Stimulus	References
1. Animals: Wild mice	anti-theta serum	Gardner et al., 1974
laboratory infected mice	graft rejection	Wu et al., 1975
" " "	mock blood transfusion	Cheung and Lang, 1977a
" " "	cyclophosphamide	Mayo et al., 1977
" " "	anti-lymphocyte serum + corticosteroid	Jordan et al., 1977
2. Tissues:		
spleen, lymph nodes)		Henson et al., 1972
) co-cultivation with		
salivary glands,) fibroblasts in vitro		Olding et al., 1975
prostate)		
)		Wise et al.,1979
)		Cheung and Lang,
)		1977b
embryos	cultivation in vitro	Chantler et al., 1979
macrophages	'activation'	Brautigam et al., 1979
3. Cell cultures:		
spleen cultures	co-cultivation with fibroblasts	Hudson et al., 1978
3T3 cells	cell cycle stimulation	Muller et al., 1978
teratocarcinoma cells	'differentiation'	Dutko and Old-stone, 1981

MCMV from persistently infected mice, tissues and cell cultures.

(i) Reactivation in Mice

It has been customary to assume that, if infectious virus cannot be detected in samples of salivary glands or some other tissues, then the animal must be latently infected (or even uninfected). As I have already argued above this assumption may not be balid, for two reasons. Firstly, it is possible that the levels of virus produced are relatively low (1-100 PFU per organ) and hence difficult to detect by standard plaque assay techniques, especially if centrifugal inoculation of indicator cells is not used. We have sometimes had to assay entire tissues in order to detect a few infectious particles. Secondly, while the virus may be truly latent in a specific tissue, it may concurrently be shed continuously (i.e. a chronic infection) from other tissues. In fact in our experience it has proven notoriously difficult to obtain persistently infected SWR/J mice which were completely free of infectious virus in all tissues assayed, especially if the mice were immature at the time of infection. Probably in the wild the mothers are relatively young adults and therefore still excrete infected saliva, which then infects the newborns. Under these conditions chronic infection would prevail. In addition to these problems, individual mice (even of the same strain) do not all exhibit the same duration of the chronic phase, and consequently the result that some mice in an experiment are entirely free of infectious virus is no guarantee that the others are also free of virus.

These arguments in no way detract from the value of the systems enumerated in Table 3, however, since the reactivation is obviously abrogating some kind of control system, so that virus replication is elevated, either simultaneously in several tissues, or in one key tissue initially followed by dissemination to others. And it still remains a possibility that certain treatments may reactivate the virus from a latent state in a specific tissue in the face of continuous shedding from another.

The point at tissue therefore is not whether the models
in Table 3 are valid or relevant, for they certainly are, but
some of them may represent models for elevating the chronic
infection rather than for reactivating a true latent
infection. With regard to the mechanism involved, the common
denominator for reactivation in mice appears to be some aspect
of the immune system, since most of these treatments are known
to be 'immunosuppressive'. However, one should bear in mind
that additional non-immunological 'side-effects' probably
accompany all of these treatments, although it is difficult at
present to envisage a common non-immunological mechanism.
Nevertheless a similar dilemma is posed in trying to deduce
the precise immunological mechanism that could be involved,
unless this simply reflects the fact that the virus is
continually controlled by a combination of immune responses.

(ii) Reactivation from Tissues

In these experiments, fragments of tissue or groups of
intact cells are co-cultivated with fibroblast indicator
cells. Reactivation is indicated by the appearance of
characteristic cytopathic effects and the emergence of
infectious virus in the indicator cells. Concurrently portions
of these tissues are assayed for free virus. It is probably
easier to ascertain the absence of infectious virus in such
individual tissues than it is for whole mice, although the
problem raised above may still exist.

Earlier experiments were done with spleens and other
lymphoid tissues, although more recently similar results have
been obtained with submaxillary glands, prostate, embryos, and
peritoneal macrophages.

The mechanism of reactivation is not understood. It is
unlikely to be a simple loss of controlling factors operating
in vivo, since the emergence of infectious virus during
cultivation in vitro usually takes many days. It appears that
virus is first released from its carrier cells in an
infectious form, rather than as a free genome or

nucleoprotein, since its appearance can be inhibited by antibody in the culture medium but not by DNase (Hudson et al., 1978; Wu and Ho, 1979). The virus then spreads in the indicator fibroblasts and possibly any fibroblasts which have grown out from the tissue sample. The initial carrier cell or latently-infected cell could itself be a fibroblast or some other cell type in which virus replication depends upon the cell cycle. Non-dividing cells from tissues frequently start dividng when cultivated in vitro.

(iii) <u>Reactivation in Cell Culture</u>

In order to study the molecular basis of reactivation, we have resorted to the use of cell culture models, as indicated in Table 3. These are described in more detail in the next section.

THE USE OF CELL CULTURE MODELS

In Table 4 is a summary of the extent of virus replication in various cultured mouse cells. The information is incomplete in the sense that few of these cultures have been tested at different phases of the cell cycle or in relation to extracellular modulators. Furthermore any of these cells could conceivably harbour a latent infection under certain conditions.

Non-murine cell types are documented in Table 5. Evidently MCMV can replicate to some degree in cultures from rat, hamster, rabbit, sheep and monkey. Also the apodemus CMV can replicate in human cells. The Smith strain of MCMV does not replicate in human cell lines, although some viral genes can be expressed (Mosmann, 1975; Walker and Hudson, unpublished). The virus does not appear to do anything in mink lung cells.

(i) <u>Spleen Cell Cultures</u>

Several years ago we set up the spleen cell culture system for MCMV infection in vitro. Although the results provided a few insights into virus-cell interactions, the long

TABLE 4   Susceptibility of Murine Cells to MCMV in
           vitro.

Cell line or tissue	Virus yield[a] (pfu per cell)	
Embryonic fibroblasts	10	100
3T3 lines (several)	"	
3T6	"	
MKSA (SV40 transformed kidney)	>10	
primary brain	>1	
tracheal epithelial cells[c]	>1	
teratocarcinoma cells (several)[b]	-to >1	
L929	<1	
Y-1 (adrenal cells)	"	
primary kidney	"	
primary spleen	"	
primary liver	"	
macrophage lines (several)	"	
T lymphocytes	–	
L5178Y (leukemic T-cells)	–	

[a]Data from Hudson, 1979: [b]Dutko and Oldstone, 1981:
[c]Nedrud et al., 1982. Other more recent data, Hudson
et al., unpublished.

term cultivation of persistently infected cells proved
difficult to achieve. We were able to demonstrate that the
virus did not replicate in T-lymphocytes, that B-lymphocytes
were generally unresponsive, and that a low level of infection
occurred in macrophage-like cells.

This system was eventually abandoned because of the
difficulty in maintaining such heterogenous cultures.
Nevertheless we did show that the results mimicked the
virus-cell interactions taking place in vivo (Loh and Hudson,
1979).

(ii) Murine Fibroblasts

The cell cycle dependance of MCMV replication in

TABLE 5   Susceptibility of Non-Murine Cells to MCMV in
           vitro.

Species of Origin	Cell Type	Virus Yield (pfu/cell)	Viral Gene Expression
Rat	Primary cerebellum	>1	+
Hamster	BHK line	<1	+
Rabbit	Primary kidney; RK13 line	<1	+
Mink	Mv1Lu line[a]	−	?
Sheep	Primary fetal brain	>1	+
Monkey	BSC-1 line	<1	+
Human	HeLa; KB lines	−	−
	Hep-2; WI-38; MRC-5[a]	−	+

Data taken from Hudson, 1979. [a]Hudson et al., unpublished.

fibroblasts has been mentioned already. This property is
illustrated in Fig. 2 for 3T3 cells. These cells quickly enter
a quiescent or G_o phase as serum growth factors are depleted.
The virus readily infects such cells but will only replicate
when fresh medium containing serum is added. Under these
conditions a substantial fraction of the cell population
initiates a cell cycle. The consequent initiation of S-phase
is followed by viral DNA replication and ultimately the
production of infectious virus (Muller, 1977).

     If the infected 3T3 cultures are maintained in the G_o
phase, infectious virus eventually disappears completely. But
the virus can be reactivated at any time, however, by simply
providing serum in fresh medium (Muller, 1977). This is
illustrated in Fig. 3, which also shows that the number of
infectious centers remains high. Thus this system furnishes a
useful short term model for studying the establishment of a
latent infection and its reactivation by manipulating the
cells' environment.

     In further studies we compared the patterns of viral DNA,
RNA and protein synthesis in S-phase and G_o phase cells. The
results are presented in the form of a composite diagram in

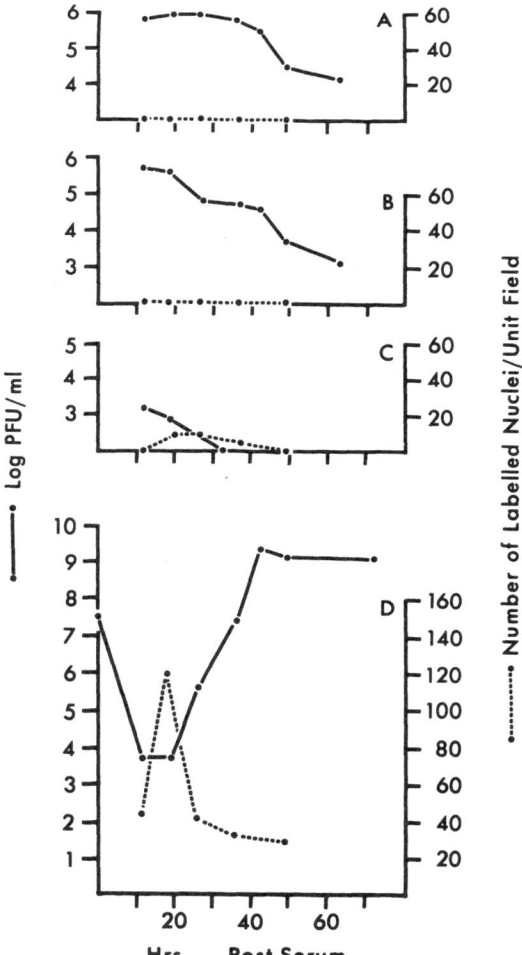

Fig. 2   Correlation between cell cycle traverse
and MCMV replication.
Cultures of 3T3 cells were left without medium
change for 9 days. They were infected with MCMV (20
pfu per cell) and, after the adsorption period, were
divided into four groups for the following
treatments: Group A, control, same depleted medium
added back to cells; Group B, depleted medium added
together with 10% fresh serum; Group C, fresh medium
only added without serum; Group D, fresh medium plus
10% serum added. All cultures were assayed for
infectious virus (pfu) and for mitotic cells (by
autoradiography following ^{3}H-thymidine pulses). Data
from Muller, 1977.

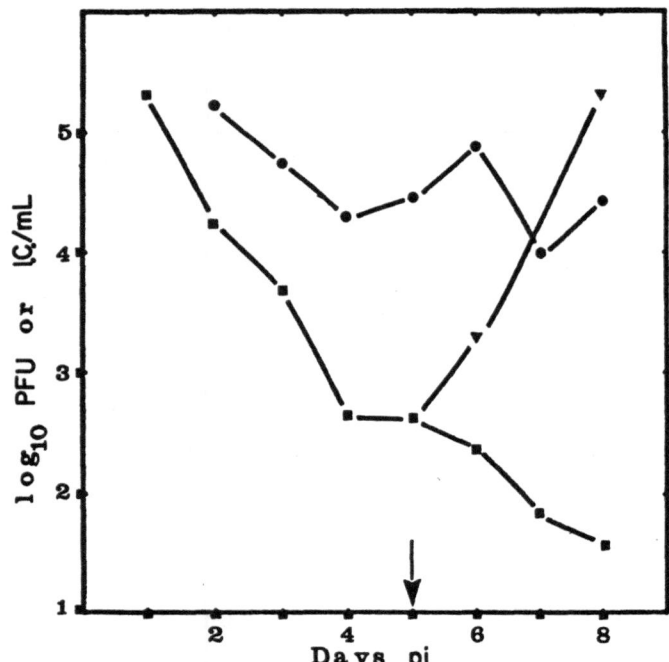

Fig. 3   Infectious virus ( ) and infectious centers
(o) in Go-phase 3T3 cells infected with MCMV on day O. At
the time indicated by the arrow, some cultures received
fresh medium plus 10% serum and were then assayed for pfu
( ).

Fig. 4. During the first four hours of infection in the
S-phase cells at least 17 viral-induced proteins are produced,
accompainied by the transcription of approximately 40% of the
viral genome (i.e. 20% of the viral DNA). Some of these
proteins, and a large fraction of the transcripts, are also
present in the G_O phase cells. In the latter, a few additional
genes are transcribed later, but no viral DNA replication can
be detected unless the cell cycle stimulus is provided. In the
S-phase cells viral DNA replication commences at 8 hpi.
accompanied by the transcription of most of the remainder of
the genome, and eventually the production of virion proteins.

Unfortunately there are two limitations to the use of
this 3T3-cell model. Firstly, cultures maintained in the G_O
phase represent dying cells, for they cannot be propagated.

Thus after continuous serum/medium deprivation the cultures become increasingly difficult to handle and accordingly experiments cannot be done after 10-14 days.

Secondly, different 3T3 cell lines vary somewhat in their response to MCMV. Thus in some of these lines it has proven

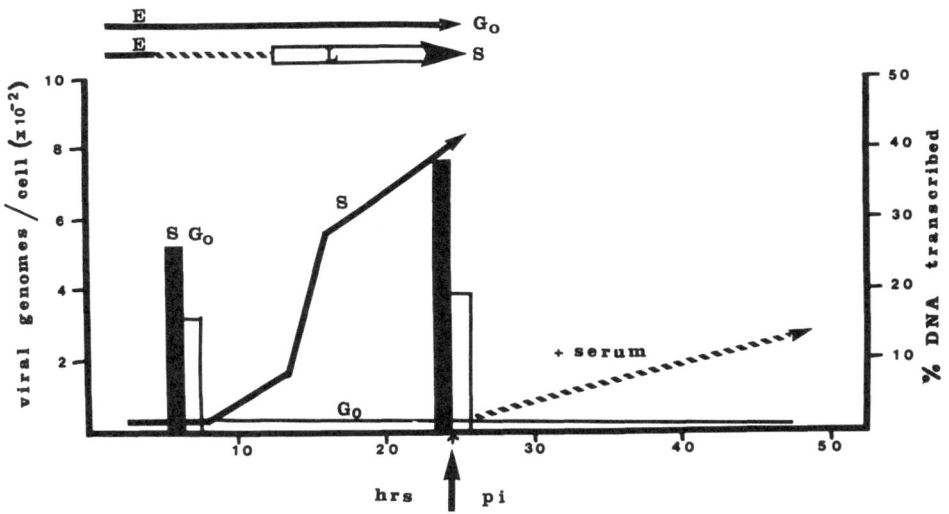

Fig. 4   MCMV gene expression in 3T3 cells.
The data have been compiled from several studies involving MCMV infected S-phase 3T3 cells (solid lines and bars) and infected Go-phase 3T3 cells (thin lines and open bars). The upper part of the diagram depicts the duration and extent of viral protein synthesis. In the graph bars represent % of DNA transcribed; lines represent number of viral genomes per cell. The broken line shows the number of viral genomes per cell following addition of fresh medium plus 10% serum to the cells.

difficult to block completely the spread of MCMV, which instead establishes a low level chronic infection. This also applies to mouse embryo cultures, although we have been able to demonstrate a correlation of cell cycle traverse with MCMV replication in the latter. This problem may be explained by the difficulty in obtaining a state of 100% G_o phase cells in such cultures.

The first of these limitations was circumvented recently in a study of teratocarcinoma cell lines (Dutko and Oldstone, 1981). The virus could be maintained in a latent state in at least one of these 'undifferentiated' cell lines. When such cells were induced to 'differentiate' viral replication ensued. This system warrants further analysis, although it is not clear how the changes taking place in teratocarcinoma cells after induction of 'differentiation' relate to infections in defined cells in vivo. But it is interesting that viral gene expression can be influenced by modulating cellular gene expression.

Another interesting model is that provided by tracheal rings cultivated in vitro. The rings can be maintained for long periods of time in vitro, and MCMV establishes a long term persistent infection in them. Of particular interest is the finding that epithelial cells serve as the reservoir of chronic virus production, and that the continuous production of infectious virus is dependent upon a continuous low turnover of dividing cells (Nedrud et al., 1982).

We have recently turned our attention to murine macrophage cell lines. One of these replicates the virus in a very low percentage of the cells, similar to that seen in spleen macrophages, but produces substantial amounts of early viral proteins. We hope that this system may be useful for further study.

CONCLUSIONS

It is clear that many factors, host and virus determined, operate and interplay during the course of acute MCMV infection. Some of these factors also influence the establishment and duration of the persistent phase of infection. The latter represents the net effect of chronic infection in tissues such as submaxillary gland and kidney, and a true latent infection in some other tissues such as spleen.

In the wild the virus seems to have adapted itself to provide for the optimal time of transmission and the greatest degree of persistence.

Reactivation of the virus in mice may represent either an enhancement of a low level chronic infection in some tissues, or a release from a latent infection imposed by constraints operating in other tissues. The immune system has been implicated as a controlling factor, although it is not clear how or at what level it may operate.

The study of several cell culture models has indicated that viral gene expression, and ultimately virus replication, can be governed by the cell cycle in fibroblasts and possibly epithelial cells, and by the cellular gene expression program in other cell types.

REFERENCES

Bancroft, G.J., Shellam, G.R. and Chalmer, J.E. 1981. Genetic influences on the augmentation of natural killer (NK) cells during murine cytomegalovirus infection: correlation with patterns of resistance. J. Immunol. 126, 988-994.

Brautigam, A.R., Dutko, F.J., Olding, L.B. and Oldstone, M.B.A. 1979. Pathogenesis of murine cytomegalovirus infection: the macrophage as a permissive cell for cytomegalovirus infection, replication and latency. J. Gen. Virol. 44, 349-359.

Chalmer, J.E. 1979. Ph. D. Thesis, University of Western Australia. Murine cytomegalovirus infection: a study of genes controlling resistance and their effects on pathogenesis.

Chalmer, J.E., Mackenzie, J.S., and Stanley, N.F. 1977. Resistence to murine cytomegalovirus linked to the major histocompatibility complex of the mouse. J. Gen. Virol. 37, 107-114.

Chantler, J.K., Misra, V. and Hudson, J.B. 1979. Vertical transmission of murine cytomegalovirus. J. Gen. Virol. 42, 621-625.

Cheung, KS. and Lang, D.J. 1977. Transmission and activation of cytomegalovirus with blood transfusion: a mouse model. J. Inf. Dis. 135, 841-845.

Dowling, J.N., Wu, B.C., Armstrong, J.A., and Ho, M. 1977. Enhancement of murine cytomegalovirus infections during graft versus host reaction. J. Inf. Dis. 135, 990-994.

Dutko, F.J. and Oldstone, M.B.A. 1981. Cytomegalovirus causes a latent infection in undifferentiated cells and is activated by induction of cell differentiation. J. Exp. Med. 154, 1636-1651.

146

Gardner, M.B., Officer, J.E., Parker, J., Estes, J.D., and
    Rongey, R.W. 1974. Induction of disseminated virulent
    cytomegalovirus infection by immunosuppression of
    naturally chronically infected wild mice. Inf. Imm. 10,
    966-969.
Henson, D., Neapolitan, C. 1970. Pathogenesis of chronic mouse
    cytomegalovirus infection in submaxillary glands of C3H
    mice. Am. J. Path. 58, 255-267.
Henson, D., Strano, A.J., Slotnick, M. and Goodheart, C. 1972.
    Mouse cytomegalovirus: isolation from spleen and lymph
    nodes of chronically infected mice. Proc. Soc. Exp. Biol.
    Med. 140, 802-806.
Hudson, J.B. 1979. The murine cytomegalovirus as a model for
    the study of viral pathogenesis and persistent infect-
    ions. Arch. Virol. 62, 1-29.
Hudson, J.B., Loh, L., Misra, V., Judd, B., Suzuki, J. 1978.
    Multiple interactions between murine cytomegalovirus and
    lymphoid cells in vitro. J. Gen. Virol. 38, 149-159.
Jordan, M.C., Shanley, J.D. and Stevens, J.G. 1977. Immuno-
    suppression reactivates and disseminates latent murine
    cytomegalovirus. J. Gen. Virol. 37, 419-423.
Loh, L. and Hudson, J.B. 1979. Interaction of murine cytomega-
    lovirus with separated populations of spleen cells. Inf.
    Immunity 26, 853-860.
Mayo, D.R., Armstrong, J.A. and Ho, M. 1977. Reactivation of
    murine cytomegalovirus by cyclophosphamide. Nature 267,
    721-722.
Mims, C.A. and Gould, J. 1978. The role of macrophages in mice
    infected with murine cytomegalovirus. J. Gen. Virol. 41,
    143-153.
Misra, V. 1977. Ph.D. Thesis, University of British Columbia.
    Structure of the murine cytomegalovirus genome and its
    expression in productive and non-productive infections.
Misra, V. and Hudson, J.B. 1980. Minor base sequence differ-
    ences between the genomes of two strains of murine cyto-
    megaloviruses differing in virulence. Arch. Virol. 64,
    1-8.
Mosmann, T.R. 1973. Ph.D. Thesis, University of British
    Columbia. Genome properties and non-productive infections
    of herpes viruses.
Muller, M. 1977. Ph.D. Thesis, University of British Columbia.
    Cell cycle dependent replication of the murine cyto-
    megalovirus.
Muller, M.T., and Hudson, J.B. 1977. Cell cycle dependency of
    murine cytomegalovirus replication in synchronized 3T3
    cells. J. Virol. 22, 267-272.
Muller, M., Misra, V., Chantler, J.K. and Hudson, J.B. 1978.
    Murine cytomegalovirus gene expression during nonproduc-
    tive infection in Gophase 3T3 cells. Virology 90,
    279-287.
Nedrud, J.G., Pagano, J.S. and Collier, A.M. 1982. Long term
    mouse cytomegalovirus infection of tracheal organ cult-
    ure: relation to host cell replication. J. Gen. Virol.
    60, 247-259.
Olding, L.B., Jensen, F.C. and Oldstone, M.B.A. 1975. Patho-
    genesis of cytomegalovirus infection. 1. Activation of

virus from bone-marrow derived lymphocytes by in vitro allogenic reaction. J. Exp. Med. 141, 561-572.

Osborn, J.E. 1982. CMV-herpesviruses of mice in: Foster H.L., Fox, J.G., Small, J.D. (ed). The mouse in biochemical research Vol. II. Academic Press, New York.

Osborn, J.E. and Walker, D.L. 1971. Virulence and attenuation of murine cytomegalovirus. Inf. Imm. 3, 228-236.

Selgrade, M.K., Nedrud, J.G., Collier, A.M. and Gardner, D.E. 1981. Effect of cell source, mouse strain, and immuno-suppressive treatment on production of virulent and attenuated murine cytomegalovirus. Inf. Immunity 33, 840-847.

Wise, T.G., Manischewitz, J.E., Quinnan, G.V., Aulakh, G.S. and Ennis, F.A. 1979. Latent cytomegalovirus infection of Balb/c mouse spleens detected by an explant culture technique. J. Gen. Virol. 44, 551-556.

Wu, B.C. and Ho, M. 1979. Characteristics of infection of B and T lymphocytes from mice after inoculation with cyto-megalovirus. Inf. Immunity 24, 856-864.

Wu, B.C., Dowling, J.N., Armstrong, J.A. and Ho, M. 1975. Enhancement of mouse cytomegalovirus infection during host versus graft reaction. Science 190, 56-58.

QUANTITATIVE ANALYSIS OF ACTIVATED CYTOLYTIC T
LYMPHOCYTES PRESENT IN VIVO AFTER INFECTION
WITH THE MURINE CYTOMEGALOVIRUS

U.H. Koszinowski, G.M. Keil, and M.J. Reddehase
Federal Research Institute for Animal Virus Diseases
P.O. Box 1149, D-7400 Tübingen

ABSTRACT
    The infection of Balb/c mice with the murine
cytomegalovirus (MCMV) served as a natural virus-host system
to study the in vivo generation of cytolytic T lymphocytes
(CTL) and their precursors (CTL-P). Two modifications of the
limiting dilution technique, the in vitro expansion of CTL-P
in medium containing interleukin only and the in vitro
activation of CTL-P in presence of interleukin and antigen
led to the detection of two distinct maturation stages of in
vivo sensitized virus specific self restricted CTL. A low
frequency set of CTL-P generated an active progeny in vitro
in absence of further antigen restimulation and was denoted
interleukin receptive CTL-P (IL-CTL-P). A high frequency set
required further antigen in vitro to generate functionally
active clones and, therefore, is denoted antigen dependent.
Both sets of cells are generated in vivo only after viral
infection and are present simultaneously at the peak of the
acute immune response. The progeny of IL-CTL-P are H-2
restricted CTL and their generation is not influenced by
selective effects of antigen in vitro. Consequently, we
consider these cells to be the best available representatives
of the genuine in vivo activated immune repertoire. The
investigation of the fine specificity of IL-CTL-P will allow
the definition of those viral determinants which are of
importance in the antiviral T cell response.

INTRODUCTION
    Most of the herpesviruses that infect man and animals
exhibit a high degree of species specificity. Only HSV 1 and
HSV 2 are less species specific and are therefore used in
animal models to study the immune response to herpesviruses.
It is, however, questionable if the immune defence mechanisms
operative in these experimental models are identical with
those operative in the natural host as a consequence of an
evolutionary acquired balance. Thus it is certainly
advantageous to study herpesvirus infections in the natural
host. The murine cytomegalovirus (MCMV) is in its main
biological features very similar to the human cytomegalovirus
(HCMV) and, therefore, appears to be an excellent model for

the human disease and for persistent and latent herpesvirus
infections in general (Hamilton, 1982). Both the human and
the murine primary cytomegalovirus infection are usually not
accompanied by major symptoms of illness. Apparent clinical
disease results only if the host is either immunologically
immature, immunodeficient or immunosuppressed. After primary
infection a delicate virus-host balance is maintained that is
characterized by viral persistency, latency and occasional
reactivation. Although it may be disputed whether a true
latency with a complete block of viral replication may result
at later stages of infection, the role of immune control is
beyond doubt because natural or experimental interference
with the immune mechanisms will cause viral reactivation and
severe disease.

Which are the immune mechanisms that maintain the
balanced virus-host interaction during infection? Recently it
has been claimed that it seems very clear that humoral
immunity is nearly irrelevant to the outcome of HCMV
infection in the clinical context of greatest interest
(Osborn, 1981). This could point to the potential role of the
cellular immune response. A specific CTL response is induced
during primary MCMV infection (Quinnan et al., 1978; Ho,
1980) and memory T cells are demonstrable later. However, it
is open to what extent the T cells contribute to the
maintainance of the persistent state. Before a central role
of T cells in the regulation of persistent and latent
herpesvirus infections can be seriously considered more
informations on the magnitude, time and place of
manifestation, and specificity of the T cell response are
required. In particular, a quantitative evaluation of the T
cell response and its correlation with stages of infection is
needed. Furthermore, only if resting T cells can be
distinguished from activated cells the role of these cells
during persistent or latent infection can be investigated.

This report focusses on the description of methods that
allow the quantification of the MCMV specific CTL response
and the distinction of different activation stages of CTL-P.

RESULTS
Frequency estimation of in vivo activated cytolytic T cell precursors

The fraction of functionally active cells generated during primary infection is usually too small to be detectable in conventional 4 h cytolytic assays. Eighteen hour assay conditions which are applied to detect the activity of small numbers of activated T cells may be obscured by the functional activity of NK cells which cannot be excluded under these conditions. Furthermore direct testing of cell populations from lymphoid organs does not allow a quantification since a given cytolytic potential may be due to very few cells with strong cytolytic activity or many cells with low activity. For the enumeration of CTL specific for MCMV the expansion of individual in vivo sensitized T cells is required until their clonal progeny is large enough to be tested.

The protocol used in our experiments is depicted in Fig.1. Mice were sensitized by footpad infection with MCMV. Few days after sensitization the draining popliteal lymph node contains both resting and MCMV sensitized T cells. During activation and differentiation in vivo a minor fraction of those T cells which are sensitized by MCMV antigens already acquire the interleukin responsive state. These T cells are considered to carry interleukin receptors. They should proliferate in vitro and maintain their functional activity provided that sufficient interleukin for proliferation is present. These conditions were obtained by culturing replicates containing variable numbers of lymph node cells in presence of pretested interleukins from a rat source. To select and expand such cells the draining popliteal lymph nodes were removed at different times after infection and the cells were distributed at various concentrations into microtiter plates in order to expand activated CTL and their precursors. Usually 24 or 36 individual microcultures per cell concentration were set up and 8 cell concentrations were tested. CTL-P that gave rise to a clonal progeny of effector cells in antigen free media

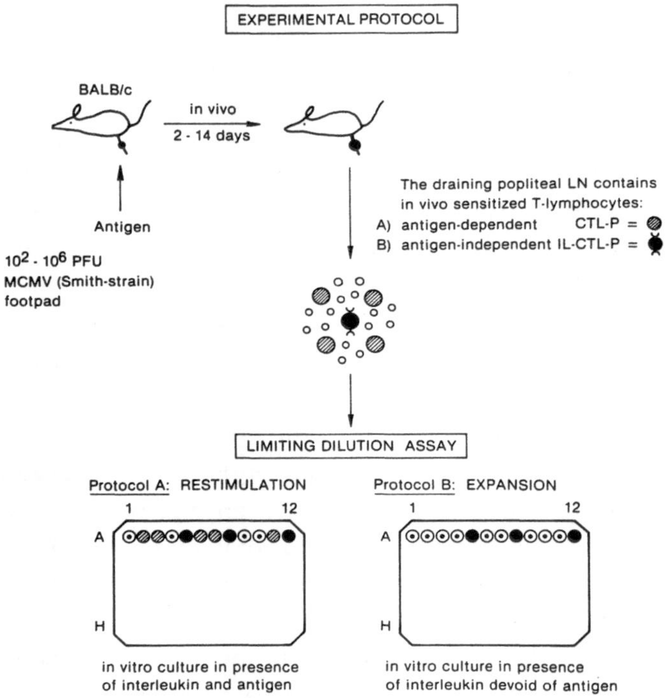

Fig. 1   Schematic description of the experimental protocol used to discriminate between different maturation stages of in vivo activated antigen specific cytolytic T lymphocyte precursors.

containing interleukin, were termed IL-CTL-P. Another set of cells was found to require antigen restimulation in order to generate a functionally active progeny. Restimulation and expansion conditions were provided by the addition of MCMV infected murine embryonic fibroblasts to in vitro cultures that also contained interleukins. These antigen dependent CTL-P also represent a primed population since in nonprimed mice no primary response to MCMV in vitro was detectable. After 5-7 days in vitro culture the functional activity of the in vitro grown T cells can be tested in conventional cytolytic assays. Precursor frequencies were calculated by two established independent methods: the maximum likelihood estimation (Fazekas de St.Groth, 1982) and the minimum Chi-square estimation (Taswell et al., 1981).

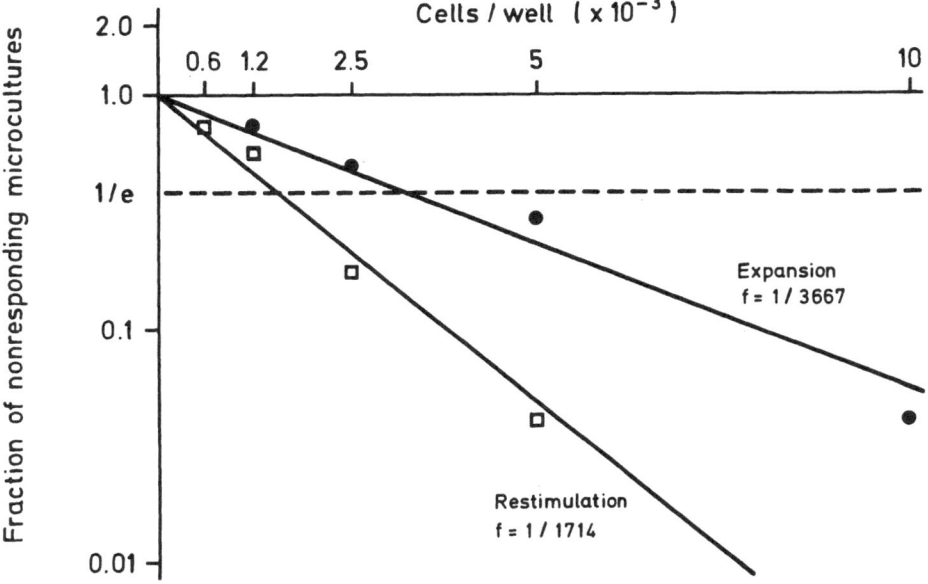

Fig. 2   After infection with 10^5 pfu MCMV day 8 immune lymphocytes were analyzed for the presence of antigen-independent and antigen-dependent cells by limiting dilution under expansion and restimulation conditions. Target cells were MCMV infected murine fibroblasts derived from day 18-21 embryos.

Peak frequencies during primary infections were observed between day 4 and 8. In the example given in Fig. 2 mice were primed with 10^5 pfu and the in vitro culture of activated cells was set up at day 5 after infection. In the expansion protocol the frequency of 1 IL-CTL-P in 4000 lymph node cells was determined and under restimulation conditions about 1 in 1700 lymph node cells could generate cytolytic activity. As to be expected the activity was a function of the infection dose. However, the increment of activation was remarkably low and the increase in relative frequency was accompanied by a

decrease in cell numbers when high concentrations of
infectious virus were used for priming (data not shown). At
the same time the contralateral lymph node contained very few
CTL-P which indicates that the primary immune response is
mainly local and there is little migration of activated
cells. Despite of the cellular immune response in the
draining lymph node, about three weeks after local infection
the virus could be detected in the salivary gland which
appears to be the privileged organ for MCMV replication
during infection. The frequency estimates for the CTL-P may
change between individual experiments due to age, sex, and
health conditions of mice. However, the detection of in vivo
activated cells that can be expanded under antigen free
conditions is reproducible and even the ratio between the
antigen-dependent and -independent cells was found to be
constant in several experiments.

The different subsets of cells that utilize interleukins are precursors of antigen specific cytolytic T cells

The in vitro antigen restimulation has been used to
reactivate cytolytic T cells from the memory state. Effector
cells generated that way are H-2 restricted and carry the Lyt
1^-, 2^+ phenotype. On the other hand, the lineage of the cells
that generate a functionally active progeny in the presence
of interleukins requires further characterization since it
has been reported that NK cells contribute to effector
mechanisms in the early response to MCMV (Quinnan et al.,
1979).

The requirement for interleukin was tested by adding
different doses of interleukin to cell cultures. It was found
that in microcultures containing low numbers of cells no
response could be generated in absence of interleukin while
at higher cell numbers some growth was seen, probably due to
interleukin produced and released from cells within the
culture. Growth and functional activity could be amplified by
additional application of interleukin. Cytolytic function
increases with increasing interleukin concentrations

TABLE 1   The generation of cytolytic activity is
           supported by interleukins.

		Target cells		
IL-dose	MCMV-MEF	Rabies-MEF	n.i.MEF	n.i.Balb 3T3
0	14	1	-	-
2.5	23	1	-	-
5	29	3	1	-
10	34	9	2	-
20	38	16	4	2

Day 6 immune lymph node cells (10^5 pfu MCMV) were expanded
for 6 days under oligoclonal conditions with various doses
(v/v) of interleukin from Concanavalin A activated rat
splenocytes. The cultures were split five-fold and tested
twice on syngeneic MCMV infected embryonic fibroblasts
(MCMV-MEF, split control) as well as on a syngeneic cell line
(Balb 3T3), noninfected target cells (MEF), and on MEF
infected with an unrelated virus (Rabies-MEF). The median
values of cytolytic activity, expressed as % specific lysis,
are given.

(Table 1). At high concentrations of interleukin some
nonspecific activity was seen also on target cells infected
with an unrelated virus which was not used for priming. The
lytic activities of cells from individual microcultures
against the two types of virus infected target cells were
analyzed by the rank correlation test and found to be not
correlated. Thus, a separate population with the capacity to
lyse irrelevant target cells proliferated in cultures that
contained high concentrations of interleukin. Indeed, it has
been reported that NK-like cells may be capable to utilize
interleukin (Dennert et al., 1981). In another set of
experiments, IL-CTL-P derived from the Balb/c and the C 57
BL/6 strain were tested for lytic activity against syngeneic
and allogeneic infected and noninfected target cells (Table
2). It was found that the IL-CTL-P derived effector cells are
self-restricted which strongly argues against NK cells.

156

TABLE 2   IL-CTL-P derived effector CTL are self
           restricted

| | Responder cells | |
Target cells (MEF)	Balb/c (H-2^d)	C57 BL/6 (H-2^b)
Balb/c-MCMV	33	5.5
C57 BL/6-MCMV	8	14.5
Balb/c not infected	0.5	4.5
C57 BL/6 not infected	1	0.5

Balb/c and C57 BL/6 day 6 immune lymph node cells were
cultivated under expansion conditions (10^5 cells/well).
After six days the cultures (N=24) were split fourfold
and tested on the four fibroblast target cells. The
median values of cytolytic activity are given.

In addition, the surface phenotype of the IL-CTL-P
derived effector cells was determined (Table 3). Effector
cells express the Thy 1$^+$, Lyt 1$^-$, 2$^+$ phenotype. Thus, by self
restriction and by Lyt phenotype IL-CTL-P could be
distinguished from activated NK cells and clearly belong to
the cytolytic T cell lineage.

TABLE 3   IL-CTL-P derived effector cells express the
Thy 1$^+$, Lyt 1$^-$, 2$^+$ phenotype

Treatment	% spec.lysis on MCMV-MEF	Sensitivity
Complement	22	
anti Thy 1.2+C	6.5	+
anti Lyt 1.2+C	22	-
anti Lyt 2.2+C	5.5	+

Effector cells grown under expansion conditions
for 6 days were treated with monoclonal antibody and
complement and then tested without correction for cell
numbers in the 4 h cytolytic test. Median values of N=24
individual microcultures in each group are given.

DISCUSSION

We have demonstrated that after infection with MCMV cytolytic T cell precursors are generated in vivo which can be expanded in vitro to generate a functionally active progeny. These precursors occur as a consequence of the priming event and are absent in normal mice. By applying different in vitro culture conditions two subsets could be discriminated which coexist in the lymph node draining the infected site (Reddehase et al., 1982). One set of low frequent antigenspecific CTL-P was defined and positively selected by the ability to utilize interleukins and the cells were therefore termed IL-CTL-P. A more frequent cell type needed in addition to interleukins stimulation by antigen to mature to functional capacity and was designated antigen dependent CTL-P. The different sets probably reflect separate maturation stages in the sequence from the virgin T cell precursor to the terminally differentiated CTL. It is open to further investigation whether those cells that require antigen stimulation in vitro to generate an active progeny represent an immature state in the maturation pathway, or whether they belong to the early memory pool. So far it is also unclear whether the antigen dependent cells, although they are specifically sensitized by MCMV, will contribute to the antiviral cellular immune response during acute infection or during the persistent stage at all. On the other hand, the IL-CTL-P show all characteristics attributed to functionally active CTL. We think, therefore, that the expansion protocol permits the best available approach to the analysis of the in vivo active CTL. Our test system offers several advantages for the analysis of the role of cytolytic T cells during acute, latent and persistent herpesvirus infections:

1. In the expansion protocol the definition of frequency and specificity of individual clones is not influenced by the selective effects of antigen restimulation in vitro. The functional activity of monoclonal or oligoclonal T cell populations is tested. Thus, the putative existence of effector cells recognizing viral

158

antigens that are correlated with the different stages of the virus replicative cycle is open for investigation.

2.	The experimental protocols allow the distinction between active and functionally inactive but sensitized T cells at all stages of infection, and hence active T cells which may be present at later stages of infection can be identified in spite of the presence of a memory cell pool.

REFERENCES

Hamilton, J.D. 1982. Monographs in Virology. (Ed. J.L. Melnick). (S. Karger, Basel).

Osborn, J.E. 1981. Cytomegalovirus: Pathology, immunology and vaccine initiatives. J. inf. Dis., 143, 618-630.

Quinnan, G.V., Manischewitz, J.E. and Ennis, F.A. 1978. Cytotoxic T lymphocyte response to murine cytomegalovirus infection. Nature, 273, 541-543.

Ho, M. 1980. Role of specific cytotoxic lymphocytes in cellular immunity against murine cytomegalovirus. Infect. Immun., 27, 767-776.

Fazekas de St.Groth 1982. The evaluation of limiting dilution assays. J. Immunol. Meth., 49, R 11-R 23.

Taswell, C. 1981. Limiting dilution assays for the determination of immunocompetent cell frequencies. I. Data Analysis. J. Immunol., 126, 1614-1619.

Quinnan, G.V., Manischewitz, J.E. 1979. The role of natural killer cells and antibody dependent cell-mediated cytotoxity during murine cytomegalovirus infection. J. exp. Med., 150, 1549-1555.

Dennert, G., Yogeeswaran, G. and Yamagata, S. 1981. Cloned cell lines with natural killer activity. Specifity, function, and cell surface markers. J. exp. Med., 153, 545-556.

Reddehase, M.J., Cox, J.H. and Koszinowski, U. 1982. Frequency analysis of cytolytic T cell precursors (CTL-P) generated in vivo during lethal rabies infection of mice. I. Distinction of CTL-P with different interleukin sensitivity. Eur. J. Immunol., 12, 519-523.

This work was supported by grant Ko 571/8 from the Deutsche Forschungsgemeinschaft

SESSION II

BOVIDE, EQUIDE AND FELIDE HERPESVIRUSES

Part 1

Chairman: P.P. Pastoret
Co-chairman: H. Ludwig

DNA OF BOVINE IPV*-VIRUS (BHV-1, IPV STRAIN) IN THE SACRAL GANGLIA OF LATENTLY INFECTED CALVES

M. Ackermann and R. Wyler

Institut für Virologie, Winterthurerstr. 266a,
CH-8057 Zürich

ABSTRACT

The trigeminal ganglia of latently BHV-1 (IBR** strain) infected calves are known to harbour viral DNA. To test if a IPV-virus strain would lead to a latent infection in sacral ganglia, two calves were inoculated intravaginally with a strain of BHV-1 known to cause IPV. The calves were treated with dexamethasone (DM) 5 weeks and 10 weeks p.i. The antibody responses to IBR and IPV were monitored throughout the experiment, and the calves were slaughtered at a latent stage of infection.

Titers of antibodies neutralizing IPV-virus but not those neutralizing IBR-virus increased after DM treatment. IPV-virus reexcretion was observed in the vaginal swabbings 8 and 9 days after the onset of DM administration. Thus, latency of IPV was verified at the time of slaughtering by seroconversion, absence of virus shedding and virus recrudescence after DM treatment.

By in situ hybridisation techniques and autoradiography, DNA of BHV-1 was detected in 10 of 20 sacral ganglia of latently infected calves. Viral DNA was restricted to the nucleus of nerve cells. The results obtained correspond to those known from nasal infections with IBR strains leading to a localisation of viral DNA in trigeminal ganglia.

*) IPV :   Infectious Pustular Vulvovaginitis
**) IBR :   Infectious Bovine Rhinotracheitis

ON THE LATENCY OF INFECTIOUS BOVINE RHINOTRACHEITIS VIRUS
INFECTION AND ITS SIGNIFICANCE, ESPECIALLY WITH
REGARD TO THE POSSIBILITY OF CONTROLLING INFECTION

V. Bitsch

The State Veterinary Serum Laboratory,
Bülowsvej 27, DK-1870 Copenhagen V

ABSTRACT
    Results of investigations performed from 1969-1971 clearly
demonstrated latency of infectious bovine rhinotracheitis (IBR)
virus infections in experimentally as well as naturally
infected cattle. It was concluded that latency after infection
is the rule rather than the exception. Persistence of
infections in herds as a result of this could readily be
demonstrated in many cases. In some herds very long periods, as
much as one to two years, elapsed between the spread of
infection, and in some cases the infection actually
disappeared. From the results obtained, it was concluded that
control and eradication of IBR virus infections would be
feasible. Some epidemiological data relating to the occurrence
and eradication of IBR virus infection in Danish AI centres are
briefly reviewed, and an attempt to eradicate the infection in
a herd of beef cattle is described: this was initiated 3 years
ago and has so far been successful.

INTRODUCTION

    Studdert et al. (1964) demonstrated virus in the prepuce
of a bull 26 days after inoculation with infectious bovine
rhinotracheitis (IBR) virus, and Snowdon (1965), who examined
an experimental genitally infected bull regularly over 19
months, found virus in its prepuce on several occasions during
the first year. He also demonstrated intermittent release of
virus from the vagina of a heifer and found virus in nasal
swabs from another one as late as 17 months after intravenous
inoculation.

    This was the current state of knowledge about the latency
of IBR virus infections in cattle when the first cases were
diagnosed in Denmark in January 1969. Virus was isolated from
semen and preputial washings of bulls at an AI centre and from
vaginal samples of cows inseminated with semen from the centre.

    The present paper will give results from investigations
subsequently undertaken with the aim of further elucidating

this phenomenon and its significance, especially with respect
to the possibility of controlling infection.

GENITAL AND RESPIRATORY INFECTION IN BULLS

Experimental infection (Bitsch, 1973)

In March 1969 a bull (Bull A) was inoculated nasally and
preputially with a Danish genital isolate of IBR virus. An
in-contact bull (Bull B) was inoculated into the prepuce after
6 weeks, as preputial washings of this bull had so far been
virus-negative. After 120 weeks the bulls were given injections
of prednisolone.

Results from examinations of preputial washings and blood
samples collected at regular intervals are illustrated in
Figure 1. After the primary infection phase virus was
demonstrated in a nasal swab from Bull B after 1 year and in
nasal samples from both bulls after more than 2 years after
prednisolone treatment.

Semen collected during periods of preputial virus release
was tested for virus and the titer was found to parallel that
of the corresponding preputial washing.

Natural genital infection (Bitsch, 1975)

Data concerning all virus-positive preputial washings from
naturally infected bulls are recorded in Table 1. Three samples
were taken during the primary phase of infection. In one bull
virus was demonstrated as late as 4 years after it had been
found serologically positive.

For the bulls from Centre B with virus-positive washings,
virus was demonstrated in 11 of 27 samples (41%) taken from
February-April 1969, in 7 of 32 samples (22%) taken from
May-October 1969 but in none of 17 samples taken in 1970 and
1971.

Conclusions

From the results obtained in the investigations of both
experimental and natural infections it was concluded that

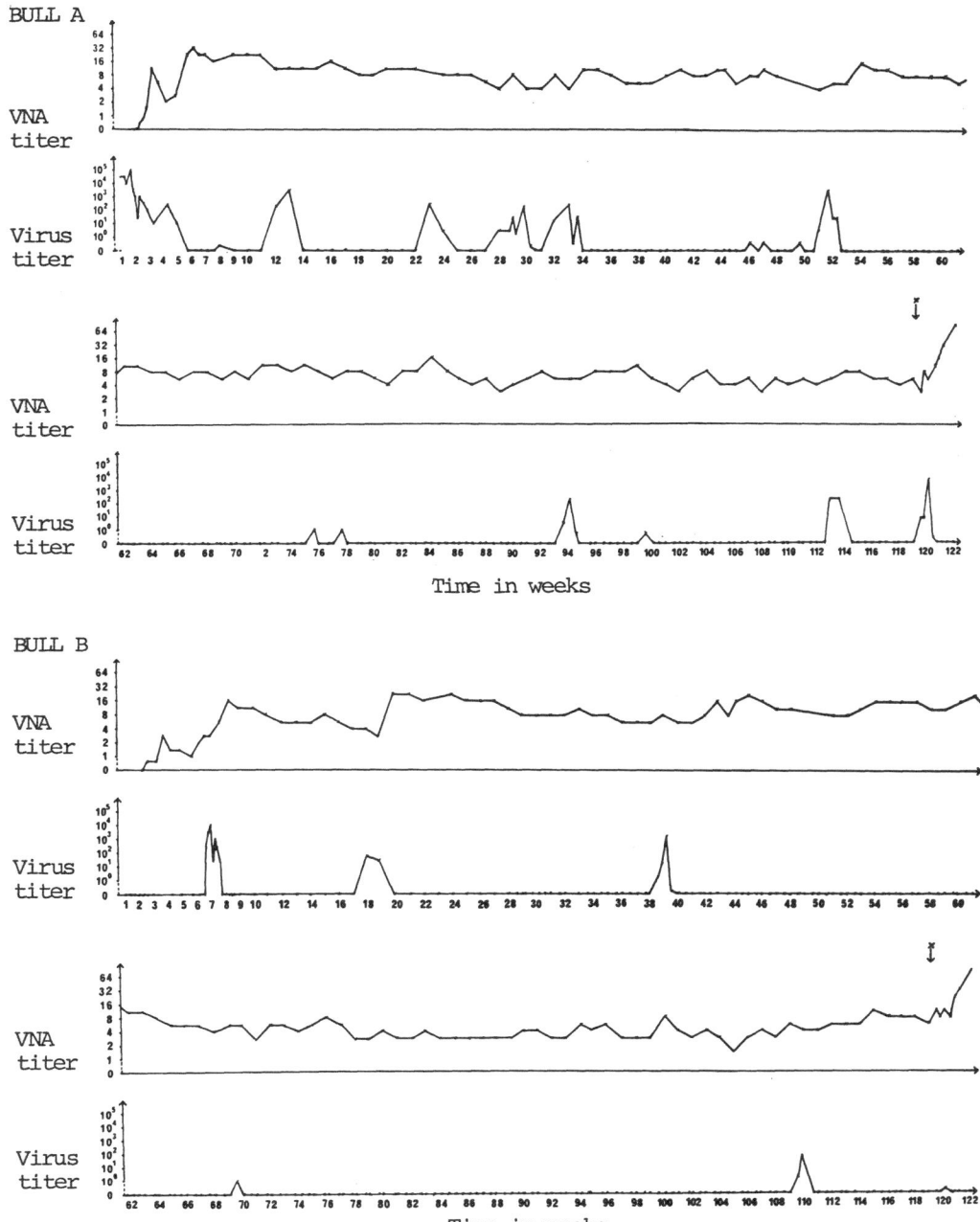

Fig. 1. Bulls A and B. Virus-neutralizing antibody (VNA) titers in serum and virus titers (TCID$_{50}$ per o.1 ml) in preputial washings(approx. 50 ml) after experimental infection. Observation period: 122 weeks. Symbol x: 500 mg of prednisolone injected intramuscularly; repeated after 1 and 3 days.

TABLE 1   Isolation of IBR virus from preputial washings of naturally infected bulls and relevant virus-neutralizing antibody (VNA) titers.

Bull	AI centre	Preputial washing		Blood sample	
		date of collection	virus titer[1]	date of collection	VNA titer[2]
TS	B	9/1 69	$10^{5.2}$	9/1 69	negative
				4/2 69	8
TN	B	9/1 69	$10^{4.5}$	9/1 69	negative
		14/3 69	$10^{1.8}$	4/2 69	8
SAt	B	9/1 69	$10^{1.8}$	9/1 69	2
		6/2 69	$10^{0.2}$	4/2 69	8
SJ	B	9/1 69	$10^{0.5}$	9/1 69	0.5
		15/4 69	$10^{0.2}$	4/2 69	4
RS	B			9/1 69	2
		6/2 69	$10^{-0.2}$	4/2 69	4
SH	B	6/2 69	$10^{1.2}$	4/2 69	5.6
SAn	B	6/2 69	$10^{-0.2}$	4/2 69	1
		13/5 69	$10^{0.5}$		
		3/6 69	$10^{0.8}$		
		27/6 69	10^{0}	1/9 69	2.8
AA	B	6/2 69	10^{0}	4/2 69	1
		14/2 69	10^{0}		
		8/3 69	$10^{-0.2}$		
		14/3 69	$10^{0.5}$	1/9 69	22
SV	B	6/2 69	$10^{2.2}$	4/2 69	2.8
		13/5 69	$10^{2.2}$	1/9 69	11
TT	B	3/6 69	10^{0}	4/2 69	5.6
SE	B			4/2 69	4
		1/9 69	10^{0}	1/9 69	5.6
SAg	B			4/2 69	5.6
		1/9 69	$10^{0.8}$	1/9 69	5.6
MF	M	9/2 71	10^{0}	28/2 70	5.6
		16/2 71	$10^{0.5}$	18/12 70	5.6
ØI	Ø	6/12 73	10^{-1}	14/11 69	2.8

1. $TCID_{50}$ per 0.1 ml

2. Virus-serum mixtures incubated at $37^{\circ}C$ for 1 hour.

latency of IBR virus infections is a life-long condition and
that any previously·IBR virus infected animal should be
regarded as a potential threat of infection to uninfected
animals. Nevertheless, some results indicated that the risk of
recurrent shedding of virus was reduced after the first 4 or 6
months.

In periods with intermittent virus production the amounts
of virus excreted were considerably lower than during the
primary infection phase. Attempts to eradicate IBR virus
infections in herds should therefore have a good chance of
success, but only if infected animals are separated from
uninfected ones and precautions are taken to prevent indirect
transmission of virus from the infected group.

It is worth emphasizing that control of IBR virus
infection is essential in AI centres in areas where this
infection is unwanted.

PERSISTENCE OF IBR VIRUS INFECTIONS IN HERDS

AI centres (Autrup and Bitsch, 1978)

All 45 Danish AI centres were tested serologically between
1969-1970. In some of the 4 centres in which the infection had
been spread to a high proportion of the bulls, observations
strongly indicated that spread had occurred on more than one
occasion.

In one centre seropositive bulls were separated from the
other animals and slaughtered shortly thereafter. In the three
other centres infected animals were kept apart from uninfected
ones, but only in the final phases were the two groups kept in
separate houses. In one of these centres, with 10 seropositive
animals out of 28 in 1970, a new reactor was found after one
year, and the circumstances indicated that it had become
infected by the respiratory route. In the other two centres, 42
of 45 animals and 64 of 96, respectively, were found infected
in 1969, but no later spread occurred, even though
epidemiological data indicated that both genital and
respiratory infections had previously occurred in one of the

centres.

From March 1974 all reactors but one have been slaughtered, and the infection could be considered to have been successfully eradicated in Danish AI centres.

Breeding herds (Bitsch, 1978a)

In many herds, where female animals were infected after AI, the infection remained in a genital form. Control of the infection in AI centres thus automatically lead to the disappearance of infection.

In other herds, which were found to have experienced respiratory infection, the later course of infection varied.

In one herd (JJu) the infection was concluded to have been spread among the animals in 1969 as a respiratory infection following introduction by AI. Only 3 'old cows', which could not be further identified, were positive in 1977, indicating no spread after 1969. (An outbreak diagnosed by virus isolation in 1982 was considered to have been caused by the introduction of an infected animal shortly before).

In another herd (PC), where in 1969 practically all animals had recently shown symptoms of IBR, only 2 of 57 animals over 6 months of age were found to be seronegative. A test of the whole herd in 1977 indicated that no spread had occurred later on.

In a third herd (KN) serological examination in 1977 (40 animals) demonstrated no further spread after the one demonstrated by testing in 1972.

In a fourth herd (SK), where in 1969 all the seropositive animals (9 of 20) were found to be the oldest animals in the herd, serological testing of 42 animals in 1977 demonstrated that no further spread had occurred.

In a fifth herd (CMø), with poor ventilation, serological tests from 1969 to 1977 clearly demonstrated respiratory infection with spread on several occasions.

In a sixth herd (JB), testing in 1974 demonstrated that extensive spread had occurred more than one year earlier. Tests in 1977 and 1980 demonstrated subsequent spread, resulting in isolated new cases of infection (1977) and infection of a proportion of the previously uninfected part of the herd (1980).

In a herd of beef cattle (CH) serological tests in 1970 and 1971 disclosed that an extensive respiratory spread had occurred before 1970. Tests in 1977 demonstrated a few later cases of infection.

In conclusion, the serological examinations described above have shown not only that IBR virus infection has persisted in several herds, but also that in others there was no further spread of infection after the initial outbreak.

Consequently, it should be practicable to eradicate respiratory infections in conventional herds. Preliminary results from such an attempt are given below.

Eradication of IBR in a herd of beef cattle

In November 1979 all 194 of 196 animals over 1 year of age compared to only 9 of 74 calves 4-10 months of age, were found to be serologically positive. Three months later, six of the positive calves were found to be negative (colostral antibody).

Seronegative calves were placed in a separate house on the same premises as positive animals. The same procedure was used for young calves the following two years. A very few calves were found to be infected and were excluded. In addition, two bull calves, which were first found to be seronegative and were thereafter kept isolated together, were later found to be seropositive. Generally, maternal antibody persisted in the calves for 3 to 7 months.

The negative part of the herd now comprises 26 cows aged 3-3 ^{1}/2 years, 42 heifers aged 2-2 ^{1}/2 years, and approximately 30 calves aged 1-1 ^{1}/2 years.

Finally it should be emphasized that for control and eradication purposes it is essential to employ a test that can be considered sensitive enough to detect all antibody carriers. The test used in Denmark is a modified virus-neutralizing antibody test described earlier (Bitsch, 1978b).

REFERENCES

Autrup, E. H. and Bitsch, V. 1978. The occurrence, control and eradication of infection with infectious bovine rhinotracheitis virus at artificial insemination centres in Denmark. Nord. Vet.-Med., 30, 169-177.

Bitsch, V. 1973. Infectious bovine rhinotracheitis virus infection in bulls, with special reference to preputial infection. Appl. Microbiol., 26, 337-343.

Bitsch, V. 1975. The infectious bovine rhinotracheitis virus infection in cattle in Denmark, with regard to distribution, epidemiology, importance, diagnosis and control. Bull. Off. int. Epiz., 84, 95-105.

Bitsch, V. 1978a. Persistence of infection with infectious bovine rhinotracheitis virus in Danish cattle herds. Nord. Vet.-Med., 30, 178-185.

Bitsch, V. 1978b. The P37/24 modification of the infectious bovine rhinotracheitis virus-serum neutralizationtest. Acta. vet. scand., 19, 497-505.

Snowdon, W. A. 1965. The IBR-IPV virus: reaction to infection and intermittent recovery of virus from experimentally infected cattle. Austr. vet. J., 41, 135-142.

Studdert, M.J., Baker, A.V. and Savan, M. 1964. Infectious pustular vulvovaginitis virus infection of bulls. Am. J. vet. Res., 25, 303-314.

HERPESVIRUSES OF BOVIDAE:

THE CHARACTERIZATION, GROUPING AND ROLE OF

DIFFERENT TYPES, INCLUDING LATENT VIRUSES

Hanns Ludwig

Institut fur Virologie
Freie Universität Berlin
(im Robert Koch-Institut)
Nordufer 20, 1000 Berlin 65
Germany

ABSTRACT
      Bovine herpesviruses have been grouped into bovid
herpesviruses types 1 to 6 (BHV-1 to 6) on the basis of
historical considerations, serological findings and restriction
endonuclease cleavage patterns of their DNAs. BHV-1 covers the
"IBR-like" and "IPV-like" genome types which correlate with
defined clinical entities. BHV-2 represents the bovine herpes
mammillitis virus. BHV-3 is the malignant catarrhal fever (MCF)
virus, representing both attenuated strains and the African
form. BHV-4 comprises a variety of strains which are either
passenger viruses or from disease outbreaks and which have
siminlar genome cleavage sites. BHV-5 stands for the
herpesvirus ovis found associated with sheep adenomatosis.
BHV-6 represents a new goat herpesvirus antigenically related
to BHV-1. All these bovine herpesviruses have the capacity to
remain latent in their host and may be reactivated.

INTRODUCTION AND HISTORICAL REMARKS

      A comprehensive view of bovine herpesviruses has recently

been given (Ludwig, 1982), which is based on clinically

oriented reports (Kokles, 1967; Plowright, 1968; McKercher,

1973; Cilli and Castrucci, 1976; Gibbs and Rweyemamu, 1977;

Straub, 1978) and which updates our present knowledge on

molecular biology and disease mechanisms. Therefore, this

present review is succinct.

      Besides their uniform morphology (Wildy et al., 1960) and

their uniqueness in using the nucleus in the process of

replication and maturation (Roizmann, 1978) all the bovine

herpesviruses may be assumed to remain latent in the infected

organism. This may occur in different ways and at different

sites.

      Based on earlier efforts to group bovine herpesviruses, I

have proposed a classification (Table 1) scheme for known

herpesviruses of bovidae. They are named bovid herpesviruses
types 1 to 6 and abbreviated BHV-1 to -6.

BHV-1 is found worldwide and is associated with different
clinical entities, the most prominent ones affecting the
respiratory or genital tracts. It should be pointed out that in
these very early reports on "Bläschenausschlag" (Zwick and
Gminder, 1913; Witte, 1933) no connection was noticed between
infectious pustular vulvovaginitis and abortions. After
isolation of a herpesvirus from infectious bovine
rhinotracheitis (Madin et al., 1956) this virus was then
reported from several other countries.

Reports on BHV-2 cam from Africa (Huygelen et al., 1960 a,
b) and from England (Martin et al., 1966) where the clinical
picture of mammillitis had been described much earlier (Hare,
1925). Since then, the virus has been recognized in several
other European countries and in North America (Cilli and
Castrucci, 1976), and its biological properties are well
established (Sterz et al., 1973/74; Ludwig, 1976, 1982).

The malignant catarrhal fever which occurs in defined
clinico-pathologicial entities as "Bösartiges Katarrhal Fieber"
(Götze und Ließ, 1929) or "Snootsiekte" (Mettan, 1923) has been
investigated intensively by Plowright's group and will be
discussed at this meeting (Plowright, 1982). We categorized
this virus as BHV-3.

Various other isolates made form cattle and buffalos which
have been identified as herpesviruses (for review, see Gibbs
and Rweyemamu, 1977), form a rather uniform group of viruses
and are classified as BHV-4 (Ludwig, 1982).

The virus which seems to be involved in "Jaagsiekte" in
sheep, known in European countries as sheep pulmonary
adenomatosis (Mackay, 1969; Verwoerd et al., 1978; De Villiers,
1979) is grouped as BHV-5.

BHV-6 comprises isolates originating from goats. This
virus has recently been separated from BHV-1 (IBR/IPV viruses),
although it is closely related to them (Engels et al., 1981).
Serological studies show that it seems to be present not only
in Switzerland and California, but that it is also latent in

TABLE 1   Classification of Bovine Herpesvirus

Virus groups[a]	Clinical entities and synonyms[c]	Abbreviations	Natural host	Criteria[d]
BHV-1d) Bovid Herpesvirus 1	"Bläschenausschlag"; exanthema coitale vesiculosum; infectious pustular vulvovaginitis/infectious bovine rhinotracheitis	IPV IBR	Cattle	g) Serology DNA pattern
BHV-2 Bovid Herpesvirus 2	Allerton Bovine Mammillitis; bovine herpes mammillitis; pseudo-lumpy skin disease	BHM	Cattle	h) Serology DNA pattern
BHV-3 Bovid Herpesvirus 3	"Bösartiges Katarrhal Fieber"e) (African) malignant catarrhal fever; "snotsiekte"	BKF MCF	Wildebeest	i) Serology pattern
BHV-4 Bovid Herpesvirus 4	Associated with various clinical forms of disease	Various strain abbreviations	Cattle	j) Serology pattern
BHV-5f) Bovid Herpesvirus 5	Sheep pulmonary adenomatosis "jaagsiekte"; herpesvirus ovis infection		Sheep	k) Serology DNA analysis
BHV-6 Bovid Herpesvirus 6	Caprine herpesvirus infection		Goat	l) Serology DNA pattern

Legend to TABLE 1

a)   These different herpesvirus groups do not cross-react by
     neutralization, except BHV-1 and 6.
b)   The term bovid was used to keep the scheme open for
     isolates from all bovidae.
c)   The established names together with abbreviations commonly
     used are given.
d)   The serological cross-reactivity of isolates or data from
     restriction endonuclease analysis of the DNA together with
     historical considerations are the basis for the above
     proposed nomenclature.
e)   No herpesvirus has unequivocally been attributed to this
     syndrome in European countries.
f)   This virus had already been proposed as bovid herpesvirus
     4 (Roizman et al., 1973), when the above various
     herpesvirus isolates from cattle were not yet
     characterized.
Reference strains:
g)   strain LA (Madin et al., 1956)
h)   strain TVA (Rweyemamu and Johnson, 1969)
i)   strain WC11 (Plowright et al., 1965)
j)   strain Movar 33/63 (Bartha et al., 1966)
k)   strain JS-3 (De Villiers, 1979)
l)   strain E/CH (Mettler et al., 1979).

---

goats in Greece, Turkey and other countries (Leiskau and
Engels, unpublished).

The most pathogenic virus for bovines is the pseudorabies
(PsR) virus which was first isolated from a fatally diseased
cow (Aujeszky, 1902). The natural host of this virus, however,
seems to be the pig, and it is therefore grouped as herpesvirus
suis.

Present knowledge on molecular biology

On the basis of all known molecular biological data and
biological criteria, BHV-1, -2 and -6 have been placed in the
subfamily alpha-herpesvirinae, BHV-4 in the beta-herpesvirinae,
and BHV-3 in the gamma-herpesvirinae.

The general principles of virus-cell-interactions known
for bovine herpesviruses are comparable to those of much better
studied groups like HSV, PsR virus, CMV, EBV or herpesvirus
saimiri. Electronmicroscopy has been a valuable tool to study
the assembly and maturation of these viruses and to identify

new isolates. This has been of special importance for viruses which could not be grouped serologically and which we now classify as BHV-4 (Fig. 1, Fig. 2).

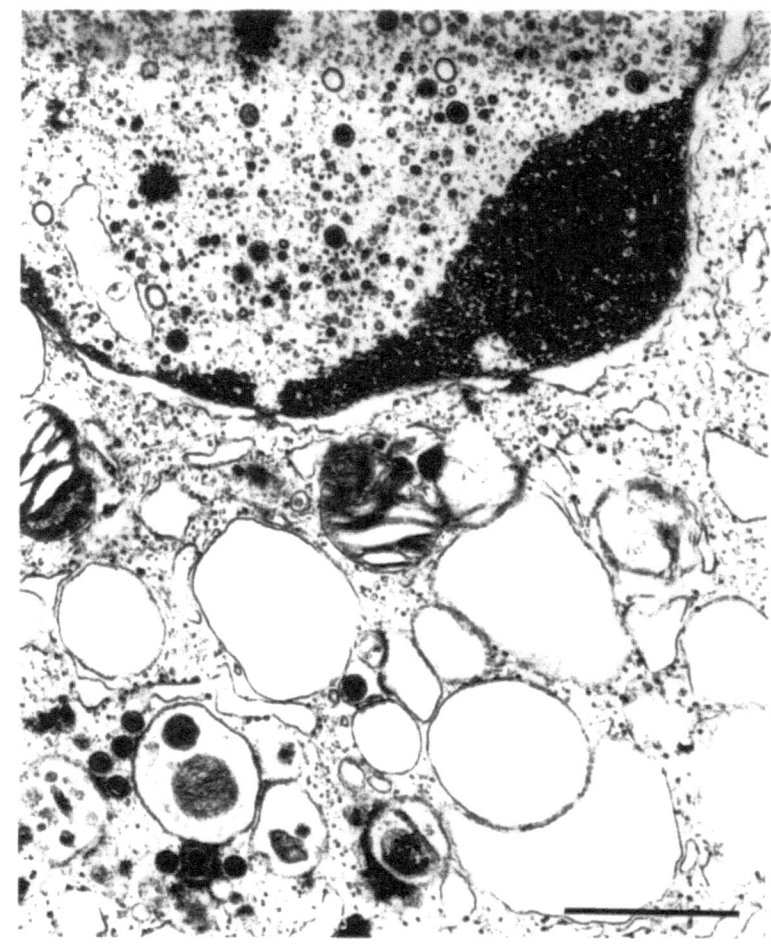

Fig. 1   A BHV-3 (malignant catarrhal fever virus, strain WC11) infected bovine fetal skin cell. Partially assembled nucleocapsides can be seen in the nucleus, and in the cytoplasm complete capsids - as judged from the typical electron dense core structure - are evident.
Magnification: 27.000; bar: 1 μm.
Courtesy: Hans Gelderblom.

As with all other double stranded DNA viruses, the use of the restriction endonuclease "fingerprinting" technique which was successfully applied in epidemiological studies of HSV-,

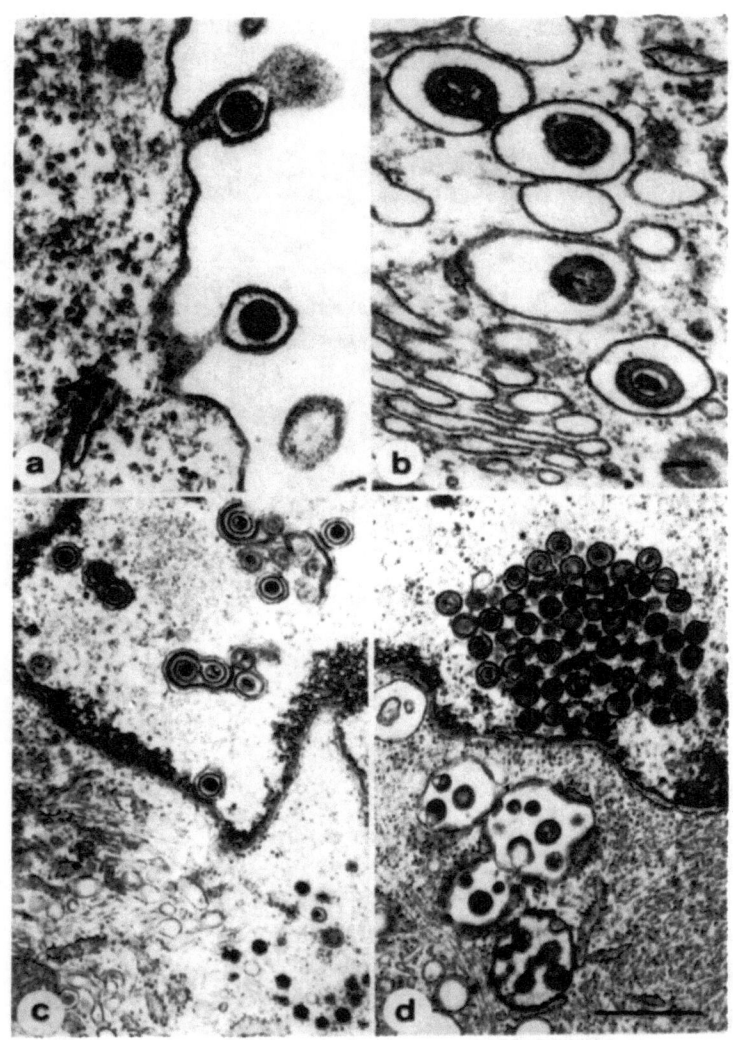

Fig. 2   Various bovine herpes viruses, showing peculiar
features in maturation, morphogenesis and egrees in bovine
fetal skin cells. (a) Capsids of BHV-1 (strain V101)
become enveloped at the plasma membrane. (b) BHV-4 (strain
ÜT) particles: one of them in progress of budding into the
endoplasmatic reticulum. Magnification: 70.000; bar : 100
nm. (c) Nuclear and cytoplasmatic distribution of
enveloped and naked BHV-2 (strain TVA) capsids.
(d) Aggregate of mature, enveloped particles of BHV-4
(strain Movar 33/63) within the nucleus. Magnification:
18.000; bar: 500 nm.

PsR- and feline herpes virus infections (Buchman et al., 1978; Ludwig et al., 1981; Herrmann et al., 1982a; Herrmann et al., 1982b) has considerably improved our knowledge about bovine herpesviruses. Physical maps for BHV-1 (Skare et al., 1975; Skare, pers. communication) and BHV-2 (Buchman and Roizman, 1978a, b) are known. They resemble those of PsR virus and HSV, respectively. BHV-6, most probably, falls into the same group as BHV-1, wheras the maps of type 3, 4 and 5 viruses have not yet been established. A summary of DNA cleavage patterns of the various bovine herpesviruses using different enzymes is given in Figs. 3 and 4. There is no doubt that restriction enzyme analysis is the method of choice for quick and accurate classification of these viruses. This allows for the separation of the goat herpesvirus (BHV-6) from BHV-1 where a close serological relationship exists. For BHV-3, and the different strains grouped together in BHV-4, this report is currently the only one which allows separation of these viruses into two groups, since several isolates in the BHV-4 group arose from MCF-like cases.

It was of special interest for us to establish the DNA pattern for MCF viruses. For this purpose, viral DNA from infected cells which showed herpesvirus particles after inoculation with WC 11 or C 500 strain was investigated. The DNA cleavage pattern shows that there are none or only a small number of similarities in the molecular weight of fragments, when BHV-3 and -4 strains are compared (Fig. 4, Table 2). The BHV-4 group seems to incorporate a variety of bovine herpesvirus isolates, from which we have investigated a few reference strains derived from less defined clinical entities or even from normal tissue culture (Ludwig, 1982).

Restriction enzyme analysis of the viral DNA seems to be an excellent tool to detect subgroups of bovine herpesviruses and even to recognize variants in different strains. In our studies we have selected enzymes specific for fewer cleavage sites, thus yielding fragments, allowing for better grouping of strains (Roizman and Tognon, 1982; Herrmann et al., 1982b).

178

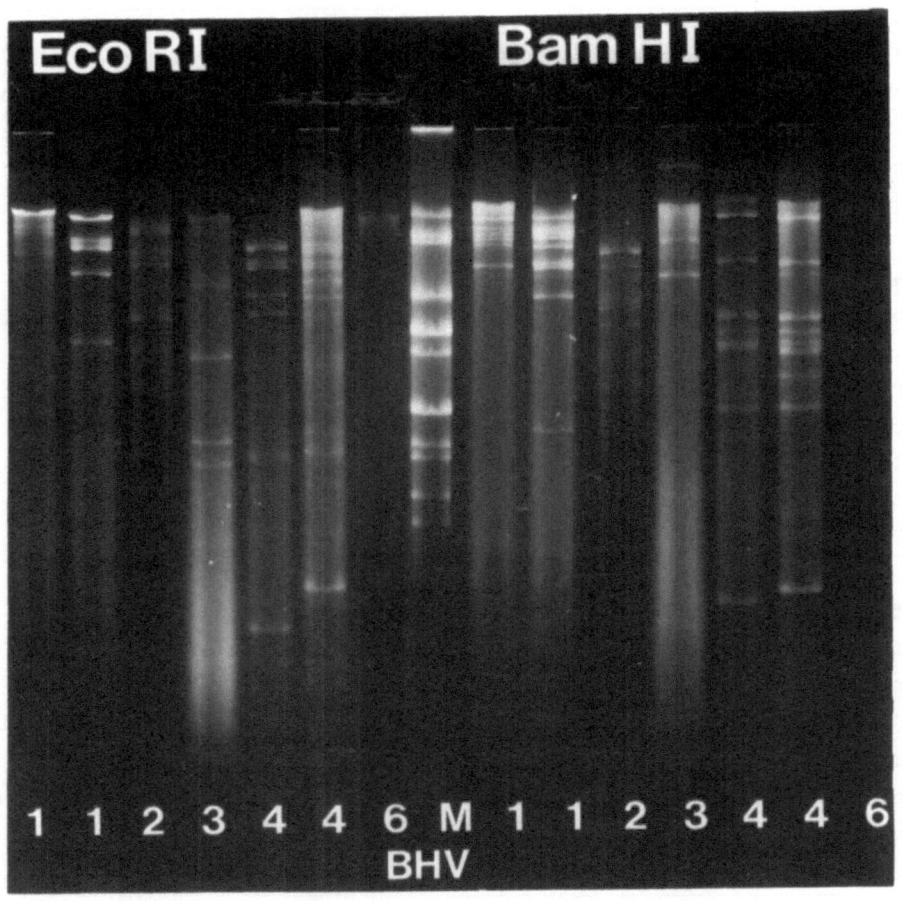

Fig. 3 A   Comparison of the Eco RI and Bam H I DNA
restriction patterns of bovine herpesviruses types 1 to 6
indicated in the lanes: 1 (left lane, BHV-1 "IBR-like"); 1
(right lane, BHV-1 "IPV-like"); 2, BHV-2 (strain TVA); 3,
BHV-3 (strain WC 11); 4, (left lane, BHV-4, strain Movar);
4 (right lane, BHV-4, strain DN-599); 6, BHV-6 (strain
E/CH); M, Pseudorabies virus (Bam H I fragments serve as
molecular weight markers). DNA-fragments were separated by
electrophoresis on 0.8% agarose slab gels at 40 V for 18
hours. Gels were stained (ethidiumbromide 1 μg/1) and
photographed under UV-transillumination (302 nm) with a
Polaroid land camera.

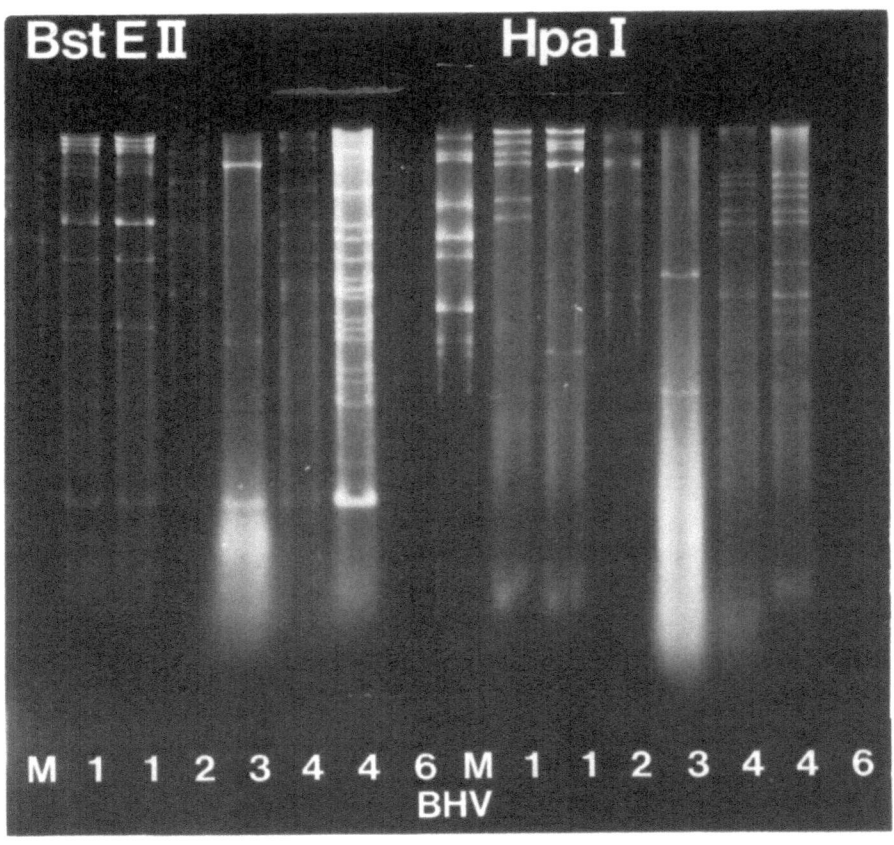

Fig. 3 B   Comparison of the Bst E II and Bam H I DNA
restriction patterns of BHV-1, -2, -3, -4 and -6; the same
strains and conditions were used as given in Fig. 4 A;
left M is PsR virus digested with Bst E II, right M is PsR
virus digsted with Bam H I.

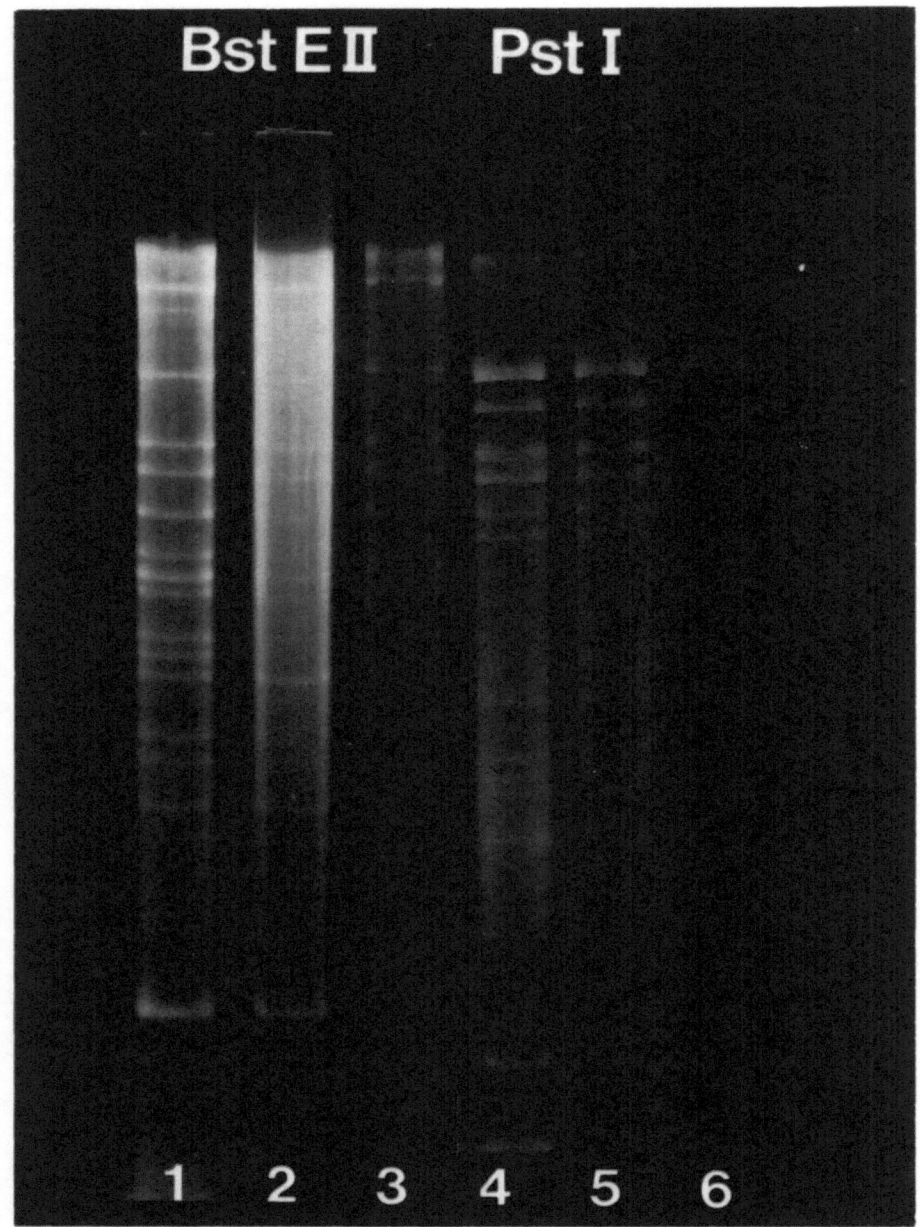

Fig. 4   Comparison of the Bst E II and Pst I DNA
restriction patterns of BHV-4 strains; lanes: 1, strain
DN-599; 2, strain Storz buff.; 3, strain Movar; the
strains used in lanes 4,5 and 6 are the same ones as in
1,2 and 3. The same conditions were used as given in Fig.
4 A.

BHV-1 strains could be separated into two groups, "IBR-like" and "IPV-like"; strains from the first group also appear to be responsible for abortion. These groupings were originally suggested as a result of studies on latent BHV-1 viruses reactivated from normal fetuses (Ludwig and Storz, 1973; Storz et al., 1980; see also, Pauli et al., 1982, this issue).

Since no serological means exist to differentiate strains which we have grouped within BHV-4, DNA analysis is the only available tool for use in shedding some light on the unity and diversity of these isolates (Fig. 4). There are slight differences in strains originating from Europe and the United States. However, with strains that have been examined so far, no clear correlation with clinical entities could be made. To our surprise these strains could convincingly be grouped together based on their DNA patterns. This suggests that these viruses are spread worldwide, and that they coexist with bovine animals and usually do not harm them. They may fill a special niche in the interaction of virus and organism and, if a comparison is sought for, they may be found to be similar to the cytomegaloviruses (CMV) of man. Although a variety of isolates seem to fall into this group their molecular biology is almost unexplored.

The only data on BHV-5 which have been reported to date stem from De Villiers (1979) but no detailed studies on the physical map of the genome exist.

The reason for designating goat herpesvirus as BHV-6 came from DNA studies performed in our laboratory (Engels et al., 1981). Previously this virus could not clearly be differentiated from BHV-1, and this was supported by our antigen and protein studies. The DNA cleavage pattern, however, sets it apart completely from the "IBR-like" and "IPV-like" genomes. Its DNA is cleaved in a unique way only at one place - at different locations though, with two different enzymes - which points to molecular properties of the DNA not known in any other herpesvirus. The sequence arrangement of the DNA, most probably comparable to that of BHV-1, remains to be established, as does its genetic relationship to BHV-1.

Like other herpesvirus groups (those of humans, horses or pigs), it is not surprising that the bovine herpesviruses do not or only insignificantly cross-react with each other. There is no overt cross-neutralization with the exception of BHV-1 and -6 (Engels et al., 1981). The antigenic cross-reactivity involves envelope structures which can be more easily defined using monospecific sera (Engels et al., manuscript in preparation). Our findings of a lack of cross-reactivity between BHV-3 and -4 support their separation into different groups (Table 3). The antigens of BHV-2 have been characterized to some extent (Sterz et al., 1973/74; Norrild et al., 1978; Ludwig, 1982). BHV-2 is the only bovine virus which closely cross-reacts with HSV and the simian B virus (Ludwig et al., 1982). Looking at the proteins involved in the immune response of BHV-1 and -2 infections, glycoproteins of apparent cular weights between 100 and 120 x 10^6 seem to play a major role. These are the only two viruses where more detailed antigen and protein studies have been reported (Sklyanskaja et al., 1977; Norrild et al., 1978; Pastoret, 1981; Ludwig, 1982). Further details on BHV-1 antigens and proteins are reported in this issue (Pauli et al., 1982).

Diagnosis of infection

The experience clinician and pathologist will be able to diagnose BHV-1, -2, -3 and -5 infections without any problems, whereas BHV-4 and -6 infections might be much more difficult (Table 5). In all cases the isolation of viruses by in vitro assay systems was successful. The different groups are characterized by their differences in host range and especially by individual growth properties in tissue culture (Fig. 5) by cytopathic effect and by virus output (Table 4). Specific antisera are available for BHV-1, -2, -3 and -6 to facilitate laboratory diagnosis. The BHV-4 group usually does not give rise to natural antibodies, and there have been no reports of experimentally prepared specific antisera.

Besides serological methods of characterizing these viruses, molecular biological techniques have, during the last

few years, considerably improved our chances of diagnosing
bovine herpesvirus infections, once isolates have been obtained

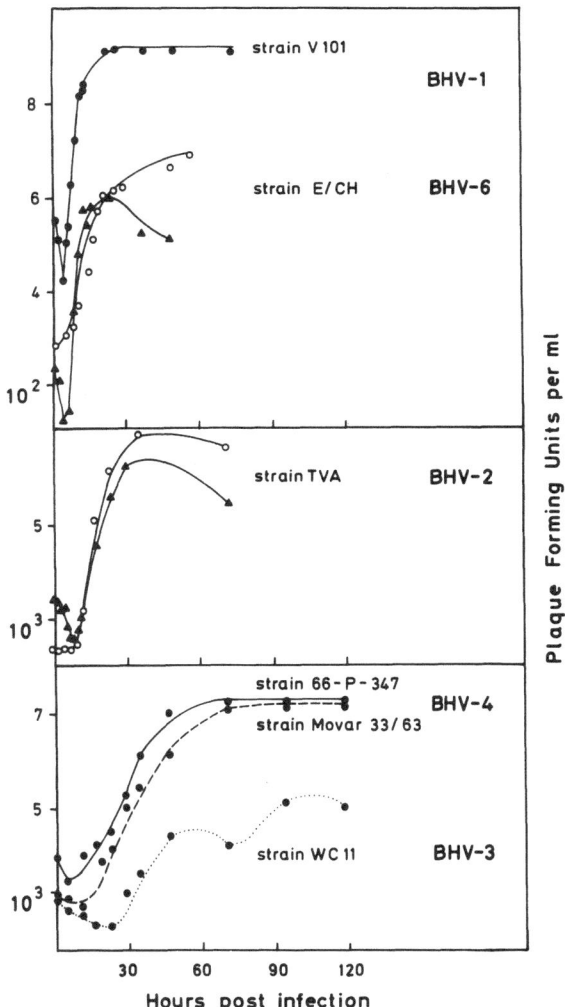

Fig. 5   Bovine herpesvirus growth curves. BHV-1 and -6
replicate quickly, whereas BHV-3 and -4 strains show a
rather slow growth (BHV-3 assayed by a fluorescent focus
assay). Open symbols (BHV-2 and -6) represent
extracellular, closed symbols represent intracellular
virus.

Clinical importance

The clinical symptoms caused by the different bovine herpesviruses are governed by a variety of factors, which have been detailed in a previous review (Ludwig, 1982) and should only briefly be mentioned here.

Certainly the virulence of the virus and the site of infection - generalized or localized to individual organs - play a role. How host defence mechanisms are involved in the clinical disease or in suppression of the disease has been studied mainly for BHV-1, -2 and -3 infections (Rouse and Babiuk, 1978; Cilli and Castrucci, 1976; Gibbs and Rweyemamu, 1977; Ludwig, 1976; Plowright, 1968).

Information of the immune response against BHV-4, -5 and -6 infections is very sparse. In general, it has been observed that even with elevated antibody levels, reactivation and shedding of virus may occur. For BHV-1 infections, it has been shown that the immune status of the host may influence virus reactivation and disease (Pastoret, 1981).

The importance of cell mediated immunity and the effect of interferon production on BHV-1 infection have been reviewed and will not be discussed here (Rouse and Babiuk, 1978).

The economic importance of the individual bovine herpesvirus infection has definitely changed in the last 30-50 years. The ways in which cattle, sheep and goats - to mention the most important reservoirs of these viruses - are treated will influence outbreaks of diseases. Crowding of animals - and by this - creation of stress situations, which may lead to immunosuppression, have led to serious outbreaks of IBR in the last years. The rapid passage of virus through a large population of animals might be one of the reasons that more virulent recombinants evolve. Other reports in this meeting may support this view.

Outlook

Investigations of bovine herpesviruses will always be governed by economic importance and not so much by academic interest. It remains a major challenge to determine the complete genomic structures of the six virus types, which have been identified so far. The best candidates for this are BHV-1 and -6 because of their quick replication and high virus yield. At the moment the possibility that the goat herpes virus (BHV-6) represents a host-restricted natural recombinant of BHV-1 cannot be excluded.

Research on BHV-2 should be carried out because of its special dermatotropism and because of its remarkable fusion activity both in vitro and in vivo. Furthermore, this virus is the only one sharing major common antigenic determinants with human and primate herpesviruses.

BHV-3 infections in cattle and rabbits could serve as excellent additional models for studying the pathogenesis of lymphoproliferative diseases. The increasing number of isolates probably falling into the BHV-4 group should attract further interest in the role these passenger viruses play in disease processes.

The bovine herpesviruses are in many ways analogous to the human and primate herpesviruses. For example, the high lytic BHV-1, -6 and BHV-2 are comparable with HSV or B virus in their natural hosts. The slow growing BHV-4 viruses have characteristics of CMV. The tumor-associated BHV-3 shares similarities with EBV, herpesviruses saimiri or ateles. Evolution of herpesviruses in one host might exclude and eliminate those herpesviruses with strong antigenic cross-reactivities.

Generally speaking, BHV-1 infections of the "IBR-like" type still seem to be of great importance. The genital form caused by the "IPV-like" viruses appears to be of less significance.

Whether vaccination with modified live virus is an adequate way to prevent BHV-1 outbreaks must be carefully considered. Inactivated vaccines or immunization with major immunogenic components may either be more reasonable alternatives.

The importance of BHV-2 infections seems to have dwindled in the last 10-20 years. This disease only appeared in localized areas, mainly in England. BHV-3 infections (malignant catarrhal fever) in European countries are becoming more and more sporadic. However, in Africa, where the virus is endemic, overt infections in ungulates can cause considerable losses.

Further studies should show whether the BHV-4 group is merely of academic interest or whether it possibly plays a greater role in large herds of animals where stress factors could contribute to activation of various diseases associated with these viruses.

BHV-6 infections seem mainly to affect young goats. There are only two reported outbreaks of this disease in the world, and this might reflect a lack of clinical importance. Little information exists about the spread of infection in goat flocks; recent studies point to the presence of BHV-6 also in Greece and Turkey.

As yet all members of the 6 groups so far seem to have the capacity to remain latent in their host and may be reactivated, although the nature of the persistent infection in BHV-3 and -4 is less clear than for the others.

Studies with bovine herpesviruses will always have the great advantage of a unique immunological situation. Large quantities of serum or immunocompetent cells and even blood or organ cells from the same animal may be used over a period of years. Since bovine cells can be grown in the animal's own sera and then injected into the original host, experiments may be done under syngeneic conditions.

REFERENCES
Aujeszky, A. 1902. Über eine neue Infektionskrankheit bei Haustieren. Zbl. Bakt. I. Orig., 32, 353.
Bartha, A., Juhász, M. and Liebermann, H. 1966. Isolation of a bovine herpesvirus from calves with respiratory disease and keratoconjunctivitis. Acta Vet. Acad. Sci. Hung., 16, 357.
Buchman, T.G. and Roizman, B. 1978a. Anatomy of bovine mammillitis DNA. I. Restriction endonuclease maps of four populations of molecules that differ in the relative orientation of their long and short components. J. Virol., 25, 395.
Buchman, T.G. and Roizman, B. 1978b. Anatomy of bovine mammillitis DNA. II. Size and arrangements of deoxy-nucleotide sequences. J. Virol., 27, 239.
Buchman, T.G., Roizman, B., Adams, G. and Stover, B.H. 1978. Restriction endonuclease fingerprinting of herpes simplex

virus DNA: A novel epidemiological tool applied to a
nosocomial outbreak. J. Infect. Dis., 138, 488.
Cilli, V. and Castrucci, G. 1976. Infection of cattle with
Bovid herpesvirus 2. Fol. Vet. Lat., 6, 1.
De Villiers, E.-M. 1979. Purification of the JS-3 isolate of
Herpesvirus ovis (bovid herpesvirus 4) and some properties
of its DNA. J. Virol., 32, 705.
Engels, M., Darai, G., Gelderblom, H. and Ludwig, H. 1981.
International Workshop on Herpesviruses. Bologna, Italy,
July 1981. p. 20.
Gibbs, E.P.J. and Rweyemamu, M.M. 1977. Bovine herpesviruses,
Part II. Bovine herpesviruses 2 and 3. Vet. Bull., 47,
411.
Götze, R. and Liess, J. 1929. Erfolgreiche Übertragungsversuche
des bösartigen Katarrhalfiebers von Rind zu Rind.
Identität mit der Südafrikanischen Snotsiekte. Dtsch.
tierärztl. Wschr., 37, 433.
Hare, T. 1925. Staphylococcal and streptococcal dermatitis of
the udder in dairy cows. Vet. Res., 5, 943.
Herrmann, S., Gaskell, R. Ehlers, B. and Ludwig, H. 1982a.
Molecular epidemiology of latent herpesvirus felinis. CEC
Symposium on "Latency of herpesviruses", Tübingen, 21.-23.
Sept. 1982.
Herrmann, S.C., Heppner, B. and Ludwig, H. 1982b. Pseudorabies
viruses from clinical outbreaks and latent infections can
be grouped in four major genome types. CEC Symposium on
"Latency of herpesviruses", Tübingen, 21.-23. Sept. 1982.
Huygelen, C. Thienpont, D. and Vandervelden, M. 1960b.
Isolation of a cytopathogenic agent from skin lesions of
cattle. Nature (London), 186, 979.
Huygelen, C. Thienpont, D., Dekeyser, P.J. and Vandervelden, M.
1960a. Allerton virus, a cytopathogenic agent associated
with lumpy skin disease. II. Inoculation of animals with
tissue culture passaged virus. Zbl. Vet. Med., 7, 754.
Kokles, R. 1967. Die infektiöse Rhinotracheitis und das
Coitalexanthem des Rindes. In "Handbuch der
Virusinfektionen bei Tieren" Bd. II (Ed. H. Röhrer). (VEB
Gustav Fischer, Jena). pp. 901-960.
Ludwig, H. and Storz, J. 1973. Activation of herpesvirus from
normal bovine fetal spleen cells after prolonged
cultivation. Med. Microbiol. Immunol, 158, 209.
Ludwig, H. 1976. Bovine herpes mammillitis (BHM) virus and its
relationship to other herpesviruses. Proc. XX. Wld. Congr.
Thessaloniki, 6.-12. July 1975. pp. 1318-1319.
Ludwig, H. 1982. Bovine Herpesviruses. In "The Herpesviruses"
(Ed. B. Roizman) I B. (Plenum Press, New York and London).
in press.
Ludwig, H., Pauli, G., Gelderblom, H., Darai, G., Koch, H.-G.,
Flügel, R.M., Norrild, B. and Daniel, M.D. 1982. B virus
(herpesvirus simiae). In "The Herpesviruses" (Ed. B.
Roizman) (Plenum Press, New York and London). in press.
Ludwig, H., Heppner, B. and Herrmann, S. 1981. The genomes of
different field isolates of Aujeszky's disease (pseudo-
rabies) virus. CEC Seminar on Aujeszky's Disease.
Tübingen, June 1981.

188

Mackay, J.M.K. 1969. Tissue culture studies of sheep pulmonary
    adenomatosis (jaagsiekte). II. Transmission of cytopathic
    effects to normal cultures. J. Comp. Pathol., 79, 147.
Martin, W.B., Hay, D., Crawford, L.V., Le Bouvier, G.L. and
    Crawford, E.M. 1966. Characteristics of bovine mammillitis
    virus. J. Gen. Microbiol., 45, 325.
McKercher, D.G. 1973. Viruses of other vertebrates. In "The
    Herpesviruses" (Ed. A.S. Kaplan) (Academic Press, New
    York, San Francisco, London). pp. 427-493.
Mettam, R.W.M. 1923. Snotsiekte in cattle. 9th and 10th Reps.
    Dir. vet. Educ. Res., Union of S. Africa. p. 395.
Mettler, F., Engels, M., Wild, P. and Bivetti, A. 1979.
    Herpesvirus-Infektion bei Zicklein in der Schweiz.
    Schweiz. Arch. Tierheilk., 121, 662.
Madin, S.H, York, C.J. and McKercher, D.G. 1956. Isolation of
    the infectious bovine rhinotracheitis virus. Science, 124,
    721.
Mohanty, S.B., Hammond, R.C. and Lillie, M.G. 1971. A new
    bovine herpesvirus and its effect on experimentally
    infected calves. Arch. ges. Virusforsch., 34, 394.
Norrild, B., Ludwig, H. and Rott, R. 1978. Identification of a
    common antigen of herpes simplex virus, bovine herpes
    mammillitis virus, and B virus. J. Virol., 26, 712.
Pastoret, P.-P. 1981. Le virus de la rhinotracheïte infectieux
    bovine (bovid herpesvirus 1): Aspects biologiques et
    moleculaires. Thesis, Université de Liège. in press.
Pauli, G., Gregersen, J.-P., Storz, J. and Ludwig, H. 1982.
    Biology and molecular biology of latent bovine herpes
    virus type 1 (BHV-1). CEC Symposium on "Latency of
    herpesviruses", Tübingen, 21.-23. Sept. 1982.
Plowright, W. 1982. Malignant catarrhal fever virus: a
    lymphotropic herpesvirus of ruminants (a review). CEC
    Symposium on "Latency of herpesviruses", Tübingen, 21.-23.
    Sept. 1982.
Plowright, W. 1968. Malignant catarrhal fever. J. Amer. Vet.
    Med. Ass., 152, 795.
Plowright, W., Macadam, R.F. and Armstrong, J. 1965. Growth and
    characterization of the virus of bovine malignant
    catarrhal fever in East Africa. J. Gen. Microbiol., 39,
    253.
Roizman, B., Bartha, A., Biggs, P.M., Carmichael, L.E.,
    Granoff, A., Hampar, B., Kaplan, A.S., Melendez, L.V.,
    Munk. K., Nahmias, A., Plummer, G., Rajcani, J., Rapp, F.,
    Terni, M., de Thê, G., Watson, D.H. and Wildy, P. 1973.
    Provisional labels for herpesviruses. J. Gen. Virol., 20,
    417.
Roizman, B. 1978. The herpesviruses. In "The Molecular Biology
    of Animal Viruses", Vol. 2. (Ed. D.P. Nayak) (Marcel
    Dekker, New York, Basel). pp. 769-848.
Roizman, B. and Tognon, M. 1982. Restriction enzyme analysis of
    herpesvirus DNA: Stability of restriction endonuclease
    patterns. The Lancet, March 20, 1982.
Rouse, B.T. and Babiuk, L.A. 1978. Mechanisms of recovery from
    herpesvirus infections - a review. Can. J. Comp. Med., 42,
    414.

Rweyemamu, M.M. and Johnson, R.H. 1969. A serological
    comparison of seven strains of bovine herpes mammillitis
    virus. Res. Vet. Sci., 10, 102.
Saito, J.K., Gribble, D.H., Berrios, P.E., Knight, H.D. and
    McKercher, D.G. 1974. A new herpesvirus isolate from
    goats: Preliminary report. Amer. J. Vet. Res., 35, 847.
Skare, J., Summers, W.P. and Summers, W.C. 1975. Structure and
    function of herpesvirus genomes. I. Comparison of five
    HSV-1 and two HSV-2 strains by cleavage of their DNA with
    EcoRI restriction endonuclease. J. Virol., 15, 726.
Sklyanskaya, E.I., Itkin, Z.B., Gofman, Y.P and Kaverin, N.V.
    1977. Structural proteins of infectious bovine rhino-
    tracheitis virus. Acta Virol., 21, 273.
Sterz, H., Ludwig, H. and Rott, R. 1973/74. Immunologic and
    genetic relationship between herpes simplex virus and
    bovine herpes mammillitis virus. Intervirology, 2, 1.
Storz, J. 1968. Comments on malignant catarrhal fever. J. Amer.
    Vet. Med. Ass., 152, 804.
Storz, J., Ludwig, H. and Rott, R. 1980. Aktivierung des
    boviden Herpesvirus 1 aus foetalem Gewebe. Proc. XI.
    Internat. Congr. on Diseases of Cattle, Tel-Aviv. (Bregman
    Press, Haifa). pp. 471-473.
Straub, O.C. 1978. Bovine Herpesvirusinfektionen. VEB Gustav
    Fischer, Jena.
Verwoerd, D.W., De Villiers, E.-M. and Coetzee, S. 1978. On the
    etiological role of Herpesvirus ovis in jaagsiekte. In
    "Oncogenesis and Herpesviruses III/2" (Ed. G. de Thê, W.
    Henle, F. Rapp). (IARC Scie. Publ. No. 24, Lyon). pp.
    869-873.
Wildy, P., Russel, W.C. and Horne, R.W. 1960. The morphology of
    herpes virus. Virology, 12, 204.
Witte, J. 1933. Untersuchungen über den Bläschenausschlag
    (Exanthema pustulosum coitale) des Rindes. Z. Hyg.
    Infekt.- Krankh., 44, 163.
Zwick, W. and Gminder. 1913. Untersuchungen über den
    Bläschenausschlag (Exanthema vesiculosum coitale) der
    Rinder. Berl. Tierärztl. Wschr., 29, 637.

INFECTIOUS BOVINE RHINOTRACHEITIS VIRUS EXCRETION AFTER VACCINATION, CHALLENGE AND IMMUNOSUPPRESSION

P.F. Nettleton, J.M. Sharp, A.J. Herring and J.A. Herring

Moredun Research Institute, 408 Gilmerton Road,
Edinburgh, Scotland

ABSTRACT

Three calves vaccinated with a live attenuated vaccine against IBR were challenged 9 weeks later with a field isolate of IBR virus. The calves were protected against clinical illness and the excretion of challenge virus was reduced compared with the control animal. Two months and seven months after challenge the 4 calves were treated with corticosteroid and all re-excreted IBR virus on both occasions. Using different biological properties of the vaccine and field virus the re-excreted isolates were shown to be principally field virus although vaccine virus was also recovered. Restriction endonuclease (RE) analysis of some of these isolates has confirmed that both virus types were re-excreted.

INTRODUCTION

Bovine herpesvirus 1 (BHV1) infection in cattle has been associated with respiratory, ocular, reproductive, central nervous system, enteric, neonatal and dermal disease (Gibbs and Rweyemamu, 1977). In Britain original reports of disease were of mild infections of the respiratory system and eye, infectious bovine rhinotracheitis (IBR) (Dawson et al., 1962; Darbyshire and Shanks, 1963), but disease of the reproductive tract, infectious pustular vulvovaginitis (IPV) and balanoposthitis (IPB) also occurred, alone (Huck et al., 1971; Deas and Johnston, 1973) or concurrently with IBR (Collings et al., 1972). A more severe form of IBR emerged in north-east Scotland during the winter of 1977-78 (Wiseman et al., 1978) and spread quickly so that the disease became a major economic problem in beef fattening units and dairy herds in many parts of Britain (Wiseman et al., 1979). This resulted in 1979 in the licensing of a live intranasal vaccine, Tracherine (SmithKline Animal Health Ltd.) wich contains a temperature sensitive (ts) mutant of IBR virus, strain RLB 106 ts. This strain of virus had been shown to be non-pathogenic, protective and genetically stable (Zygraich et al., 1974) and vaccine prepared from the virus is protective and non-abortigenic (Kucera et al., 1978).

IBR field virus is known to become latent in cattle following primary infection and periodically can be re-excreted naturally (Snowdon et al., 1965) or following administration of corticosteroids (Davies and Duncan, 1974). Such carrier animals are important reservoirs of virulent virus and the long-term success of vaccination will partially depend on whether the proportion of carrier animals in the population can be reduced. Vaccination after exposure to field virus does not lead to virus-free animals (Straub, 1979) while animals vaccinated with modified live virus and later exposed to virulent virus have been shown to re-excrete virus of un-determined pathogenicity following corticosteroid treatment (Sheffy and Davies, 1972). Ts IBR vaccine virus can establish latent infections (Pastoret et al., 1980) but there was no information as to whether or not vaccinated cattle were sufficiently protected to prevent the establishment or latent infections by wild type virus. This experiment, a preliminary report of which has already been published (Nettleton and Sharp, 1980) was carried out to address this question.

MATERIALS AND METHODS

Cells and virus

Secondary bovine embryonic kidney (BEK) cells and Madin-Darby bovine kidney (MDBK) cells of unknown passage level were grown in Eagle's minimal essential medium supplemented with 10% lactalbumin hydrolysate (LAH) and 10% adult bovine serum. A semicontinuous cell line of embryonic bovine trachea (EBTR) was grown in Eagle's 59 supplemented with 10% LAH and 10% foetal calf serum and used between the 8th and 35th passage. All cell cultures were screened for the presence of contaminating bovine virus diarrhoea virus using an indirect immunofluorescence test (Nettleton, Herring and Corrigall, 1980). BEK and EBTR cells were free of virus but the MDBK cells were found to be infected and were used only for growth of viral stocks for restriction endonuclease analysis. Following infection all cells were maintained in serum free '199' medium supplemented with 0.5% bovine serum albumin (BSA), 0.1% LAH and 0.1% yeast extract and

containing 100 i.u./ml penicillin, 100 µg/ml streptomycin, 50
i.u./ml polymixin-B and 2 µg/ml amphotericin B deoxycholate.

Tracherine vaccine, kindly supplied by SmithKline Animal
Health Ltd., was used for vaccination of the calves and
laboratory stocks of ts virus were grown from the vaccine over
2 passages in EBTR cells. Virulent IBR virus (strain 6660) was
recovered from the retropharyngeal lymph node of a calf dying
of respiratory disease in Aberdeenshire in March, 1978; it was
passaged twice in BEK cells and once in EBTR cells.

Animals

Two pairs of Jersey calves aged six months which were
seronegative for IBR were housed in separate loose boxes. Three
calves were vaccinated with Tracherine according to the
manufacturer's instructions and the fourth kept as an in-
contact control. Calves were examined clinically before
infection and daily for the next 12 days. Following examination
nasal, ocular, preputial and rectal swabs were each collected
into separate bottles of 4 ml Hank's BSS containing 1% BSA, 300
i.u./ml penicillin, 300 µg/ml streptomycin, and 50 i.u./ml
polymixin B (VTM). Nine weeks after vaccination all 4 calves
were challenged by intranasal instillation of 8.0 $\log_{10}$ $TCID_{50}$
of strain 6660. The calves were examined as before and nasal
and ocular swabs collected into separate bottles of VTM. Two
months after challenge all calves were injected intravenously
with corticosteroid (Dexadresson: Intervet Laboratories) at a
daily dose rate of 0.1 mg per kg for 5 days and 7 months after
challenge all calves received further corticosteroid (Betsolan
soluble: Glaxovet) at the same dose rate and again for 5 days.
The calves were examined clinically and nasal swabs collected
into VTM.

Six 3 to 8 week old Jersey bull calves free of antibodies
to IBR virus were used to test the pathogenicity of 3 IBR
viruses recovered from challenged vaccinates following the
first course of corticosteroid, the viruses having been
passaged three times at terminal dilution in BEK cells and
stocks prepared in EBTR cells. Two calves, aged 6 and 8 weeks
received 6.7 $\log_{10}$ $TCID_{50}$ of virus recovered from calf 3 on day

12, three calves aged 3, 4 and 8 weeks, received 6.9 $\log_{10}$ $TCID_{50}$ of virus recovered from calf 2 on day 5 and one calf aged 4 weeks received 6.9 $\log_{10}$ $TCID_{50}$ of virus from calf 3 on day 5. Virus was given as a 5 ml intranasal dose divided equally between each nostril, and nasal swabs were collected daily into VTM for 8 days.

Virus isolation

Swabs in VTM were sonicated for 30 seconds in an ultrasonic water bath (Engisonic Ltd., model B32) and 0.2 ml volumes of $\log_{10}$ dilutions of medium were inoculated on to duplicate tubes of BEK cells (original 4 calves) or EBTR cells (6 calves used for comparative pathogenicity). After 1 hour at $37^{o}C$ the inoculum was washed off with Hank's BSS containing antibiotics and 1 ml of maintenance medium was added to each tube. The cultures, incubated at $37^{o}C$ or $40^{o}C$, were examined for up to 6 days to detect virus cytopathic effect and the concentration of virus in the starting material was calculated according to the method of Spearman and Karber (Lennette and Schmidt, 1969).

Plaque sizing of recovered isolates, which had received 1 pass at terminal dilution in BEK cells, was carried out on confluent monolayers of EBTR cells grown in 60 mm plastic petri dishes. Virus dilutions were adsorbed for 1 hour at $37^{o}C$, the inoculum removed and 8 ml of maintenance medium supplemented with 10% horse serum and containing 1.5% carboxy methyl cellulose added. After 4 days incubation at $37^{o}C$ in a 5% CO_2 incubator the cells were fixed with 10% buffered formol saline and stained with crystal violet. Plates with well separated plaques were selected and minimum plaque diameters were measured using a graticule in an inverted microscope giving x 25 magnification. 50-20 plaques were measured for each isolate and the plaque sizes compared by an analysis of variance. Ts and 6660 viruses were included in every test and the relationship between the calf isolates and the vaccine and challenge viruses was obtained from T values using means and standard errors derived from the analysis of variance.

Neutralisation tests

The levels of IBR antibody in nasal secretions, collected by tampon, and serum were measured in a microtitre test in which duplicate dilutions of test fluid were mixed with approximately 40 $TCID_{50}$ of the 'Oxford' strain of IBR and incubated at 37°C for 1 hour before EBTR cells were added. Tests were read after 48 hours and results expressed as the reciprocal of the highest serum dilution neutralising virus in both wells.

Restriction endonuclease analysis of IBR isolates

Virus stocks tested for pathogenicity in calves were further purified by plaque picking three times. Plaque picked virus was used to infect either EBTR cells or MDBK cells at a multiplicity of infection of approximately 1. The cells were incubated at 37°C for 48 hours after which viral cytopathic effect was complete. The medium was harvested, chilled to 4°C, clarified by centrifugation for 10 minutes at 2,400 g and the virus pelleted at 40,000 g for 1 hour.

Viral DNA was prepared from the crude viral pellets by digestion with 200 µg/ml Proteinase K (Sigma Chemical Co. Ltd.) in 50 mM Tris-HCl buffer pH 8.3 containing 1 mM EDTA and 2% w/v SDS for 1 to 2 h at 37°C followed by extraction with an equal volume of 'phenol'-chloroform mixture (6:4 by volume). 'Phenol' consisted of a mixture of 500 g of phenol with 70 g m-cresol, 200 g of water and 0.5 g 8-hydroxyquinoline. Nucleic acid from the aqueous phase of the extraction was precipitated with two volumes of ethanol at -20°C and further purified by CsCl density gradient centrifugation for 40 h at 70,000 g in a Beckman type 65 rotor. The starting solution was 20 mM Tris-HCl pH 7.5 containing 1 mM EDTA and 5.82 M CsCl. The gradients were fractionated by upward displacement using an ISCO model 185 density gradient fractionator with UV monitor and the viral DNA was found in a sharp peak at a density of 1.73. Examination of the absorption profiles from a number of preparations of DNA showed that there was no detectable peak at the position expected for contaminating host cell DNA and thus the CsCl gradients were omitted in later experiments.

Restriction endonuclease digests were performed with a
five fold excess of enzyme for between 2 and 3 h, the
conditions used being those recommended by the suppliers (Sigma
Chemical Co. Ltd. for Eco R1 and Hind 111 and New England
Biolabs Inc. for Mbo 1). The resulting digests were analysed by
polyacrylamide gel electrophoresis using either 7.5% gels or
6.0 to 12% gradient gels (acrylamide to bis-acrylamide ratio of
37.5:1). The buffers used were those described by Laemmli
(1970) but the stacking gel was omitted. The gels had the
dimensions 14 x 19 x 0.15 cms and electrophoresis was carried
out for 16 h at 25 mA. The separated restriction fragments were
visualised by silver staining which is considerably more
sensitive than ethidium bromide fluorescent detection. The
method used was based on that developed by Sammons et al.
(1981) for polypeptide detection and is described in full in
Herring et al. (1982).

RESULTS

Cultural characteristics of the vaccine and challenge virus

a)   Growth at $37^{\circ}C$ and $40^{\circ}C$. The geometric mean and standard
deviations of three matched titrations at the two different
temperatures are shown in Table 1. It was clear that while the
titre of the vaccine virus was reduced by more than 4.0 $\log_{10}$
$TCID_{50}$ at $40^{\circ}C$ that of the challenge virus was not significantly reduced at the higher temperature.

TABLE 1   Titration of vaccine and challenge viruses at
two temperatures

Virus	Incubation temperature	
	$37^{\circ}C$	$40^{\circ}C$
Vaccine (ts)	6.66[*]	2.5
	$\pm$ 0.76	$\pm$ 0.5
Challenge (6660)	6.66	6.33
	$\pm$ 0.76	$\pm$ 0.58

[*]Virus titre ($\log_{10}$ $TCID_{50}$/0.2 ml $\pm$ S.D.)

b)   Plaque size. Analysis of variance showed that the mean
plaque sizes of the vaccine and challenge virus were significantly different (p < 0.001). Results from three tests are
shown in Table 2 and demonstrate the test to test variation in
absolute plaque sizes encountered. For this reason both viruses were included alongside the unknown calf isolates in every
test.

TABLE 2   Mean diameter ($\pm$ S.E.) of 50 plaques each of
the vaccine and challenge viruses in three
tests.

	Vaccines virus (ts)	Challenge virus (6660)
Test 1	22.46 $\pm$ 0.92	39.96 $\pm$ 1.20
Test 2	20.62 $\pm$ 0.77	31.04 $\pm$ 1.36
Test 3	36.78 $\pm$ 1.27	45.60 $\pm$ 1.46

Calf vaccination, challenge and immunosuppression

Following vaccination virus was only detected in nasal
secretion of 2 of 3 calves over an 8 day period (Fig. 1). All

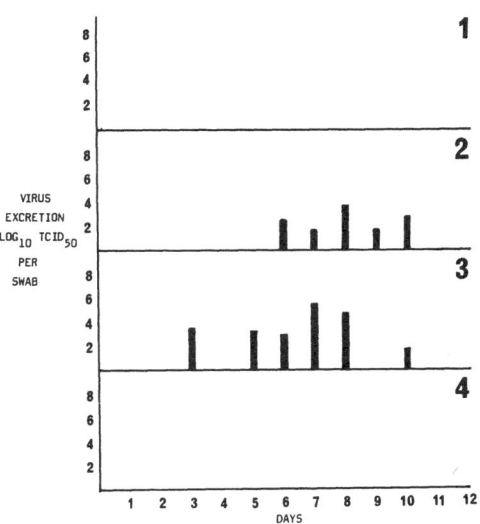

Fig. 1   Virus excreted by vaccinated animals. Calves 1,
2 and 3 given 6.2 $\log_{10}$ $TCID_{50}$ 'Tracherine'

isolates had temperature growth and plaque size characteristics of the vaccine virus.

Virus was not recovered from ocular, rectal or preputial swabs from th 3 calves nor from any sample taken from the incontact calf. Neutralising antibody was not detected in serum or nasal secretions of any of the calves over the next eight weeks.

Following challenge the unvaccinated calf developed pyrexia (> 40°C) from day 3 to day 6, coinciding with a serous nasal discharge. Nasal ulceration with a mucopurulent discharge developed on day 7 but by day 9 the ulcers were healing and there was no nasal discharge. Calf 1 had pyrexia on day 3 but otherwise no clinical symptoms were seen in the 3 vaccinated calves. The virus excretion patterns of the calves are shown in Fig. 2.

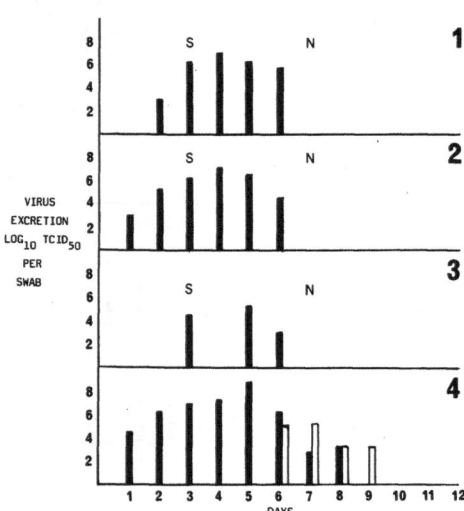

Fig. 2   Virus excreted by animals challenged with 8.0 $\log_{10}$ $TCID_{50}$ IBR strain 6660.   virus from nasal swabs.   virus from ocular swabs. Neutralising antibodies first detected in the serum-S and nasal secretion-N.

The vaccinates excreted virus only from the nose for between 3 to 6 days whereas the unvaccinated calf excreted high levels of virus from the nose for 8 days and virus from the eye on days 6 to 9. Five selected isolates had temperature growth and plaque size characteristics of the challenge virus. Neutralising antibodies were detected in the sera of the vaccinated calves within 3 days of challenge and in the control calf after 13 days. Neutralising activity was detected in nasal secretions of the vaccinates one week after challenge but did not develop in the control calf (see Table 3).

TABLE 3   Neutralising activity of nasal mucous (NM) and serum (S) of the 4 calves.

Time	Calf 1		Calf 2		Calf 3		Calf 4	
	NM	S	NM	S	NM	S	NM	S
Pre-vaccination	< 2	< 2	< 2	< 2	< 2	< 2	< 2	< 2
Pre-challenge	< 2	< 2	< 2	< 2	< 2	< 2	< 2	< 2
Post challenge (3 days)	ND	4	ND	4	ND	4	ND	< 2
" " (1 week)	2	16	4	64	4	64	< 2	< 2
" " (2 weeks)	2	64	4	64	8	64	< 2	8
Pre corticosteroid	4	64	8	128	4	64	< 2	512
Post corticosteroid	8	256	16	512	16	64	2	512

Corticosteroid treatment two months after challenge had no clinical effect on the calves but all yielded IBR virus at some time from the fourth day of corticosteroid treatment onwards. Growth of excreted virus at 37°C and 40°C showed both vaccine and wild type virus were recovered from calf 3 while virus from the other calves grew equally well at both temperatures implying that it was challenge virus (Fig. 3).

Plaque assay results confirmed these findings except that the mean plaque size of virus recovered from calf 2 although closer to that of the challenge virus was significantly smaller (Table 4).

Further characterisation of 3 recovered isolates was achieved by testing their pathogenicity in 3 to 8 week old calves. Virus recovered from calf 3 on day 5 which appeared to

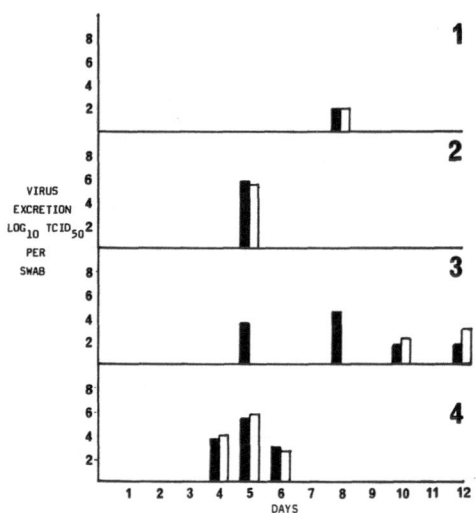

Fig. 3 Nasal excretion of virus following corticosteroid 2 months after challenge   virus growth at 37°C
     virus growth at 40°C.

TABLE 4 Comparison of mean plaque sizes of isolates from
        immunosuppressed calves with those of the vaccine
        and challenge strains. Results are shown as pro-
        bability levels of isolates having plaques sizes
        different to the 2 original strains. N.S $p > 0.05$;
        * $p < 0.05 > 0.01$; ** $p < 0.01 > 0.001$;
        *** $p < 0.001$

Virus	Calf No.							
	1	2		3			4	
	Day	Day		Day			Day	
	8	5	5	8	10	12	4	6
Vaccine (ts)	***	***	N.S.	N.S.	***	***	***	***
Challenge (6660)	N.S.	**	***	***	N.S.	N.S.	N.S.	N.S.

be vaccine virus was apathogenic and caused no clinical illness
in the calf which subsequently received it. By contrast virus
isolated on day 12 from calf 3 which appeared to be wild type
was fully virulent causing depression, nasal ulceration and
discharge, and pyrexia for 3 and 4 days in the 2 calves that
received it. Virus from calf 2 did not cause pyrexia in any of

the three calves receiving it and the only clinical sign of
infection was discrete ulceration of the nasal mucosae from day
6 onwards accompanied by slight mucopurulent discharge. The
mean virus excretion levels from the 6 calves are shown in Fig.
4 and further confirm that both vaccine and challenge virus
were recovered from calf 3 following immunosuppression. The
isolate from calf 2, although it had temperature growth characteristics identical to the challenge virus and a plaque size
closer to that of the challenge virus, was excreted at intermediate titres.

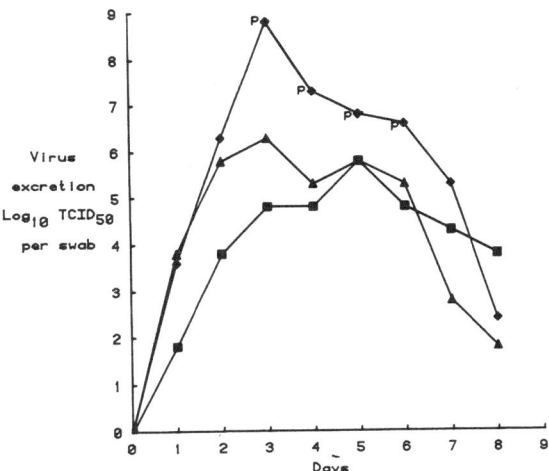

Fig. 4 . Virus excreted by calves used to test the
pathogenicity of isolates from immunosuppressed challenged
vaccinates —— isolate from calf 3 day 5; ▲——▲ isolate from calf 3 day 12; ◆——◆ isolate from calf 2 day
5.   P = Pyrexia

As further verification of the above findings restriction
endonuclease digests of vaccine and challenge viruses and the
same 3 recovered isolates were examined using Eco R1 and Hind
III enzymes for which mapping data was available (J. Skare and
I. Skare, personal communication). The only differences observed in these digests were in the mobility of a Hind III fragment which was known to be terminal and to exhibit high variab-

ility when many strains were compared. We therefore extended
the analysis using MbO1, an enzmye with a four base recognition
sequence which cleaves IBR DNA into more than 80 fragments
varying in size from approximately 2×10^6 daltons downwards.
These fragments were resolved using polyacrylamide gradient
gels and visualised by silver staining. Again the overall fragment patterns were very similar but this fine analysis revealed
several small difference between the isolates, some of which
are indicated by numbers in Figure 5.

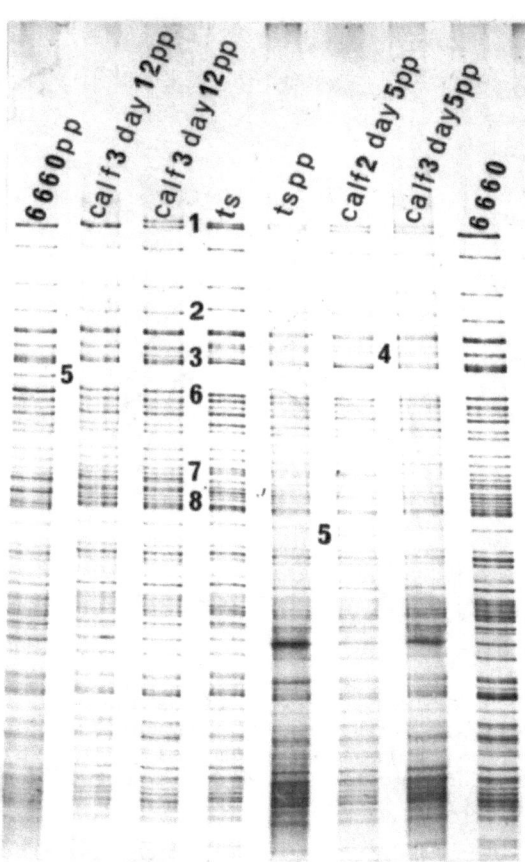

Fig. 5   MbO1 restriction endonuclease digests of DNA
from plaque purified (pp) virus recovered from corticosteroid treated calves compared with digests of unpurified and plaque purified vaccine and challenge viruses.
2 separate plaque picked stocks of calf 3 day 12 are
shown. See text for numbers showing differences in the
gel pattern.

Difference 1 was in the largest band which was shown to be hypervariable when a large number of strains was compared and so was not a reliable strain marker. This effect was very clear with agarose gels which resolved the two largest bands in all these strains. The bands marked 5 appeared only after plaque purification, and in the case of strain 6660 resulted from amplification of a minor component. The bands marked 2, 3, 6, 7 and 8 are those which distinguish the vaccine and challenge strain. It is notable that the isolates recovered after corticosteroid treatment resemble either the challenge virus (6660) or the vaccine strain (ts) in their fragment pattern at these sites and that their relationship as judged by these criteria are consistent with their biological typing as described above. Thus calf 3 day 12 resembles 6660 and was virulent, calf 3 day 5 and calf 2 day 5 resemble ts and were avirulent. However of these last two avirulent isolates only calf 3 day 5 showed the temperature sensitivity of the vaccine strain. Slight differences between the fragment pattern of these 2 isolates were seen (marked 4 on Fig. 5).

In summary, from the four properties of the three isolates selected for further characterisation there was strong evidence that both vaccine (day 5) and challenge virus (day 12) were recovered from calf 3. Virus recovered from calf 2, however, was not the same as either but the available evidence suggests that it originated from the vaccine virus, remained avirulent but lost its temperature sensitivity marker.

To investigate further the extent of latent infections the four original calves were retreated with corticosteroid 7 months after challenge. This caused depression only in the control animal for 2 days with pyrexia (40.8°C) on the day after corticosteroid administration had stopped. Small discrete ulcers of the nasal mucosa were first seen in all calves on the same day but these healed quickly and were not associated with increased mucous discharge. All calves again excreted virus as shown in Fig. 6 with the vaccinates excreting less than the control. All viruses had, temperature growth characteristics of the challenge virus.

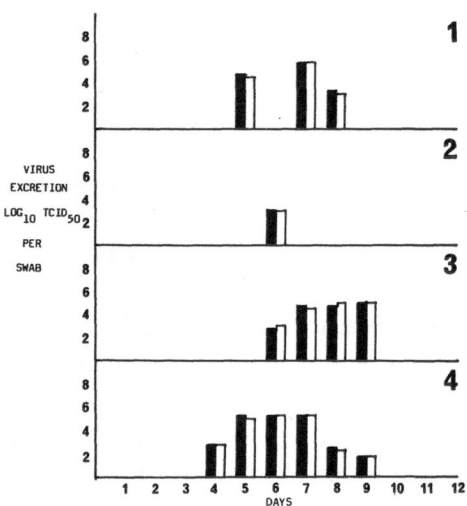

Fig. 6   Nasal excretion of virus following corticosteroid 7 months after challenge. ■ virus growth at 37°C; □ virus growth at 40°C.

Plaque sizes of these recovered isolates confirmed that the one from calf 2 and 2 of 3 from calf 1 were indistinguishable from the challenge virus, but although other isolates were closer to the challenge virus in vivo passage had caused a reduction in plaque size which was shown to be significant by the analysis of variance (Table 5). The fact that virus recovered from calf 4 which had received challenge virus only,

TABLE 5   Comparison of mean plaque sizes of isolates from immunosuppressed calves with those of the vaccine and challenge strain. Results are expressed as described in Table 4.

	Calf No.									
	1			2	3			4		
	Day			Day	Day			Day		
Virus	5	7	8	6	6	7	8	4	5	6
Vaccine (ts)	***	***	***	***	***	***	***	***	***	***
Challenge (6660)	NS	*	NS	NS	**	*	*	**	NS	**

on 2 of 3 days tested also gave a reduced plaque size suggests
that this property may not be a wholly reliable property for
comparing primary infecting virus and that re-excreted after
a period of latency.

Further characterisation of these isolates has not yet
been carried out.

DISCUSSION
The ts vaccine produced no clinical symptoms in any of the
three calves and viral multiplication, as demonstrated by the
excretion of low levels of virus from day 3 post-infection
onwards from only 2 of 3 calves, was slow and limited to the
nasal mucosa. Although no viral replication was detected in
calf 1 this was as well protected as the other vaccinates when
they were challenged. Compared to the control animal vaccinated
calves excreted lower levels of virus for fewer days after
challenge. Virus was excreted only from the nose of the
vaccinates there being no viral spread to the eye, a common
sequel to experimental intranasal infection with virulent virus
(McKercher, 1963). Further evidence of successful vaccination
was given by the rapid humoral antibody response following
challenge. Our results, therefore, provided further evidence to
that already reported (Zygraich et al., 1974; Kucera et al.,
1978; Frerichs et al., 1982) of the safety and efficacy of the
ts vaccine in protecting against respiratory disease caused by
IBR virus.

We have also shown that vaccination reduced but did not
prevent the establishment of latent infections as judged by the
re-excretion of virus following corticosteroid treatment two
and seven months after challenge. In a comparable study
Pastoret et al. (1980) showed that 7 of 8 animals vaccinated
with ts IBR virus excreted virus for up to 8 days following
dexamethasome treatment suggesting that ts IBR virus could
produce latency. No virus was recovered from the same animals,
however, after they had been challenged with virulent virus
and then subjected to a further treatment of dexamethasone.
This failure to recover virus was considered to be due to the
high levels of immunity arising from the two dexamethasone
treatments and challenge whithin 3 months of vaccination. The

increased time-scale of our experiment and omission of dexamethasone after vaccination resulted in virus recovery from animals latently infected following ts IBR vaccination and challenge with virulent virus.

Characterisation of recovered isolates using the properties of relative growth at $37^{\circ}C$ and $40^{\circ}C$ and plaque size both of which had been shown to be stable markers in vitro and following primary animal infection, suggested that both vaccine and challenge virus were recovered two months after challenge but that only challenge virus was recovered seven months after challenge. Of these two characteristics there was evidence that the plaque size was not a wholly reliable marker for comparing primary infecting virus and that re-excreted after a period of latency, an observation which has been made by other workers (Pastoret et al., 1979). Further characterisation of 3 selected isolates recovered two months after challenge was carried out by testing their pathogenicity in calves. These results confirmed that both avirulent vaccine virus and fully virulent challenge virus were recovered from one of the vaccinated calves, but that an isolate, from another calf, which had a temperature growth pattern similar to the challenge virus was of very low virulence in calves. Since it has been shown that IBR virus does not undergo any significant modification in its pathogenicity following reactivation (Castrucci et al., 1980) there was no immediate explanation for the derivation of this isolate. In order to investigate this finding further purified stocks of the 3 selected isolates and the vaccine and challenge virus were prepared and restriction endonuclease (RE) analysis of their DNA carried out. Investigations of herpes simplex virus strains using this technique have shown not only that types 1 and 2 can be readily discriminated, but also that unrelated isolates of HSV1 can be distinguished on the basis of minor differences in the fragment pattern (Lonsdale et al., 1979). Our RE analysis of UK isolates of BHV-1 has revealed 2 broad types exemplified by the 'Cooper' strain (Summers et al., 1975) and the 'K22' strain (Skare et al., 1975). A report on 7 strains from Switzerland and Germany (Engels et al., 1981) classifies those with 'Cooper' RE profiles as IBR viruses and those with 'K22' RE profiles as IPV viruses irrespective of the disease syndrome from which they were isolated. This classific- ation may be premature since the vaccine virus, originally isolated from a case of IPV in Belgium in 1969 (N. Zygraich, personal communication) and the challenge virus, isolated from a case of IBR in Scotland in 1978 were both 'Cooper' types and were only distinguishable when an enzyme was used which cleaves the DNA into many fragments. Results from these experiments further showed that both vaccine and challenge viruses were recovered from vaccinated calf number 3 and that virus isolated from calf number 2 had an RE profile similar to the vaccine virus, even though it was no longer temperature sensitive. The fact that it failed to produce disease in calves showed that maintenance of the ts marker was not necessary to ensure non pathogenicity and suggests that multiple mutation has occurred during attenuation. The origin of this isolate is unlikely to be ascertained. As the ts mutation has been shown to be genetically stable (Zygraich et al., 1974) it is unlikely that this non-virulent strain has arisen by reversion. It would seem more likely that the isolate originated from recombination with the challenge virus either 'in vivo' or 'in vitro' following reisolation.

These findings have shown that both ts vaccine virus and virulent challenge virus can establish latent infections in vaccinated calves, and that possible interaction between the viruses may occur necessitating careful characterisation of all recovered isolates.

REFERENCES

Castrucci, G., Wada, E.M., Ranucci, S., Frigeri, F., Cilli, V., Pedini, B., Tesei, B. and Arush, M.A. 1980. Reactivation of latent infection by infectious bovine rhinotracheitic virus in calves. Microbiologica, 3, 307-318.
Collings, D.F., Gibbs, E.P.J. and Stafford, L.P. 1972. Con- current respiratory and genital disease associated with infectious bovine rhinotracheitis/infectious pustular vulvovaginitis (IBR/IPV) virus in a dairy herd in the United Kingdom. Vet. Rec., 91, 214-219.
Darbyshire, J.H. and Shanks, P.L. 1963. The isolation of infectious bovine rhinotracheitis virus in Scotland. Vet. Rec., 75, 897-899.

208

Davies, D.H. and Duncan, J.R. 1974. The pathogenesis of recur-
    rent infections with infectious bovine rhinotracheitis
    virus induced in calves by treatment with corticosteroids.
    Cornell vet., 64, 340-366.
Dawson, P.S., Darbyshire, J.H., Loosmore, R.M., Paterson, A.B.
    and Faull, W.B. 1962. Infectious bovine rhinotracheitis
    (IBR). A clinical condition of cattle occurring in the
    United Kingdom. Vet. Rec., 74, 1379-1383.
Deas, D.W. and Johnson, W.S. 1973. The isolation and trans-
    mission of the virus of infectious bovine rhinotrache-
    itis/infectious pustular vulvovaginitis. Vet. Rec., 92,
    636-639.
Engels, M., Steck, F. and Wyler, R. 1981. Comparison of the
    genomes of infectious bovine rhinotracheitis and in-
    fectious pustular vulvovaginitis virus strains by restric-
    tion endonuclease analysis. Arch. Virol., 67, 169-174.
Frerichs, G.N., Woods, S.B., Lucas, M.H. and Sands, J.J. 1982.
    Safety and efficacy of live and inactivated infectious
    bovine rhinotracheitis vaccines. Vet. Rec., 111, 116-122.
Gibbs, E.P.J. and Rweyemamu, M.M. 1977. Bovine herpesviruses
    Part I. Bovine Herpesvirus I. Vet. Bull., 47, 317-343.
Herring, A.J., Inglis, N.F., Ojeh, C.K., Snodgrass, D.R. and
    Menzies, J.D. 1982. Rapid diagnosis of rotavirus in-
    fection by direct detection of viral nucleic acid in
    silver stained polyacrylamide gels. J. Clin. Micro.,
    16, 473-477.
Huck, R.A., Millar, P.G., Evans, D.M., Stables, J.W. and Ross,
    A. 1971. Penoposthitis associated with infectious bovine
    rhinotracheitis/infectious pustular vulvovaginitis
    (IBR/IPV) virus in a stud of bulls. Vet. Rec., 88, 292-
    297.
Kucera, C.J., White, R.G. and Beckenhauer, W.H. 1978. Evaluat-
    ion of the safety and efficacy of an intranasal vaccine
    containing a temperature sensitive strain of infectious
    bovine rhinotracheitis virus. Am. J. Vet. Res., 39, 607-
    610.
Laemmli, U.K. 1970. Cleavage of structural proteins during the
    assembly of the head of bacteriophage T4. Nature (Lond.),
    227, 680-685.
Lennete, E.H. and Schmidt, N.J. 1969. Diagnostic procedures for
    viral and rickettsial infections. 4th Edition. (American
    Public Health Association Inc.).
Lonsdale, D.M., Brown, S.M., Subak-Sharp, J.H., Warren, K.G.
    and Koprowski, H. 1979. The polypeptide and the DNA
    restriction enzyme profiles of spontaneous isolates of
    herpes simplex virus type 1 from explants of human
    trigeminal, superior cervical and vagus ganglia. J. Gen.
    Virol., 43, 151-171.
McKercher, D.G., Wada, E.M. and Straub, O.C. 1963. Distribution
    and persistence of infectious bovine rhinotracheitis virus
    in experimentally infected cattle. Am. J. Vet. Res., 24,
    510-514.
Nettleton, P.F., Herring, J.A. and Corrigall, W. 1980. Isolat-
    ion of bovine virus diarrhoea virus from a Scottish red
    deer. Vet. Rec., 107, 425-426.

Nettleton, P.F. and Sharp, J.M. 1980. Infectious bovine rhino-
    tracheitis virus excretion after vaccination. Vet. Rec.,
    107, 379.
Pastoret, P.P., Babiuk, L.A., Misra, V. and Griebel, P. 1980.
    Reactivation of temperature-sensitive and non-temperature-
    sensitive infectious bovine rhinotracheitis vaccine virus
    with dexamethasone. Infect. Immun., 29, 483-488.
Pastoret, P.P., Jetteur, P., Aguilar-setien, A., Leroy, P.,
    Godart, M., Schoenars, F. (1979). Etude par une méthode
    de comparison de la moyenne des plages de souches du
    virus IBR (Bovid herpesvirus 1) isolées chez les bovins
    après injection de dexaméthasome. Ann. Med. vet., 123,
    203-207.
Sammons, D.W., Adams, L.D. and Nishizawa, E.E. 1981. Ultra-
    sensitive silver-based color staining of polypeptides in
    polyacrylamide gels. Electrophoresis, 2, 135-141.
Sheffy, B.E. and Davies, D.H. 1972. Reactivation of a bovine
    herpes virus after corticosteroid treatment.
    P.S.E.B.M., 140, 974-976.
Skare, J., Summers, W.P. and Summers, W.C. 1975. Structure and
    function of herpesvirus genomes. I. Comparison of five
    HSV-1 and two HSV-2 strains by cleavage of their DNA with
    ECORI restriction endonuclease. J. Virol., 15, 726-732.
Snowdon, W.A. 1965. The IBR-IPV virus:reaction to infection
    and intermittent recovery of virus from experimentally
    infected cattle. Austr. Vet. J., 41, 135-142.
Straub, O.C. 1979. Persistence of infectious bovine rhino-
    tracheitis-infections pustular vulvovaginitis virus in
    the respiratory and genital tract of cattle. Comp. Immun.
    Microbiol. Infect. Dis., 2, 285-294.
Summers, W.C., Fickel, T., Skare, J., Summers, W.P. and
    Wagner, M. 1975. Use of restriction endonucleases to
    analyse the DNA of herpesviruses. In Oncogenesis and
    Herpesviruses II. Ed. G. de Thé., M.A. Epstein and
    H. zur Hausen. W.H.O. International Agency for Research
    on Cancer, pp. 139-143.
Wiseman, A., Msolla, P.M., Selman, I.E., Allan, E.M., Cornwell,
    H.J.C., Pirie, H.M. and Imray, W.A. 1978. An acute severe
    outbreak of infectious bovine rhinotracheitis: clinical,
    epidemiological, microbiological and pathological aspects.
    Vet. Rec., 103, 391-397.
Wiseman, A., Selman, I.E., Msolla, P.M., Pirie, H.M. and
    Allan, E. 1979. The financial burden of infectious bovine
    rhinotracheitis. Vet. Rec., 105, 469.
Zygraich, N., Lobmann, M., Vascoboinic, E., Berge, E. and
    Huygelen, C. 1974. In vivo and in vitro properties of a
    temperature sensitive mutant of infectious bovine rhino-
    tracheitis virus. Res. Vet. Sci., 16, 328-335.

THE ROLE OF LATENCY IN THE EPIZOOTIOLOGY
OF INFECTIOUS BOVINE RHINOTRACHEITIS

P.-P. Pastoret, E. Thiry, B. Brochier,
G. Derboven, H. Vindevogel
Department of Virology,
Faculty of Veterinary Medicine,
University of Liège,
45, rue de Vétérinaires,
B-1070 Brussels, Belgium

ABSTRACT

Latency is one of the major problems associated with the infection of cattle by the virus of Infectious Bovine Rhinotracheitis/Infectious Pustular Vulvovaginitis, or Bovineherpesvirus 1 (BHV 1). Both wild virulent strains and the attenuated vaccine strains can remain latent in cattle and may be reactivated by several stimuli including the use of glucocorticoids, such as dexamethasone.

Several problems arise due to BHV 1 latency, in the epizootiology of the infection:

a) first of all, one may consider that all the animals become latent carriers after a primary infection with a virulent strain;

b) all the attenuated strains remain latent after vaccination;

c) we cannot really control the dissemination of attenuated strains;

d) vaccination does not prevent the establishment of a virulent strain in a latent state;

e) it is still not determined whether recombination between attenuated strains and field virus occurs or not in an animal latently infected with both of these strains;

f) the immune status of the latently infected animal influences the pattern of reexcretion.

An animal latently infected with a virulent strain or with an attenuated one still pathogenic for the foetus is a permanent threat for the other animals of its surroundings, since the reactivated strains seem to be identical to the original ones.

The introduction of a latent, silent carrier in a herd free of the infection is the best way to introduce the disease, especially under certain circumstances or with the use of certain drugs. Latency also allows BHV 1 to persist in a restricted herd without new introduction of exogenous virus.

As the animal latently infected with a field strain or an inadequately attenuated one is a permanent threat for the

animals of its surroundings and since those strains can be
disseminated by duly vaccinated animals, vaccination gives a
false impression of safety.

The emphasis of the studies in medical prophylaxis of the
disease must not only be given to the measures or the
mechanisms that help the vaccinated animal to overcome the
disease resulting from a contact with a field virulent strain,
but also on the measures or the mechanisms that enable the
animal to overcome or to control reactivation and reexcretion.

Since the attenuated strains remain as latent as virulent
ones and as reactivated strains in a singly infected animal
remain stable, restriction analysis of the DNA of BHV 1
isolates will be an important tool for the study of the
epizootiology of infection with BHV 1).

INTRODUCTION

Latency is one of the major problems associated with the
infection of cattle by the virus of Infectious Bovine
Rhinotracheitis/Infectious Pustular Vulvovaginitis, or
Bovine herpesvirus 1 (BHV 1).

Infectious rhinotracheitis may be a severe disease,
especially when aided by some bacteria (Asso, 1976; Yates,
1982). The clinical lesions are usually restricted to the
anterior respiratory tract, with nasal exudation and
tracheitis, but may also extend to the posterior respiratory
tract, with bronchitis and pneumonia.

Infectious bovine rhinotracheitis is often associated with
numerous other symptoms, such as conjunctivitis, abortion,
metritis after caesarian section, encephalitis in young calves,
and rare cases of enteritis (Pastoret, 1979; Straub, 1978;
Wellemans et al., 1977). The great variety of the symptoms
stems from the pathogenesis of the disease and from the
privileged relationships that exist between the virus and the
organism.

PATHOGENESIS

The genesis of the local form of the disease after primary
infection such as rhinotracheitis or conjunctivitis can easily
be explained; the other forms of the disease follow
generalization of the local infection.

The role of the infectious dose on clinical signs is not
well known for Bovine herpesvirus 1 infection (Gaskell and

Povey, 1979).

Generalization of the infection is generated in three different ways:

a)   viraemia;

b)   neural spread;

c)   cell-to-cell transmission of the virus through intercellular bridges, even in the presence of specific antibodies.

a)   Viraemia

After primary infection, a very transient viraemia may take place before the appearance of specific antibodies in the serum of the animal.

In adult cattle, viraemia is, in fact, very seldom followed by a secondary localization of the disease. It is not true for the newborn calf, which suffers from acute generalized disease provoked by viraemia. This pathogenesis can explain why passive immunization of the newborn conferred by colostral antibodies is effective and protects it from the worse effects of the infection (Rosner, 1968; House and Baker, 1968).

b)   Neural spread

The virus multiplies intensively at the local site of infection and contaminates the peripheral nerves, and by that route reaches the central nervous system, where some strains may cause encephalitis (Johnson et al., 1964; Straub and Böhm, 1965; Hall et al., 1966; Bagust and Clark, 1972).

Both intranasal or intravaginal experimental inoculation of the virus produce generalization of the infection by the nervous pathway. In both cases, the distribution of the virus is quite similar, despite differences in localization within the nervous system: the virus can be found both in the brain and in the spinal cord when the animals are inoculated by the intravaginal route, but remains confined to the brain when they are inoculated by the intranasal route. This should be the consequence of the distribution of the sensory nerves to the peripheral organs which are affected by intense viral multiplication.

The major part of the macroscopic or microscopic lesions are observed at the initial site of contamination, and the extension to the nervous system produces no important damages, except within the Gasserian ganglions (Narita et al., 1976, 1978a and b).

c) Spread through intercellular bridges

Bovine herpesvirus 1, like other Herpesviridae, can use intercellular bridges to propagate itself from cell to cell, avoiding therefore the extracellular fluid. This explains why the virus can be disseminated to other cells in the presence of high titres of specific antibodies.

This kind of viral spread may be important for viral propagation after reactivation.

LATENCY

After the invading period that follows the primary infection, virus maintains itself in the organism in a latent date.

The persistence of Bovine herpesvirus 1 in the infected animal after recovery has been investigated very early on, since Storch, in Germany, had already suggested it in 1910 for infectious pustular vulvovaginitis.

The actual site of BHV 1 latency is not yet known, but it is well known that the latent virus remains localized near the site of its first multiplication and will be reexcreted in the organ primary infected (Davies and Carmichael, 1973; Davies and Duncan, 1974; Narita et al., 1978c; Pastoret et al, 1980a; Rossi et al, 1982).

Local lesions observed during reexcretion periods are either due to a viral reactivation in the epithelial cells themselves, or to a reinfection of those cells occuring after viral reactivation in the sensitive nervous system innervating those tissues (Rock and Reed, 1982); it has also been suggested that independent viral recrudescences take place at both sites (Davies and Duncan, 1974; Rossi et al., 1982).

BHV 1 can be isolated from the trigeminal ganglion of clinically normal cattle (Homan and Easterday, 1980), viral DNA can be detected in the same organ (Ackermann et al., 1981, 1982) during the latent period, and trigeminal ganglionitis can be observed during recrudescence (Narita et al., 1981); but the finding that a thermosensitive vaccine strain unable to invade nervous system (Zygraich et al., 1974a, b and c) can be reactivated by dexamethasone treatment of cattle (Pastoret al., 1980b) seems to indicate that the virus remains latent in the epithelial cells as well (Thiry et al., 1981). It is also possible, but not yet determined, that lymphocytes can be latently infected (Pastoret et al., 1980b; Ludwig and Storz, 1973).

The virus may thus be later reactivated and sometimes reexcreted since certain endogenous or exogenous stimuli may unmask it from time to time.

Latency is a phenomenon particularly interesting to study in cattle infected with BHV 1 for several reasons. First of all, BHV 1 can be experimentally reactivated by the use of glucocorticoids (dexamethasone) and furthermore, the phenomenon can be studied in the correct host species in its own natural environment. Finally, BHV 1 latency has important epidemiological significance.

The virus remains latent and can be reactivated in at least two species of the family Bovidea: cattle (Bos taurus) and wildebeest (Connochaetes taurinus) (Karstad et al., 1974), and also in English ferrets (Mustela putorius furo L) (Smith, 1978) and rabbits (Oryctolagus cuniculus) (Rock and Reed, 1982).

PERSISTENCE, REACTIVATION AND REEXCRETION

Persistence, reactivation and reexcretion of BHV 1 under natural conditions are well recorded (Storch, 1910; Parsonson, 1964; Studdert et al., 1964; Saxegaard, 1966; Hyland et al., 1975; Bitsch, 1973). Snowdon (1964, 1965) reported long-term intermittent excretion of BHV 1. Persistence of BHV 1 in cattle was investigated by McKercher et al. (1963) and Straub und Böhm

(1964) at the same period.

Frequent recurrence of clinical BHV 1 is seen in closed herds (Hyland et al., 1975), and reactivation of BHV 1 can be provoked several times in the same animal by dexamethasone treatment (Pastoret et al., 1979a, 1980b; Narita et al., 1981; Kabelik et al., 1976).

Reexcreted strains do not seem to differ from the original ones from the biochemical point of view (Pastoret et al., 1978b, 1980b and c), but some biological differences have been described (Pastoret et al., 1979b; Pastoret, 1979; Homan and Easterday, 1981); they may be related to the fact that reactivated strains are sometimes rather difficult to isolate (Saxegaard, 1966, 1970). However, Castrucci and coworkers (1980) have shown that BHV 1 does not undergo significant modifications in its pathogenicity when reactivated from latently infected animals for the first time.

It is also well known for other herpesviruses that latency ensures the durability of the infection.

LATENCY AND EPIZOOTIOLOGY

a)   Introduction

As reactivated and reexcreted strains do not differ in their pathogenicity after reactivation, latency is one of the major problems associated with the infection of cattle with BHV 1 from the epizootiological point of view:

1)   first of all, one may consider that all the animals become latent carriers after a primary infection with a virulent strain;

a)   all the attenuated strains so far studied remain latent after vaccination (Pastoret et al., 1980b; Frerichs et al., 1982);

3)   we cannot really control the dissemination of attenuated strains;

4)   vaccination does not prevent the establishment of a virulent strain in a latent state;

5)   it is still not determined whether recombination between attenuated strains and field virus occurs or not in an

animal latently infected by both of these strains (Straub, 1975);

6) the immune status of the latently infected animal influences the pattern of reexcretion.

It is yet unknown whether or not the immune status of the animal following a primary infection influences the ability of another strain to establish latency in the same animal; especially if the dose of virus and its previous multiplication is important for the establishment of latency.

An animal latently infected with a virulent strain or with an attenuated one still pathogenic for the foetus is a permanent threat for other animals in its surroundings.

b) Latency, reactivation and reexcretion of field virulent virus

It is yet unknown if the dose of BHV 1 that infects cattle plays a role in the establishment of latency.

Most of the authors agreed that only around 60% of the infected animals were latent carriers, since only 60% of them shed infectious virus after dexamethasone treatment, but we have shown that one could not always recover infectious particles by dexamethasone treatment of latently infected animals.

Two and a half months after primary infection with virulent virus, cattle were intravenously injected with six consecutive daily doses of dexamethasone (0.1 mg/kg body weight). Nasal swabs were collected daily for two weeks. This procedure was repeated twice later, using double doses of dexamethasone on the last occasion (Pastoret et al., 1978a and d, 1979a). The infectivity of the swabs was tested daily and physical particles were counted in electron micrographs after negative staining, according to the pseudoreplication technique.

After the first treatment with dexamethasone, the animals excreted high levels of physical particles, whether or not physical particles were detected following the second or the third course of dexamethasone; infectious particles appeared after a lag period after the first treatment and infectious virus was detected at low levels in only one animal after the second and the third treatment.

This feature of reactivation can be explained keeping in mind that immunity influences the level of reexcretion after reactivation. The techniques used may be not sensitive enough to detect thre reexcretion even if reactivation occurs.

c) Latency, reactivation and reexcretion of vaccine strains (ts and non-ts) intranasally administered

Nine month old, healthy, male or female, Hereford cattle were randomly divided into two groups of eight animals.

One group was vaccinated intranasally with ts-IBR and the other group with non-ts IBR (Con-IBR). Six weeks later, animals were treated for five consecutive days with dexamethasone. Nasal swabs were taken daily for virus isolation and titration (Pastoret et al., 1980b). Three weeks after the end of the first dexamethasone treatment, the ts group was challenged with virulent virus (strain 108) and the non-ts group was treated with dexamethasone for a second time, as described above. Four weeks after challenge with virulent virus, the ts-IBR group was once again treated with dexamethasone and monitored for virus excretion.

Following the first dexamethasone treatment, 6 out of 8 non-ts and 7 out of 8 ts-IBR animals excreted infectious virus. However, once again, all the animals were probably latently infected and reexcreted virus, since all of them exhibited a rise in specific anti-IBR antibody levels. Furthermore, in the Con-IBR group, animals that did not excrete detectable virus after the first dexamethasone treatment did so after a second treatment with dexamethasone.

The ts-IBR vaccinated animals, on average, excreted more virus (5.25 log vs 3.75 log) and over a longer period of time, suggesting that ts-IBR vaccines produced latency as readily as did the non-ts ones. The virus isolated from the ts-IBR vaccinated animals was indeed temperature-sensitive, since the plaquing efficiency was very low at 39°C. Furthermore, in all cases, the restriction enzymes cleavage pattern of the reactivated ts virus was similar to that of the original ts vaccine strain and differed from the non-ts attenuated strain (Pastoret et al., 1980b; Thiry et al., 1982). Since the attenuated strains remain as latent as virulent ones and as reactivated strains in a singly infected animal remain stable, restriction analysis of the DNA of BHV 1 isolates will be an important tool for the study of the epizootiology of BHV 1 infection (Taylor et al., 1982). When the ts-vaccinated animals were infected with the virulent strain 108, they excreted this virus for up to 6 days after infection. When this group was later treated a second time with dexamethasone, no virus excretion could be detected. It was therefore not possible to determine whether recombination between attenuated and virulent field virus occurs or not.

Since attenuated strains are excreted after intranasal administration and can be reactivated and reexcreted later on, one cannot really control the dissemination of attenuated strains.

IMMUNE CONTROL OF REEXCRETION

First of all, reactivation must be differentiated from reexcretion, since reactivation may occur in some animals where no excretion of infectious particles can be detected.

After a primary infection with a non-ts attenuated strain, the animals have a normal amount of neutralizing antibodies, but a lower amount of antibodies participating in the ADCC reaction and a low blastogenesis index.

After a first reactivation by dexamethasone treatment, there is an increase in neutralizing antibodies and a steady increase in both ADCC and blastogenesis index, together with an important viral reexcretion. When a second treatment with dexamethasone is given, there are less infectious particles which are reexcreted, no increase in neutralizing antibodies or in ADCC antibodies, but still an increase in blastogenesis index.

If, between the two dexamethasone treatments, some animals

are boosted with a virulent strain of IBR virus, the second
dexamethasone treatment is unable to provoke reexcretion of
infectious particles, there is no change in the amount of
neutralizing or ADCC antibodies, but still an increase in
blastogenesis index.

The sequence of events may be interpreted as follows.
After a primary infection, the animal has an immune status that
enables it to prevent the clinical effects of a reinfection
with a virulent field virus, but is not sufficient to control
an episode of reexcretion.

The first viral excretion provoked by dexamethasone
treatment reinforces the immune status of the animal and the
efficiency of some immune mechanisms such as ADCC and
cell-mediated ones (Aguilar-Setién et al., 1979b, 1980; Davies
and Carmichael, 1973). These kinds of mechanisms can control
the reactivation better and prevent the production of viral
particles before their spread. If the immune mechanisms are
even better reinforced, for instance by the booster effect of
the infection by a virulent strain, the animal is able to
completely control the induced reactivation, and no reexcretion
occurs.

Sufficiently immunized animals are quite able to
completely control the reexcretion and therefore the
dissemination of the virus, even if reactivation occurs
(Pastoret et al., 1980b, 1982a and b). Thus Straub and Wagner
(1977) hyperimmunized bulls to avoid contamination of the semen
by BHV 1.

The reason why, for instance, the mean level of
reexcretion is higher in the ts-vaccinated animals and the
virus shed for a longer period may be that these animals have a
lower level of immunity following primary vaccination.

CONSEQUENCES OF LATENCY ON MEDICAL PROPHYLAXIS
First of all, vaccination of cattle, either with
inactivated vaccines or with attenuated strains, does not
prevent the further establishment of a virulent strain in a
latent state (Pastoret et al., 1982a, Nettleton and Sharp,

1980; Sheffy and Rodman, 1973; Zuffa and Feketeova, 1980).

Conversely, vaccination either with an inactivated vaccine or with an attenuated strain does not prevent the further excretion of a field virus latently carried by the animal before vaccination (Straub, 1979). Moreover, as already mentioned, it has been known for a long time that at least one attenuated strain given intramuscularly and still pathogenic for the foetus remains latent after vaccination, and the same is true for at least two attenuated strains given intranasally (Darcel le Q. and Dorward, 1975; Pastoret et al., 1980b).

As the animal latently infected with a field strain or an inadequately attenuated one is a permanent threat to its surroundings and since those strains can be disseminated by duly vaccinated animals, vaccination gives a false impression of safety (Nettleton and Sharp, 1980).

Finally, since the specific immunity impedes the reexcretion, there is a certain lapse of time between the induction of reactivation and the appearance of infectious particles in the nasal secretions; when several animals from different origins are gathered together, it is therefore, among other reasons, advisable to vaccinate the animals as soon as possible after their arrival, to give them a chane to built up as early as possible a protective immunity (Imray, 1980) and to produce interferon (Straub and Ahl, 1976; Cummins and Rosenquist, 1982). It is also advisable to vaccinate the heifers before pregnancy (Chow, 1972; Saunders et al., 1972).

CONCLUSIONS

Latency ensures the durability of BHV 1 infection.

An animal latently infected with a virulent strain or with an attenuated one still pathogenic for the foetus is a permanent threat to the other animals in its surroundings.

The introduction of a latent, silent carrier in a herd free of the infection is the best way, if not the only one, to introduce the disease. Uncontrolled therapeutic or zootechnic measures can enhance the risk (Duchatel et al., 1981).

The presence of bulls latently infected with BHV 1 (IPV)

is also a major concern for artificial insemination (Schultz et al., 1976; Straub, 1978).

However, if the animals are sufficiently immunized, they are quite able to completely control the reexcretion and therefore the dissemination of the virus, even if reactivation occurs (Pastoret et al., 1980b).

The practitioner must know that he cannot really control the dissemination of attenuated strains. Thus the emphasis of the studies on medical prophylaxis of the disease must not only be given to the measures and the mechanisms that help the vaccinated animal to overcome the disease resulting from a contact with a field virulent strain, but also on the measures and the mechanisms that enable the animal to overcome or to control reactivation and reexcretion.

For hygienic prophylaxis, it would be very useful to have good diagnostic procedures, not only to ascertain clinical diagnosis of BHV 1 infection in cattle, but also for the detection of the latent carriers of the virus, to prevent the introduction of such animals.

A good test should be simple, reliable, specific and not rely on too transient phenomena. The delayed hypersensitivity test is perhaps a good candidate, for several reasons (Aguilar-Setién et al., 1978, 1979a).

DNA recombinant technology will, in the near future, provide us with better tools for the study and the diagnosis of animal herpesvirus latency.

REFERENCES
Ackermann, M., Peterhans, E. and Wyler R. 1981. DNA of bovine herpesvirus type 1 (BHV-1) is present in the trigeminal ganglia of latently infected calves. Abstract. Fifth international congress of Virology. Strasbourg, France, August 27, 1981.
Ackermann, M., Peterhans E. and Wyler, R. 1982. DNA of bovine herpesvirus type 1 in the trigeminal ganglia of latently infected calves. Am. J. Vet. Res., 43, 36-40.
Aguilar-Setién A., Pastoret O.P., Burtonboy, G. and Schoenaers, F. 1978. Test d'hypersensibilité retardée au virus de la rhinotrachéite infectieuse bovine (Bovid herpesvirus 1), avec du virus purifié. Ann. Méd. Vét., 122, 193-199.
Aguilar-Setién, A., Pastoret, P.P., Jetteur, P., Burtonboy, G. and Schoenaers, F. 1979a. Excrétion du virus de la

rhinotrachéite infectieuse bovine (IBR, <u>Bovid herpesvirus</u>
<u>1</u>). après injection de dexaméthasone, chez un bovin
réagissant au test d'hypersensibilité retardée, mais
dépourvu d'anticorps neutralisant ce virus. Ann. Méd.
Vét., <u>123</u>, 93-101.

Aguilar-Setién, A., Pastoret, P.P., Michaux, C., Burtonboy, G.,
Jetteur, P. and Schoenaers, F. 1979b. Inhibition, en
présence de l'antigène homologue, de la migration de
leucocytes circulants provenant de bovins inoculés ex-
périmentalement avec le virus de la rhinotrachéite infectieuse bovine (<u>Bovid herpesvirus 1, BHV 1</u>). Ann. Méd.
Vét., <u>123</u>, 249-255.

Aguilar-Setién, A., Pastoret, P.P. and Schoenaers, F. 1980.
L'immunité envers le virus de la rhinotrachéite
infectieuse bovine (<u>Bovid herpesvirus 1</u>). Ann. Méd. Vét.,
<u>124</u>, 103-122.

Asso, J. 1976. Problèmes posés par l'existence de la rhinotrachéite bovine en France. Bull. Soc. Vét. Prat., <u>2</u>,
105-111.

Bagust, T.J. and Clark, L. 1972. Pathogenesis of meningoencephalitis produced in calves by infectious bovine rhinotracheitis herpesvirus. J. Comp. Path., <u>82</u>, 375-383.

Bitsch, V. 1973. Infectious bovine rhinotracheitis virus infection in bulls, with special reference to preputial
infection. Appl. Microbiol., <u>26</u>, 337-343.

Castrucci, G., Wada, E.M., Ranucci, S., Frigeri, F., Cilli, V.,
Pedini, B., Tesei, B. and Arush, M.A. 1980. Reactivation
of latent infection by infectious bovine rhinotracheitis
virus in calves. Microbiologica, <u>3</u>, 307-318.

Chow, T.L. 1972. Duration of immunity in heifers inoculated
with infectious bovine rhinotracheitis virus. J. Amer.
Vet. Med. Ass., <u>160</u>, 51-54.

Cummins, J.M. and Rosenquist, B.D. 1982. Partial protection
of calves against parainfluenza-3 virus infection by
nasalsecretion interferon induced by infectious bovine
rhinotracheitis virus. Am. J. Vet. Res., <u>43</u>, 1334-1338.

Darcel le Q., C. and Dorward, W.J. 1975. Recovery of
infectious bovine rhinotracheitis virus following
corticosteroid treatment of vaccinated animals. Can. Vet.
J., <u>16</u>, 87-88.

Davies, D.H. and Carmichael, L.E. 1973. Role of cell-mediated
immunity in the recovery of cattle from primary and recurrent infections with infectious bovine rhinotracheitis
virus. Infect. Immun., <u>8</u>, 510-518.

Davies, D.H. and Duncan, J.R. 1974. The pathogenesis of recurrent infections with infectious bovine rhinotracheitis
virus induced in calves by treatment with corticosteroids.
Cornell Vet., <u>64</u>, 340-366.

Duchatel, J.P., Evrard, P. and MaghuinRogister, G. 1981.
Analyse qualitative de préparations anabolisantes
clandestines. Ann. Méd. Vét., <u>125</u>, 405-408.

Frerichs, G.N., Woods, S.B., Lucas, M.H. and Sands, J.J. 1982.
Safety and efficacy of life and inactivated infectious
bovine rhinotracheitis vaccines. Vet. Rec., <u>111</u>, 116-122.

Gaskell, R.M. and Povey, R.C. 1979. The dose response of cats
to experimental infection to feline viral rhinotracheitis

virus. J. Comp. Path., 89, 179-191.

Hall, W.T.K., Simmons, G.C., French, E.L., Snowdon, W.A. and Asdell, M. 1966. The pathogenesis of encephalitis caused by the infectious bovine rhinotracheitis virus. Aust. Vet. J., 42, 229-237.

Homan, E.J. and Easterday, B.C. 1980. Isolation of bovine herpesvirus-1 from trigeminal ganglia of clinically normal cattle. Am. J. Vet. Res., 41, 1212-1213.

Homan, E.J. and Easterday, B.C. 1981. Further studies of naturally occuring latent bovine herpesvirus infection. Am. J. Vet. Res., 42, 1811-1813.

House, J.A. and Baker, J.A. 1968. Comments on combination vaccines for bovine respiratory diseases. J. Amer. Vet. Med. Ass., 152, 893-894.

Hyland, S.J., Easterday, B.C. and Pawlisch, R. 1975. Antibody levels and immunity to infectious bovine rhinotracheitis virus (IBR) infections in Wisconsin dairy cattle. International Symposium on Immunity to infections of the respiratory system in Man and Animals, London, 1974. Develop. biol. Standard., 28, 510-525.

Imray, W.S. 1980. Use of a modified live infectious bovine rhinotracheitis vaccine in the field. Vet. Rec., 107, 511-512.

Johnson, L.A.Y., Simmons, G.C. and McGavin, M.D. 1964. Studies on the transmissibility of a viral meningoencephalitis of calves. Aust. Vet. J., 40, 189-194.

Kabelik, V., Horyna, B. and Trunkat, J. 1976. The corticoid-activation of the infectious bovine rhinotracheitisinfect-ious pustular vulvovaginitis (IBRIPV). Vet. Med. (Praha), 21, 449-460.

Karstad, L., Jessett, D.M., Otema, J.C. and Drevemo, S. 1974. Vulvovaginitis in wildebeest caused by the virus of in-fectious bovine rhinotracheitis. J. Wildl. Dis., 10, 392-396.

Ludwig, H. and Storz, J. 1973. Activation of herpesvirus from normal bovine fetal spleen cells after prolonged culti-vation. Med. Microbiol. Immunol., 158, 209-217.

McKercher, D.G., Wada, E.M. and Straub, O.C. 1963. Distribution and persistence of infectious bovine rhinotracheitis virus in experimentally infected cattle. Am. J. Vet. Res., 24, 510-514.

Narita, M., Inui, S., Namba, K. and Shimizu, Y. 1976. Trigeminal ganglionitis and encephalitis in calves intranasally inoculated with infectious bovine rhinotracheitis virus. J. Comp. Path., 86, 93-100.

Narita, M., Inui, S., Namba, K. and Shimizu, Y. 1978a. Neural changes in calves intravaginally inoculated with infectious bovine rhinotracheitis virus. J. Comp. Path., 88, 381-386.

Narita, M., Inui, S., Namba, K. and Shimizu, Y. 1978b. Neural changes in calves after intraconjunctival inoculation with infectious bovine rhinotracheitis virus. J. Comp. Path., 88, 387-394.

Narita, M., Inui, S., Namba, K. and Shimizu, Y. 1978c. Neural changes in recurrent infection of infectious bovine rhino-tracheitis virus in calves treated with dexamethasone. Am.

J. Vet. Res., 39, 1399-1403.
Narita, M., Inui, S., Namba, K. and Shimizu, Y. 1981. Recrudescence of infectious bovine rhinotracheitis virus and
   associated neural changes in calves treated with dexamethasone. Am. J. Vet. Res., 42, 1192-1197.
Nettleton, P.F. and Sharp, J.M. 1980. Infectious bovine rhinotracheitis virus excretion after vaccination. Vet. Rec.,
   107, 379.
Parsonson, I.M. 1964. Infectious pustular vulvovaginitis in
   dairy cattle in Victoria. Aust. Vet. J., 40, 257-260.
Pastoret, P.P. 1979. Le virus de la rhinotrachéite infectieuse
   bovine (Bovid herpesvirus 1). Aspects biologiques et molé-
   culaires. Thèse, Université de Liège.
Pastoret, P.P., Aguilar-Setién, A., Burtonboy, G., Lamy, M.E.
   and Schoenaers, F. 1978b. Comparison of several strains
   of infectious bovine rhinotracheitis virus. Abstracts
   International Virology IV, The Hague, p. 526.
Pastoret, P.P., Aguila-Setién, A., Burtonboy, G., Mager, J.,
   Jetteur, P. and Schoenaers, F. 1979a. Effect of repeated
   treatment with dexamethasone on the reexcretion pattern of
   infectious bovine rhinotracheitis virus and humoral immune
   response. Vet. Microbiol., 4, 149-155.
Pastoret, P.P., Aguilar-Setién, A., Burtonboy, G. and
   Schoenaers, F. 1978a. Mesure de la réexcrétion du virus
   de la rhinotrachéite infectieuse bovine après injection de
   dexaméthasone. Ann. Méd. Vét., 122, 449-456.
Pastoret, P.P., Aguilar-Setién, A., Burtonboy, G. and Schwers,
   A. 1980a. Effet de la cyclophosphamide sur la latence du
   virus de la rhinotrachéite infectieuse bovine (Bovid
   herpesvirus 1). Ann. Méd. Vét., 124, 55-67.
Pastoret, P.P., Aguilar-Setién, A. and Schoenaers, F. 1978d.
   Le virus de la rhinotrachéite infectieuse bovine. Ann.
   Méd. Vét., 122, 371-391.
Pastoret, P.P., Babiuk, L.A., Misra, V. and Griebel, P. 1980b.
   Reactivation of temperaturesensitive and non temperature-
   sensitive infectious bovine rhinotracheitis vaccine virus
   with dexamethasone. Infect. Immun., 29, 483-488.
Pastoret, P.P., Burtonboy, G., Aguilar-Setién, A., Godart, M.,
   Lamy, M.E. and Schoenaers, F. 1980c. Comparison between
   strains of infectious bovine rhinotracheitis virus (Bovid
   herpesvirus 1), from respiratory and genital origins,
   using polyacrylamide gel electrophoresis of structural
   proteins. Vet. Microbiol., 5, 187-194.
Pastoret, P.P., Jetteur, P., Aguilar-Setién, A., Leroy, P.,
   Godart, M. and Schoenaers, F. 1979b. Etude par une
   méthode de comparaison de la moyenne des plages de souches
   du virus IBR (Bovid herpesvirus 1) isolées chez les bovins
   après injection de dexaméthasone. Ann. Méd. Vét., 123,
   203-207.
Pastoret, P.P., Thiry, E. and Vindevogel, H. 1982a. Problèmes
   liés à la latence lors de vaccination contre le virus de
   la rhinotrachéite infectieuse bovine (Bovid herpesvirus
   1). Herpesvirus of man and animal, Lyon, 1981. Develop.
   Biol. Stand., Karger ed., in press.
Pastoret, P.P., Thiry, E., Brochier, B. and Derboven, G. 1982b.
   Bovid herpesvirus 1 infection of cattle: pathogenesis,

226

latency, consequences of latency. Ann. Rech. Vêt., in
press.
Rock, D.L. and Reed, D.E. 1982. Persistent infection with
bovine herpesvirus type 1: rabbit model. Infect. Immun.,
35, 371-373.
Rosner, S.F. 1968. Infectious bovine rhinotracheitis. A
clinical review, immunity and control. J. Amer. Vet. Med.
Ass., 153, 1631-1638.
Rossi, C.R., Kiesel, G.K., Rumph, P.F. 1982. Association between route of inoculation with infectious bovine rhinotracheitis virus and site of recrudescence after dexamethasone treatment. Am. J. Vet. Res., 43, 1440-1442.
Saunders, J.R., Olson, S.M. and Radostits, O.M. 1972. Efficacy
of an intramuscular infectious bovine rhinotracheitis
vaccine against abortion due to the virus. Can. Vet. J.,
13, 273-278.
Saxegaard, F. 1966. Problems connected with the diagnosis of
subclinical infection with infectious pustular vulvovaginitis virus (IPV virus) in bulls. Nord. Vet. Med., 18,
452-459.
Saxegaard, F. 1970. Infectious Bovine Rhinotracheitis/Infect-
ious Pustular Vulvovaginitis (IBR/IPV) virus in cattle
with particular reference to genital infections. Vet.
Bull., 40, 605-611.
Schultz, R.D., Hall, C.E., Sheffy, B.E., Kahrs, R.F. and
Bean, B.H. 1976. Current status of IBR-IPV virus
infection in bulls. United States Animal Health
Association's 80th Annual Meeting, Miami Beach, Florida.
Sheffy, B.E. and Rodman, S. 1973. Activation of latent infect-
ious bovine rhinotracheitis infection. J. Amer. Vet. Med.
Ass., 163, 850-851.
Smith, P.C. 1978. Experimental infectious bovine rhinotrache-
itis virus infections of english ferrets (Mustela putorius
furo L.). Am. J. Vet. Res., 39, 1369-1372.
Snowdon, W.A. 1964. Infectious bovine rhinotracheitis and
infectious pustular vulvovaginitis in australian cattle.
Aust. Vet. J., 40, 277-288.
Snowdon, W.A. 1965. The IBR-IPV virus: reaction to infection
and intermittent recovery of virus from experimentally
infected cattle. Aust. Vet. J., 41, 135142.
Storch. 1910. Dtsch. tierärztl. Wschr., 18, 130.
Straub, O.C. Les possibilités de mise en oeuvre de vaccins
anti IBR/IPV. Bull. Off. int. Epiz., 84, 83-93.
Straub, O.C. 1978. Bovine Herpesvirusinfektionen. VEB. Gustav
Fischer Verlag, Jena, Band 17.
Straub, O.C. 1979. Persistence of infectious bovine rhino-
tracheitis-infectious pustular vulvovaginitis virus in the
respiratory and genital tract of cattle. Comp. Immun.
Microbiol. infect. Dis., 2, 285-294.
Straub, O.C. and Ahl, R. 1976. Lokale Interferonbildung beim
Rind nach intranasaler Infektion mit avirulentem IBRIPV-
Virus und deren Wirkung auf eine anschließende Infektion
mit Maul und Klauenseuche-Virus. Zbl. Vet. Med. B., 23,
470-482.
Straub, O.C. and Böhm, H.O. 1964. Untersuchungen über die
Lokalisation und Persistenz des Virus des infektiösen

Rhinotracheitis und des Bläschenausschlages in
experimentell infizierten Rindern. Berl. Münch. Tierärztl.
Wschr., 77, 458-462.
Straub, O.C. and Böhm, H.O. 1965. Experimentelle Infektionen
des Zentralnervensystem durch das Virus der bovinen Rhino-
tracheitis. Dtsch. tierärztl. Wschr., 72, 124-128.
Straub, O.C. and Wagner, K. 1977. Die Sanierung einer
Besamungsstation von IBRIPV-Virusausscheidern durch einen
Einsatz von IBR-IPV-LebendImpfstoff. Dtsch. tierärztl.
Wschr., 84, 259-261.
Studdert, M.J., Barker, C.A.V. and Savan, M. 1964. Infectious
pustular vulvovaginitis virus infection of bulls. Am. J.
Vet. Res., 25, 303-314.
Taylor, R.E.L., Seal, B.S. and Jeor, S. St. 1982. Isolation
of infectious bovine rhinotracheitis virus from the
soft-shelled Tick, Ornithodoros coriaceus. Science, 216,
300-301.
Thiry, E., Pastoret, P.P., Brochier, B., Kettman, R. and Burny,
A. 1982. Différenciation de souches du virus de la
rhinotrachéite infectieuse bovine (Bovine herpesvirus 1)
par l'analyse de l'ADN viral après digestion par Eco RI.
Ann. Méd. Vét., 126, in press.
Thiry, E., Pastoret, P.P., Dessy-Doizé, C., Hanzen, C.,
Calberg-Bacq, C.M., Dagenais, L., Vindevogel, H. and
Ectors, F. 1981. Réactivation d'un herpesvirus en culture
de cellules testiculaires prélevées chez un taureau
atteint d'orchite et d'azoospermie. Ann. Méd. Vét., 125,
207-214.
Wellemans, G., Strobbe, R. and Leunen, J. 1977. Les troubles
respiratoires des bovins en Belgique. Bull. Off. int.
Epiz., 88, 61-68.
Yates, W.D.G. 1982. A review of infectious bovine rhinotracheitis, shipping fever pneumonia and viralbacterial syner-
gism in respiratory disease of cattle. Can. J. Comp. Med.,
46, 225-263.
Zuffa, A. and Feketeova, N. 1980. Protection of cattle
vaccinated with inactivated Oiladjuvant IBR-Vaccine
against experimental infection. Zbl. Vet. Med. B, 27,
725-733.
Zygraich, N., Huygelen, C. and Vascoboinic, E. 1974a.
Vaccination of calves against infectious bovine
rhinotracheitis using a temperature sensitive mutant. 13th
International Congress of IABS, Budapest 1973, Part B:
selected veterinary vaccines. Develop. Biol. Stand., 26,
8-14.
Zygraich, N., Lobmann, M., Vascoboinic, E., Berge, E. and
Huygelen, C. 1974b. In vivo and in vitro properties of a
temperature sensitive mutant of infectious bovine rhinotracheitis virus. Res. Vet. Sci., 16, 328-335.
Zygraich, N., Vascoboinic, E. and Huygelen, C. 1974c. Replication of a temperature sensitive mutant of infectious bovine rhinotracheitis virus in the tissues of inoculated
calves. Zbl. Vet. Med., B, 21, 138-144.

BIOLOGY AND MOLECULAR BIOLOGY OF LATENT
BOVINE HERPES VIRUS TYPE 1 (BHV-1)

G. Pauli[1], J.-P. Gregersen[1], J. Storz[2], H. Ludwig[1]

[1]Institut für Virologie, Freie Universität Berlin, Nordufer 20 (im Robert Koch-Institut), 1000 Berlin 65, Federal Republic of Germany, and [2]Department of Microbiology, Colorado State University, Fort Collins, Colorado, USA.

ABSTRACT
The major antigen involved in neutralization of BHV-1 was a glycoprotein with an apparent molecular weight of 93,000 in SDS polyacrylamide gels. Although antigen analysis did not allow differentiation between BHV-1, a differentiation into "IBR-like" and "IPV-like" strains was possible using restriction enzyme analysis (HpaI). Eight BHV-1 isolates from normal foetuses belonged to the "IBR-like" viruses. From the data available it was concluded that only "IBR-like" strains have the information for induction of abortion.

INTRODUCTION

BHV-1 shares essential properties with other members of the herpesvirus group. Besides morphological and biochemical similarities, one of the most striking features of these viruses is the ability to induce latent infections even without causing clinically overt diseases. BHV-1 can be isolated from various clinical entities, e.g. infectious bovine rhinotracheitis (IBR), infectious pustular vulvovaginitis (IPV), conjunctivitis, encephalitis and abortion (reviewed by Straub, 1978; Ludwig, 1982). Although separation of isolates by serological methods is impossible, a clear difference in pathogenicity for animals seems to exist between various isolates. IBR viruses induce severe infections of the respiratory tract which may be associated with further complications, such as, encephalitis, conjunctivitis and abortion, whereas infections with IPV virus seem to be clinically milder and are mainly restricted to the genital tract. As already mentioned, infections of pregnant cows with IBR virus can cause abortion (McKercher and Wada, 1964). The foetus shows a systemic infection characterized by focal necrotic lesions of the liver, kidney lymph nodes and the digestive tract. Infections of heifers with IPV virus does not seem to induce abortion (Witte, 1933; Snowdon, 1965).

Based on this information it was of interest to investigate the biochemical and biological properties of BHV-1 viruses isolated from apparently normal foetuses (Ludwig and Storz, 1973; Storz et al., 1980). As little was known about the antigenic composition of BHV-1, this investigation analyses the major antigens of BHV-1, especially those antigens which are involved in neutralization of the viruses.

Besides the antigen studies, restriction enzyme analysis of the different isolates was performed. It was anticipated that this would provide more information about these isolates, since it is known that BHV-1 strains may be grouped into "IBR-like" and "IPV-like" strains using restriction enzyme patterns of the DNA (Engels et al., 1981; Pauli et al., 1981; Ludwig, 1982).

MATERIALS AND METHODS
Growth of virus

BHV-1 was grown in GBK cells using Eagle's medium Dulbecco's modification (EDM) supplemented with 2% heat inactivated foetal calf serum. For immunization of rabbits a permanent rabbit kidney cell line (RR), (Pauli, unpublished), was used for virus and antigen production. For stock virus, production cells were inoculated with a multiplicity of infection (MOI) of 10^{-3}. Cell free virus was harvested 24-36 hrs post infection (hpi).

Preparation of hyperimmune sera in rabbits

Individual sera were prepared against three BHV-1 strains with an "IPV-like" restriction enzyme pattern (B1, B4, Mo6; see Table 1) and against one BHV-1 strain with an "IBR-like" genome pattern. RR cells grown for at least five days in the presence of 2% rabbit serum were infected with an MOI of one. At 24-36 hpi, approximately 2×10^7 cells suspended in one ml PBS were mixed with an equal volume of Freund's adjuvant and injected intradermally. After the first immunization using complete Freund's adjuvant, all booster injections were done with

incomplete Freund's adjuvant. Ten days after each immunization
the animals were bled.

TABLE 1   BHV-1 strains and isolates

		restriction enzyme pattern (Hpa I)
LA	IBR reference strain Los Angeles	"IBR-like"
K22	IPV reference strain	"IPV-like"
B1	vaccination strain	"IPV-like"
B4	vaccination strain	"IPV-like"
Mo3	IBR-isolate (1)	"IBR-like"
Mo6	IPV-isolate (1)	"IPV-like"
S2	IPV-isolate	"IPV-like"
Gi-1 - Gi-5	isolated from foetuses (spleen, 2)	"IBR-like"
BFN-1H	isolated from foetus (testicles, 3)	"IBR-like"
BFN-IIN	isolated from foetus (kidney, 3)	"IBR-like"
BFN-2D	isolated from foetus (kidney, 3)	"IBR-like"

(1): Engels et al., 1981
(2): Ludwig and Storz, 1973
(3): Storz et al., 1980

Preparation of antisera directed against individual
precipitation bands obtained by crossed immunoelectrophoresis
was done essentially as described by Vestergaard (1975).
Besides rabbit sera, bovine sera from naturally infected or
hyperimmunized animals were employed.

Serum neutralization tests
Neutralization assays were performed using microtiter
plates and overlay medium containing carboxymethyl cellulose in
EDM. Plaques were counted 40 hpi and the antibody titers
calculated (80% plaque reduction, Pauli and Ludwig, 1977).

Analysis of BHV-1 antigens on PAGE
GBK cells were infected with a MOI of ten and labelled
from 5-20 hpi with $(6-^3H)$-glucosamine (25 µCi/ml) or a mixture

of amino acids (leucine, lysine, valine 10 µCi/ml each).
Solubilization of antigens and the immunoprecipitation followed
procedures which were described earlier (Pauli and Ludwig,
1977). Precipitates were analysed on gradient slab gels (5-12%
acrylamide) using the electrophoresis system described by
Lämmli (1971). Gels were stained with Coomassie brilliant blue.
[3]H-labelled proteins were visualized by fluorography utilizing
the fluorographic cocktail "En[3]Hance" (New England Nuclear)
followed by autoradiography.

Restriction enzyme analysis

GBK cells infected with a MOI of ten were harvested 20-24
hpi. The extraction of the viral DNA was essentially that
described by Pignatti et al. (1979). DNA was digested with
restriction enzymes and analysed as described by Herrmann et
al., (this issue).

RESULTS

In crossed immunoelectrophoresis bovine sera with high
neutralizing antibody titers (1:200) precipitated only a
limited number of antigens. Usually one to two distinct
precipitation bands were visible (Fig. 1). Rabbit hyperimmune
sera directed against BHV-1 infected cells, however, recognized
up to eight different antigens. Five of them seemed to
represent the major immunogenic components (Fig. 2). No
differences in the precipitation pattern were obvious when the
different BHV-1 strains were investigated. This demonstrates
that the major antigens of these viruses cannot be
differentiated by this technique.

To answer the question whether bovine sera and rabbit
hyperimmune sera precipitate the same or different antigens,
the crossed immunoelectrophoresis with intermediate gels was
applied. The reduction of precipitation bands shows that
antigens recognized by this rabbit serum were also detected by
bovine antibodies (Fig. 1).

To further analyse the biological function of the
antigens, antisera directed against individual precipitation

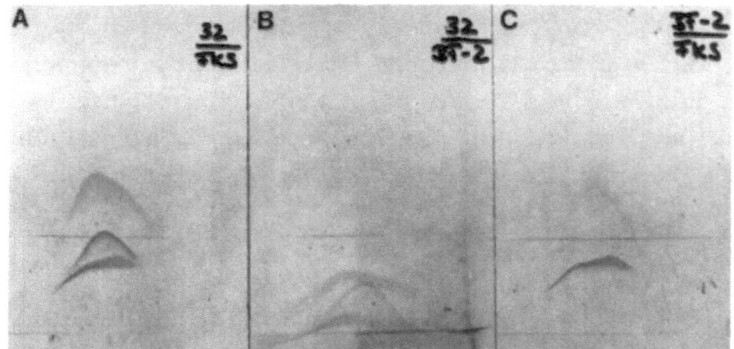

Fig. 1 BHV-1 antigens detected by rabbit hyperimmune serum and by bovine serum in crossed immunoelectrophoresis A,B: antigens precipitated with polyspecific rabbit hyperimmune serum. The intermediate gels contained either fetal calf serum (A, 15 µl/cm²) or bovine serum taken from a cow recovered from an IBR infection (B, 15 µl/cm²). C: the same antigen preparation electrophoresed into the bovine serum also used in B (15 µl/cm²). The intermediate gel contained fetal calf serum (15 µl/cm²).

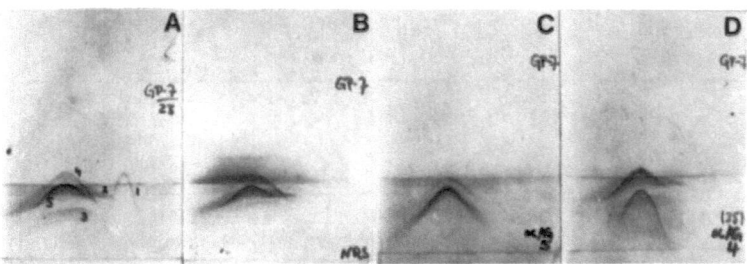

Fig. 2 Crossed immunoelectrophoresis of BHV-1 antigens. BHV-1 antigens prepared from infected cells were electrophoretically separated in the first dimension and run in the second dimension into antibody-containing agarose gels A: code numbers of BHV-1 antigens. The upper gel contained a rabbit hyperimmune serum directed against BHV-1 (15 µl/cm²). B-D: crossed immunoelectrophoresis of BHV-1 antigens into rabbit hyperimmune serum (upper gel, 15 µl/cm²) with intermediate gels containing either normal rabbit serum (B, 15 µl/cm²); rabbit anti-Ag5 serum (C, 15 µl/cm²) or rabbit anti-Ag4 serum (D, 20 µl/cm²).

bands were prepared and investigated: the specificity of the sera was tested in crossed immunoelectrophoresis (Fig. 2). In neutralization tests sera directed against Ag4 or Ag5 inactivated the virus (Table. 2). Anti-Ag4 sera showed only low neutralization titers, whereas anti-Ag5 serum was as potent as the sera directed against all virus antigens. The specificity of neutralizing activity was shown by adsorbing the sera with

uninfected cells. Only in anti-Ag4 sera was a significant loss
of neutralizing anitbodies found. The adsorption experiments
show that anti-Ag4 sera contain anitbodies recognizing antigens
on the surface of uninfected cells. The use of complement
increased the neutralization titers by a factor of 3-5.

TABLE 2   Serum neutralization tests

	rabbit anti BHV-1	rabbit anti Ag4	rabbit anti Ag5
C, inactive	340	3	150
C, active	1200	16	530
C, inactive preadsorbed	160	< 2	160
C, active preadsorbed	450	< 2	500

The table shows the mean values of three experiments (reciprocal serum dilutions at 80% plaque reduction). C, in-
active means guinea pig complement inactivated for 30 min at
$56^{\circ}C$. Preadsorption of the sera was done as described elsewhere (Pauli and Ludwig, 1977).

Identification of antigens in PAGE

PAGE analysis of precipitates received with rabbit hyperimmune sera resolved up to 25 different antigens, eight of them
glycosylated (Fig. 3). No significant differences could be observed when six strains were investigated. The monospecific
antisera directed against Ag4 and Ag5 were used in the same
technique. Both sera reacted with glycoproteins with apparent
molecular weights of 80,000 (gp80) and 83,000 (gp83). Anti-Ag5,
however, precipitated an additional glycoprotein with an
apparent molecular weight of 93,000 (gp93) (Fig. 4). The
observation that these antisera react monospecifically in

immunoelectrophoresis, while also recognizing several identical proteins in the immunoprecipitation assay is not yet fully understood.

In immunoprecipitation, bovine antisera gave the same pattern as the anti-Ag5 serum. Gp93 appeared to be the most prominent antigen precipitated (Fig. 4). This glycoprotein was previously described using a different electrophoresis system as a 128,000 glycoprotein (Pauli and Aguilar-Setién, 1980).

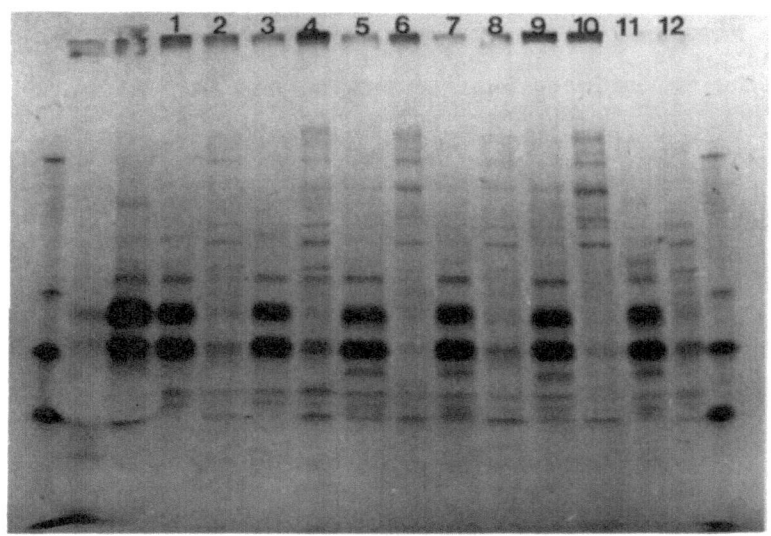

Fig. 3   PAGE analysis of immune precipitates.
³H-glucosamine (odd numbers) or ³H-amino acids (even numbers) labelled BHV-1 antigens prepared from infected cells were incubated with rabbit hyperimmune serum. Antigen-antibody-complexes were precipitated with Staph. aureus protein A and analysed on gradient slab gels (5-12 % acrylamide). The following strains were investigated: B1, lanes 1 and 2; B4, lanes 3 and 4; Mo3, lanes 5 and 6; Mo6, lanes 7 and 8; K22, lanes 9 and 10; LA, lanes 11 and 12. As molecular weight markers, phosphorylase a (94,000), bovine serum albumin (67,000), ovalbumin (45,000) and ß-lactoglobulin (18,000) were used.

Analysis of viral DNA by restriction enzymes

The antigen and protein analysis did not allow a differentiation of BHV-1 strains. The different isolates, however, could be grouped in "IBR-like" and "IPV-like" strains using restriction enzyme analysis (Engels et al., 1981; Pauli et al., 1981; Ludwig, 1982). This technique was therefore used

236

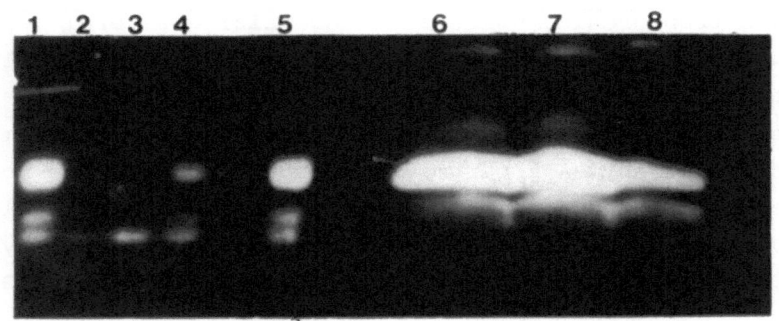

Fig. 4 PAGE analysis of ^{3}H-glucosamine-labelled BHV-1 antigens.
The following antisera were investigated: lane 1, 5, rabbit hyperimmune serum (polyspecific); lane 2, rabbit anti-Ag4 (1); lane 3, rabbit anti-Ag4 (2); lane 4, rabbit anti-Ag5. Antigen-antibody-complexes were precipitated with Staph. aureus protein A. Lane 6, bovine anti-BHV-1 hyperimmune serum (1), lane 7, bovine anti-BHV-1 hyperimmune serum (2); lane 8, serum from a cow taken three weeks after abortion.

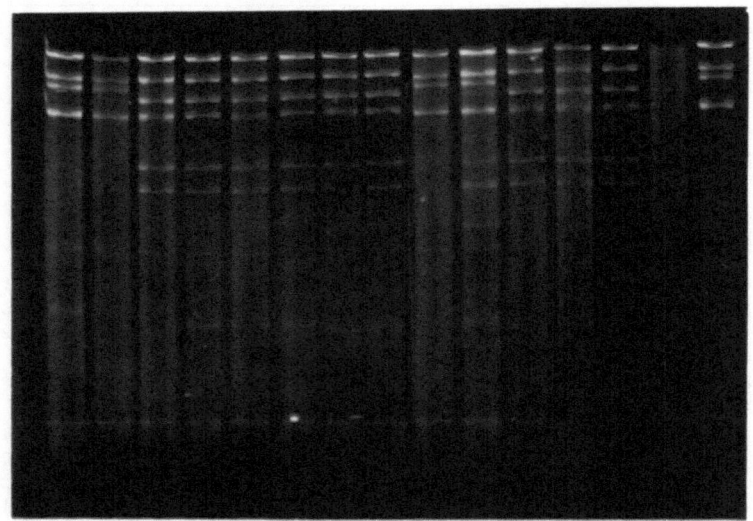

Fig. 5 Analysis of DNA fragments on agarose gels.
Purified viral DNA was digested with the restriction enzyme Hpa I and the DNA fragments analysed on 0.6% agarose gels. The following strains or isolates were investigated (see also table 1): B1 (lane 1), K22 (lane 2), Mo3 (lane 3), Gi-2 (lane 4), Gi-3 (lane 5), Gi-4 (lane 6), BFN-IIN (lane 7), BFN-1H (lane 8), S2 (lane 9), Mo6 (lane 10), BFN-2D (lane 11), Gi-1 (lane 12), Gi-5 (lane 13), LA (lane 14), B4 (lane 15).

to study the isolates obtained from apparently normal foetuses (Ludwig and Storz, 1973; Storz et al., 1980). All eight isolates investigated had a restriction enzyme pattern similar to the pattern of "IBR-like" viruses (Fig. 5), regardless of the fetal organ from which they were isolated (Table 1).

Field studies using fetal isolates

To study the virulence of such isolates, two strains which had been characterized by antigen and DNA analysis were selected. Isolate Gi-5 inoculated into the respiratory tract produced a mild disease accompanied by fever similar to the known IBR virus infection. When isolate BFN-1H was inoculated into two pregnant heifers (171 and 211 days of gestation), the 171 days old foetuses (the animal had twins) were aborted eleven days later. The 211 days old foetus was found alive 30 days later.

DISCUSSION

In agreement with others and our earlier reports from this laboratory, a differentiation of BHV-1 isolates by serological methods is not possible (Ludwig, 1982). In this investigation, detailed information is presented that various BHV-1 strains had a comparable antigen make-up. The most prominent antigen involved in neutralization seems to be a glycoprotein with an apparent molecular weight of 93,000 (gp93). When the DNA of viruses isolated from normal foetuses was analysed by the "fingerprinting technique", it could be shown that all eight isolates belonged to the "IBR-like" group of BHV-1. The isolation procedure and the organs from which the viruses were isolated, suggested that these viruses are present in a latent form in the foetus. Although nothing is known about the event of infection, our results show that foetuses can become latently infected in utero without any clinical signs.

The virulence of such isolates (especially their aborto-genic capacity) could be shown in vivo experiments, since one of those isolates, which had the "IBR-like" genome pattern, induced abortion in a pregnant heifer.

These field studies further underline our proposal (Pauli et al., 1981; Ludwig, 1982) that BHV-1 isolates can be divided into "IBR-like" viruses, which cause a variety of clinical symptoms and which, additionally, are responsible for abortion, and into "IPV-like" isolates, which do not induce abortion. This view of varying pathogenicity of BHV-1 strains is supported not only by earlier observations (Witte, 1933; Snowdon, 1965) but also by the outcome of vaccination programme.

There are reports that some vaccines, which originate from "IBR-like" virus strains, and which are used in the United States, have been found to be associated with abortion (Kahrs, 1977), whereas no abortions have been observed in animals which received BHV-1 vaccines of the "IPV-like" genome type (Ludwig, 1982).

The DNA analysis of BHV-1 strains represents a successful application of the genome "fingerprinting technique" to an old, pending problem, the IBR-IPV virus differentiation. Starting with the data that BHV-1 strains of different pathogenicity can be recognized by restriction enzyme analysis, further in vivo experiments using BHV-1 viruses with a defined genome structure are necessary to substantiate our hypothesis.

REFERENCES

Engels, M., Steck, F. and Wyler, R. 1981. Comparison of the genomes of infectious bovine rhinotracheitis and infectious pustular vulvovaginitis virus strains by restriction endonuclease analysis. Arch. Virol., 67, 169.

Kahrs, R.F. 1977. Infectious bovine rhinotracheitis: A review and update. J. Amer. vet. med. Ass., 171, 1055.

Lämmli, U.K. 1970. Cleavage of structural proteins during the assembly of the head of bacteriophage T_4. Nature (London), 227, 680.

Ludwig, H. 1982. Bovine herpesviruses. Comprehensive Virology, Plenum Press, New York (in press).

Ludwig, H. and Storz, J. 1973. Activation of herpesvirus from normal bovine fetal spleen cells after prolonged cultivation. Med. Microbiol. Immunol., 158, 209.

McKercher, D.G. and Wada, E.M. 1964. The virus of infectious bovine rhinotracheitis as a cause of abortion in cattle. J. Amer. vet. med. Ass., 144, 136.

Pauli, G. and Aguilar-Setién, A. 1980. The major immunogenic components of IBR virus. Intern. Conference on Human Herpesviruses. Workshop: Animal models for human herpesvirus infecti (Hsiung and Ludwig), Atlanta, Georgia, March 17-21.

Pauli, G. and Ludwig, H. 1977. Immunoprecipitation of herpes
    simplex virus type 1 antigens with different antisera and human
    cerebrospinal fluids. Arch. Virol., 53, 139.
Pauli, G. Darai, G., Storz, J. and Ludwig, H. 1981. IBR-IPV
    viruses: Genomes structure and disease. Med. Microbiol.
    Immunol., 169, 129.
Pignatti, P.F., Cassai, E., Meneguzzi, G., Chenciner, N. and
    Milanesi, G. 1979. Herpes simplex virus DNA isolation from
    infected cells with a novel procedure. Virology, 98, 260.
Snowdon, W.A. 1965. The IBR-IPV virus: Reaction to infection and
    intermittent recovery of virus from experimentally infected
    cattle. Aust. vet. J., 41, 135.
Storz, J., Ludwig, H. and Rott, R. 1980. Aktivierung des bovinen
    Herpesvirus 1 aus foetalem Gewebe. Proc. XI. Intern. Congr. on
    Diseases of Cattle, Tel-Aviv, pp 471-473, Bregman Press, Haifa
Vestergaard, B.F. 1975. Production of antiserum against a specific
    herpes simplex type 2 antigen. Scand. J. Imm., 4, Suppl.
    2, 203.
Witte, J., 1933. Untersuchungen über den Bläschenausschlag (Exan-
    thema pustulosum coitale) des Rindes. Z. Hyg. Infekt. Krankh,.
    44, 163.

THE ESTABLISHMENT OF IBR-IPV VIRUS LATENCY IN CATTLE
FOLLOWING THE APPLICATION OF AN INACTIVATED
IBR-IPV VACCINE

O.C. Straub

Federal Research Institute for Animal Virus Diseases,
P.O.Box 1149, D-7400 Tübingen, Federal Republic of Germany

ABSTRACT
    Ten head of cattle were vaccinated with an inactivated
IBR-IPV virus vaccine, either twice subcutaneously, once
subcutaneously and once intranasally, or twice intranasally.
After challenge with 10^5 $TCID_{50}$ IBR-IPV field virus, 8 became
latent carriers.

INTRODUCTION

    Live attenuated IBR-IPV virus vaccines have been used
widely for many years (f. review s. Straub, 1978); inactivated
vaccines have been more recently introduced. The results of
experiments with inactivated vaccines vary considerably
(Straub, 1977 & 1979; Nettleton and Sharp, 1980; Msolla et al.,
1979; Lazarowicz et al., 1980; Frerichs et al., 1982; Brun et
al., 1982). The first attenuated live virus vaccines were
administered parentally, as are the inactivated vaccines. The
newer generation of live attenuated vaccines however, from 1970
onwards (Straub, 1970; Todd et al., 1971; Zygraich et al.,
1974) could also be administered intranasally and
intragenitally resulting in a local as well as a humoral
immunity. Nevertheless, the demand for better inactivated
vaccines continued. Based on positive results obtained when
cattle were immunized intranasally with an inactivated
trivalent foot-and-mouth-disease vaccine (Straub and Bauer,
1971; unpublished data) experiments were carried out in which
an inactivated IBR-IPV vaccine was administered by different
routes.

MATERIALS AND METHODS

(1) Vaccination and Treatment Programme
    Three groups of female cattle (in total 10 animals), aged
1-2 years, free of IBR-IPV virus antibodies and housed in
isolation units in groups of 3 or 4, were used in the

experiment. They were vaccinated twice at an interval of 40 days as shown in Table 1. Two months later the animals were challenged by intranasal inoculation of 5×10^5 $TCID_{50}$ IBR-IPV field virus and 80 days later treated with prednisolon for 6 days (50 mg per dt).

TABLE 1   Vaccination Programme

Group	no. of animals	mode of application	challenge 2 months later
I	3	2 times subcutaneous	intranasally
II	3	once sub-cutaneous once intranasal	intranasally
III	4	2 times intranasal	intranasally
controls			
(1)	2	intranasal (field virus - $10^{7.5} TCID_{50}$)	intranasally
(2)	1	-	intranasally (first inoculation with field virus - $5 \times 10^{5.0} TCID_{50}$)

Antibodies in serum and nasal secretions were determined prior to the inoculation with field virus.

Swabs for virus isolation were taken daily after the virus challenge, and from the day of treatment with the immunosuppressive drug until in the last virus shedding animal virus could no longer be detected for at least two consecutive days. Body temperatures were taken twice daily during these periods and the animals checked for the presence of clinical symptoms.

(2) Virus Inactivation

A mixture of two field virus strains an IBR and an IPV strain low passage level were used for the vaccine. They were inactivated using ethylenimine as described previously in detail (Straub, 1977 and 1979). Before inactivation, the virus suspensions had a titer of 10^8 $TCID_{50}$.

(3) Virus Neutralization Test

This was carried out as usual (Straub and Wizigmann, 1968) but using 10 $TCID_{50}$ per ml without the addition of complement.

(4) Controls

Two animals were inoculated with $10^{7.5}$ $TCID_{50}$ field virus (strain C-BFA, 3rd passage). At the time of challenge a third animal received the same dosage as the vaccinated or inoculated control animals, namely 5 x $10^{5.0}$ $TCID_{50}$.

(5) Isolation of the Virus

The swabs taken were treated as described previously and the tissue cultures consisted throughout the experiment of bovine kidney cells (Straub, 1978).

RESULTS

The vaccinated animals did not show any clinical symptoms or lack of food intake; the two controls however, developed severe typical symptoms of IBR. The showed a distinct rise in temperature starting on day 2 p.i., with a maximum of $40.6^{\circ}C$ and $41.5^{\circ}C$ on days 3 and 10 respectively. Virus was shed from day 1 to 16 by both animals and the maximum virus titers in the nasal secretions reached 10^{10} $TCID_{50}$ on the third day.

All animals developed serum neutralizing antibodies and some also had provable antibodies in the nasal mucus. The results are presented in detail in Table 2.

TABLE 2 Results of the virus neutralizing tests of 10
vaccinated animals and 2 controls 40 days after the
second vaccination (prior to challenge)

Group	animal no	mode of application	serum[0] titer	antibodies in nasal mucus[0]
I	1	2 times subcutaneous	2.85	0
	2	"	2.55	0.15
	3	"	2.10	0.15
II	4	once sub-cutaneous	1.80	0
	5	once intra-nasal	1.95	0
	6	"	1.50	0
III	7	2 times intranasal	1.80	0.15
	8	"	1.65	0.15
	9	"	1.80	0
	10	"	1.65	0.30
controls	11	intranasal (field virus)	2.85	0.15
	12	"	2.85	0.15

0 in -log 10

Following challenge, only one animal from each of groups I
and II exhibited light symptoms of the disease. Two animals of
group III reacted with marked rises in temperature and an
increased nasal serous discharge but all of them shed virus for
various periods as indicated in Table 3. Three animals from
groups I and II did not shed any virus. Only one of the
controls shed virus. The challenge control developed typical
clinical symptoms of IBR and shed virus from day 1 to 12 p.i.
with a maximum of 10^{10}TCID$_{50}$ on day 5.

TABLE 3 Results of the virus recovery tests from swabs taken after the animals were challenged by the intranasal inoculation of 5×10^5 $TCID_{50}$ (field virus)

Group	animal no.	mode of application	clinical symptoms[3]	virus recovery positive from days__to__	maximum titer in nasal mucus[1]	on day p.i.
I	1	2 times subcutaneous	0	4 – 12	8.5	9
	2	"	–	– [2]		
	3	"	0	5 – 16	7.5	10
II	4	once subcutaneous once intranasal	0	3 – 12	9.25	7
	5	"	–	– [2]		
	6	"	–	– [2]		
III	7	2 times intranasal	T[4]	16 – 20	5.25	18
	8	"	–	11 – 20	5.00	14
	9	"	T	5 – 20	7.25	11
	10	"	T	9 – 20	7.50	14
controls	11	once i.n. (field virus)	–	– [2]		
	12	"	–	4 and 9	1.5	4 & 9

1) in log 10 $TCID_{50}$
2) Virus could not be recovered during the whole period
3) 0 distinct clinical symptoms
4) marked rise in temperature

Following the administration of an immunosuppressive drug all but two animals shed virus. The first animal started

shedding virus on day 4 and the last on day 12. The excretion
lasted for various periods of time and the virus titers in the
nasal secretions differed. The last day with a successful virus
recovery was day 21. The results are presented in detail in
Table 4.

TABLE 4   Results of the virus recovery test from nasal swabs
taken after the administration of prednisolon

Group	animal no.	mode of vaccine application	virus recovery positive from days __ to __	maximum titer in nasal mucus1)	on day
I	1	2 x sbc.	11 - 13	3.5	11
	2	"	- 2)		
	3	"	8 - 11	6.75	10
II	4	1 x sbc 1 x i.n.	on day 9	1.50	9
	5	" "	12 - 21	7.50	16
	6	" "	-		
III	7	2 x i.n.	8 - 12	4.75	10
	8	"	5 - 17	4.75	15
	9	"	6 - 10	8.00	9
	10	"	6 - 11	4.25	9
controls	11	once field virus i.n. plus challenge	5 - 8	5.25	7
	12	"	5 - 12	8.00	10
challenge control	13	one inoculation with $5 \times 10^5 TCID_{50}$ field virus	4 - 9	7.25	8

1) in $log10TCID_{50}$
2) Virus could not be recovered during the whole period

DISCUSSION

There can be hardly any doubt that the vaccination was unsuccessful in preventing a virus carrier state, even though two animals appeared to remain virus free. If the virus challenge dose had been higher it is possible that they would also have become latent carriers. The relatively low dosage was chosen because it had been known from earlier experiments that latently infected animals in general shed lower doses than newly infected ones. It must be stated, however, that 6 animals from the 13 shed more virus per ml of nasal mucus than was contained in the challenge dosis.

The results also demonstrate once again that there is no relationship between antibody titer and length of virus excretion or virus concentration in the nasal mucus.

Furthermore it appears that humoral antibodies alone - most probably of the IgG class - do not offer a better protection than local antibodies - presumably of the Ig A class.

It is interesting to note however, that animals vaccinated twice parenterally develop approximately the same antibody titers as animals inoculated locally with field virus (as reported previously, Straub, 1977).

Better results could perhaps be expected if inactivated vaccine is administered simultaneously both locally and systemically. It is of course of utmost importance to know the ultimate aim of a vaccination programme. If the sole purpose of a vaccine consists in disease prevention, inactivated vaccines obviously function. If disease occurs in a herd, attenuated live vaccines appear to be advantageous since they can almost stop the spread of field virus to animals that have not contacted the virus. It is also an advantage that live attenuated vaccines act as interferon inducers. In herds latently infected with IBR-IPV viruses, a combination of live and inactivated vaccine application has been proved to lead to a seronegative progeny (Straub et al., 1982). This is so provided inactivated vaccines are used repeatedly to maintain a high level of humoral antibodies, which are passed via the colostrum to the newborn. Using this procedure and strict separation methods, it will be possible to attain a virus free region.

If a programme of this nature is impossible to conduct, live attenuated vaccines can still be useful, especially in the light of results presented at this symposium, where studies with Herpes simplex have shown that only the first virus will become latent and that subsequent infections do not lead to another strain latency. If this proves true for IBR-IPV viruses it will be advantageous to use live attenuated vaccines rather than inactivated ones. Special attention should then also be paid to the possibly different behaviour of thymidine kinase positive and negative virus strains.

REFERENCES

Brun, A., Dubourget, Ph., Soulebot, J.P. 1982. Durée d'immunité conférée par un vaccin inactivé en adjuvant huileux de la rhinotrachéite infectieuse bovine. Proc. XIIth World Congress on Diseases of Cattle, RAI Amsterdam, Vol. 1, 156-161.

Frerichs, G.N., Woods, S.B., Lucas, M.H. and Sands, J.J. 1982. Safety and efficacy of live and inactivated infectious bovine rhinotracheitis vaccines. Vet. Rec., 111, 116-122.

Lazarowicz, M., Steck, F., Kihm, U. and Bommeli, W. 1980. Versuche mit Impfstoffen gegen die Infektiöse Bovine Rhinotracheitis (IBR) an Rindern. Proc. XIth Intern. Congr. Diseases of Cattle (E. Mayer, ed.), Tel Aviv, I, 298-304.

Msolla, P.M., Wiseman, A., Selman, I.E., Pirie, H.M. and Allan, E.M. 1979. Vaccination against infectious bovine rhino tracheitis. Vet. Rec., 104, 535-536.

Nettleton, P.F. and Sharp, J.M. 1980. Infectious bovine rhino-tracheitis virus excretion after vaccination. Vet.Rec., 107, 379.

Straub, O.C. 1970. Vaccination against coital exanthema. In G.E. Morse & E.J. Williams Report of the Intern. Meeting on Diseases of Cattle, Philadelphia, Pa. (Am. Assoc. of Bov. Pract.), 265-268.

Straub, O.C. 1977. Die abwechslungsweise Verwendung von inaktiviertem und attenuiertem Impfstoff zur Bekämpfung der infektiösen Balanoposthitis (IBP) bei Besamungsbullen. Berl. Münch. Tierärztl. Wschr., 90, 273-276.

Straub, O.C. 1978. Bovine Herpesvirusinfektionen. VEB Gustav Fischer Verlag, Jena.

Straub, O.C. 1979. Persistence of infectious bovine rhino-tracheitis - infectious pustular vulvovaginitis virus in the respiratory and genital tract of cattle. Comp. Immun. Microbiol. infect. Dis., 2, 285-294.

Straub, O.C. und Wizigmann, G. 1968. Die Laboratoriumsdiagnose der Infektiösen Bovinen Rhinotracheitis (IBR). Berl. Münch. Tierärztl. Wschr., 81, 108-109.

Straub, O.C., Schmidt, B. und Liebke, H. 1982. Ein Beispiel zur Sanierung IBR-IPV-Virus-verseuchter Bestände. Tierärztl. Umschau, 37, 319-324.

Todd, J.D., Volenec, F.J. and Paton, I.M. 1971. Intranasal vaccination against infectious bovine rhinotracheitis: Studies on early onset of protection and use of the vaccine in pregnant cows. J. Amer. Vet. Med. Ass., 159, 1370-1374.

Zygraich, N., Huygelen, C. and Vascoboinic, E. 1974. Vaccination of calves against infectious bovine rhinotracheitis using a temperature sensitive mutant. Develop. biol. Stand., 26, 8-14.

USE OF RESTRICTION ANALYSIS FOR THE STUDY OF
BOVID HERPESVIRUS 1 LATENCY

E. Thiry[o], P.-P. Pastoret[o], R. Kettmann[*], A. Burny[*].
[o]Department of Virology, Faculty of Veterinary Medicine,
University of Liège, rue des Vétérinaires, 45, B-1070
Bruxelles, Belgium.
[*]Department of Molecular Biology, Free University of Brussels,
rue des Chevaux, 67, B-1640 Rhode-St-Genèse, Belgium

ABSTRACT
    Cattle, free from Bovid herpesvirus 1 infection, were
intranasally infected with a plaque purified Belgian BHV 1
isolate. Latent viruses were reactivated by dexamethasone
treatment of the animals using standard procedures.
    The genomes of the strain used for primary infection and
reactivated viruses were compared after digestion with the
restriction endonuclease Eco RI.
    After discussion of these preliminary results, the use of
restriction analysis to determine if recombinant viruses appear
after reactivation in cattle previously infected with two
different BHV 1 strains will also be discussed.

INTRODUCTION

    One of the main problems encountered in the study of
latency is to know whether or not a latent virus remains stable
in a carrier animal.

    Several attempts were made in order to check the stability
of various Bovid herpesvirus 1 (BHV 1) strains: for example,
the measurement of the mean plaque size showed in certain cases
that plaques produced by reactivated strains were smaller than
those produced by the initial ones (Pastoret et al., 1979a). A
biochemical approach, using polyacrylamide gel electrophoresis
of structural proteins, revealed no difference between the
patterns of a wildtype strain and of a reactivated strain
isolated from a bovine latently infected with the previous
wildtype strain (Pastoret et al., 1980a).

    Studying the viral genome seems to be a more direct
approach: the use of restriction analysis provides this new
tool. In a previous report, Pastoret et al. (1980b) did not
show any difference between the restriction patterns of two

vaccine strains (ts strain and Connaught vaccine strain) and the reactivated strains isolated from cattle experimentally infected with these strains.

In this preliminary study, we compare the Eco RI restriction patterns of a Belgian field strain of BHV 1, isolated from a typical respiratory case and of the reactivated viruses isolated from cattle latently infected with this strain.

MATERIAL AND METHODS

Cell cultures

GBK (Georgia Bovine Kidney) cells, kindly provided by Prof. L.A. Babiuk, Saskatoon, Canada, were cultured in Roux flasks (175 cm^2, 10^8 cells) or roller bottles (850 cm^2, 5×10^8 cells) as previously described (Thiry et al., 1981).

Viruses

Strain IBR Cu5 was isolated in Belgium in 1976 from a typical respiratory case. It had been plaque purified three times. Strains IBR Cu5G1JO6 and IBR Cu5T1JO6 were isolated on day 6 after the first dexamethasone treatment from, respectively, a heifer and a bull calf infected with plaque purified IBR Cu5. Strain IBR Cu5G3JO6 was isolated from the same heifer, but on day 6 after the third dexamethasone treatment.

Restriction analysis was performed using these strains passaged three times on GBK cells.

Animals, infections, reactivation procedures

The two cattle used in this experiment were free of antibody to BHV 1. At 6 months of age, both animals received 1 ml of a viral suspension containing 8×10^5 plaque forming units (pfu) into each nostril. At 8.5 months of age, animals were intravenously inoculated with six consecutive daily doses of dexamethasone (0.1 mg per kg body weight). Nasal swabs were collected daily for 16 days. The procedure was repeated at 11 months and 14 months of age, using double the dosage of

dexamethasone on the last occasion. The strains described
before were isolated during this experimental procedure
(Pastoret et al., 1979b).

Virus multiplication, purification and restriction analysis

GBK cells were infected with virus and incubated at 37°C.
After 48 h., when the cythopatic effect was generalized, cell
culture supernatant was collected and BHV 1 purified from this
by the technique described by Talens and Zee (1976). Briefly,
after removing cell fragments and pelleting the virus, the
virus suspension was centrifuged at 150.000 g (SW 50.1) during
1 h. through a sucrose cushion (25%, w/w). The viral pellet was
resuspended and centrifuged through a potassium tartrate
preformed gradient (10%/40%, w/w). Viral bands were collected
and pelleted again. The pellet was resuspended in tris HCl
10^{-2}M, pH 8.3 (final volume: 3 ml). Purified virus suspension
was kept at 4°C.

The suspension was deproteinized by incubating overnight
with proteinase K (200 µg/ml) and SDS (0.2%). SDS was added to
a final concentration of 0.4% and NaCl to 0.25 M. Proteins were
removed by phenol-chloroform extraction. After adding NaCl to a
final concentration of 0.35 M, DNA was precipitated with
ethanol at -20°C and dissolved in TE (10^{-3}M EDTA, 10^{-2}M tris,
pH 7.5) to get a final concentration of 2 µg DNA/10 µl.

The DNA solution (10 µl) was then digested by the
restriction endonuclease Eco RI: the reaction mixture contained
viral DNA, 100 mM NaCl, 5 mM $MgCl_2$, 50 mM tris HCl (pH 7.5) and
2 U. of Eco RI (Boehringer). After incubating for 1 h. at 37°C,
the reaction was terminated by the addition of 50% Glycerol, 25
mM EDTA and 0.12% bromophenol blue.

DNA samples were loaded onto wells in a horizontal 0.8%
agarose slab and electrophoresed for 15 h. at 75 V. The
electrophoresis buffer contained 20 mM sodium acetate, 2 mM
EDTA, 40 mM tris, pH 7.8. After staining gel with ethidium
bromide (1 mg per 500 ml distilled water) for 1 h., the gel was
illuminated with an ultraviolet light and photographed with a
Polaroid MP4 camera.

RESULTS

The electrophoresis pattern of IBR Cu5 is slightly different from conventional BHV 1 respiratory strains (IBR Los Angeles, IBR Cu7): C+D band seems to be a composite of two fragments (Figure 1; Table 1).

The strains IBR Cu5T1JO6 and G1JO6 did not differ from IBR Cu5 (Figure 2). Moreover, IBR Cu5G3JO6 was similar to IBR Cu5G1J6 and IBR Cu5. Therefore with Eco RI, no difference was found between viruses isolated after successive reactivations in the same bovine.

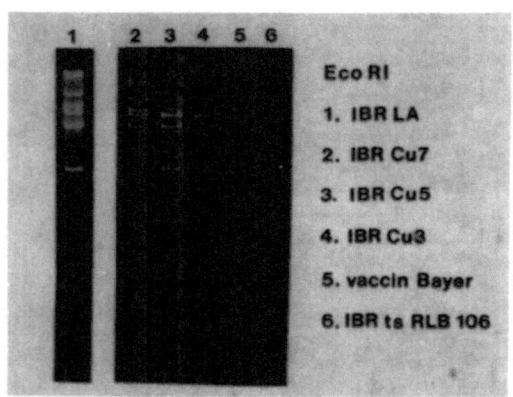

Fig. 1   Eco RI Restriction pattern of several bovide herpes virus 1 strains.

TABLE 1   Molecular weights of restriction endonuclease digests of BHV 1 strains (Eco RI) Mol wt $X10^6$

	IBR LA	IBR Cu7	IBR Cu5	IBR Cu3	IBR//IPV vaccine Bayer	IBR ts RLB 106
A	(35)	(35)	(35)	(35)	(35)	(35)
B	13.7	13.7	13.7	13.7	13.7	13.7
C	11.5	11.5			11.7	11.5
C+D			10.5	11		
D	11	10.9			10.2	10.8
E	9.2	9.3	9.5	9.3	9.3	9.2
F	5.6	5.7	5.5	5.7	5.6	5.6
G	1.6	1.6	1.6	1.6	2.5	1.6

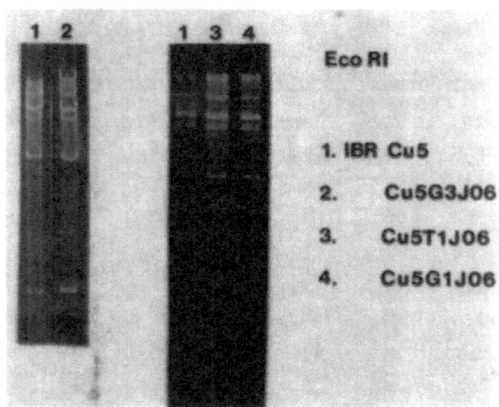

Fig. 2   Eco RI Restriction pattern of recativated
viruses and parent IBR Cu5 strains.

DISCUSSION

The results presented here are preliminary: only Eco RI
restriction patterns are studied. They must be confirmed by
using other restriction endonucleases such as Bam H1 and Hind
3.

No difference in the cleavage pattern was observed between
two reactivated viruses isolated from two distinct animals and
the strain used for primary infection of these animals, and
between two isolates obtained after two different successive
reactivation in the same animal.

Even if it finally appears that latent BHV 1 strains are
stable in the bovine carrier, another problem may arise if a
bovine animal latently infected with two different strains of
BHV 1 reexcretes a recombinant virus. In some cases,
recombinant genomes may be detected by restriction analysis:
this is well documented for intertypic recombinant between
herpes simplex virus 1 and 2 (Morse et al., 1979), where the
gain or loss of restriction sites and the production of novel
DNA fragments are generated (Amundsen, personal communication).
The detection of recombinant genomes of BHV 1 is difficult
because the genomic variation between strains, as shown by
restriction analysis, is already very slight (Engels et al.,
1981; Pastoret et al., 1980b; Pauli, 1981; Rziha et al., 1981).

If recombination could occur between two field strains, and even if the recombinant virus is infectious and leads to clinical disease, the significance of recombination would be less important than if recombination occurs between a field strain and a vaccine strain or between two vaccine strains.

REFERENCES

Engels, M., Steck, F. and Wyler, R. 1981. Comparison of the genomes of infectious bovine rhinotracheitis and infectious pustular vulvovaginitis virus strains by restriction endonuclease analysis. Arch. Virol., 67, 169.

Morse, L.S., Pereira, L., Roizman, B. and Schaffer, P.A. 1979. The use of intertypic recombinants for analysis of gene organization in herpes simplex virus. In "Oncogenesis and herpesviruses 3, part 1" (Ed. G. de The, W. Henle, F. Rapp). (IARC scientific publication). p. 41.

Pastoret, P.-P., Jetteur, P., Aguilar-Setién, A., Leroy, P., Godart, M. and Schoenaers, F. 1979a. Etude, par une méthode de comparaison de la moyenne des plages, de souches du virus IBR (Bovid herpesvirus 1) isolées chez les bovins après injection de dexaméthasone. Ann. Méd. Vét., 123, 203.

Pastoret, P.-P., Aguilar-Setién, A., Burtonboy, G., Mager, J., Jetteur, P. and Schoenaers, F., 1979b. Effect of repeated treatment with dexamethasone on the reexcretion pattern of infectious bovine rhinotracheitis virus and humoral immune response. Vet. Microbiol., 4, 149.

Pastoret, P.-P., Burtonboy, G., Aguilar-Setién, A., Godart, M., Lamy, M.E. and Schoenaers, F. 1980a. Comparison between strains of infectious bovine rhinotracheitis virus (Bovid herpesvirus 1) from respiratory and genital origins, using polyacrylamid gel electrophoresis of structural proteins. Vet. Microbiol., 5, 187.

Pastoret, P.-P., Babiuk, L.A., Misra, V. and Griebel, P. 1980b. Reactivation of temperature-sensitive and non-temperature-sensitive infectious bovine rhinotracheitis vaccine virus with dexamethasone. Infect. Immun., 29, 483.

Pauli, G. 1981. Attempts to correlate genom structure and pathogenesis of BHV 1 isolates. International Workshop on herpesviruses, Bologna, Italy, July 27-31.

Rziha, J., Döller, P. and Bachmann, P. 1981. Comparison of the DNA of Bovid herpesvirus type 1 isolates (IBR/IPV). Fifth International Congress of Virology, Strasbourg, France, August 2-7.

Talens, L.T. and Zee, Y.C. 1976. Purification and buoyant density of infectious bovine rhinotracheitis virus. PSEBM, 151, 132.

Thiry, E., Pastoret, P.-P., Dessy-Doizé, C., Hanzen, C., Calberg-Bacq, C.M., Dagenais, L., Vindevogel, H. and Ectors, F. 1981. Réactivation d'un herpèsvirus en culture de cellules testiculaires prélevées chez un taureau atteint d'orchite et d'azoospermie. Ann. Méd. Vét., 125, 207.

SESSION II

BOVIDE, EQUIDE AND FELIDE HERPESVIRUSES

Part 2

Chairlady: Rosalind M. Gaskell
Co-chairman: R. Burrows

RECOVERY OF BHV2 FROM THE NERVOUS SYSTEM OF EXPERIMENTALLY
INFECTED CALVES

F.M.M. Scott, J.S. Gilmour and W.B. Martin
Moredun Research Institute, 408 Gilmerton Road, Edinburgh

ABSTRACT
Five calves were infected intravenously with bovid
herpesvirus 2 (BHV2). Three of the calves were killed at the
acute stage of infection and BHV2 was recovered from skin
nodules, brain, ganglia and cutaneous nerve thus confirming the
results of other workers (Castrucci et al., 1977; Castrucci et
al., 1982). The remaining two calves were kept for 16 months
during which time skin nodules persisted but became
non-reactive. The calves were then given a course of
corticosteroid intravenously and one calf was killed on each of
days 3 and 5 after the last corticosteroid injection. BHV2 was
recovered only from skin lesions reactivated post
corticosteroid administration and not from the peripheral or
central nervous system. The evidence presented suggests that in
these two calves the skin was an important site of virus
latency.

INTRODUCTION

BHV2 is associated with a number of syndromes in cattle

(Gibbs and Rweyemamu, 1977). In the United Kingdom the virus is

known to cause severe herpetic lesions on the teats and udders

of cows and heifers shortly after calving (Martin et al.,

1966). Outbreaks occur only in the autumn, often with dramatic

suddenness and sometimes unassociated with the introduction of

animals to the herd. Such outbreaks often occur in herds with

no previous history of infection with BHV2. One explanation for

this could be that an earlier previously subclinical infection

had remained latent till reactivated following a reduction in

cell-mediated immunity associated with late pregnancy and

parturition (Martin et al., 1975). BHV2 has been shown to be

capable of latent infection and virus has been recovered from

reactivated skin lesions (Martin and Scott, 1979) and more

recently from nerve tissue (Castrucci, 1982). As this

phenomenon of latency could be important in the epidemiology of

the disease the experiment described was undertaken in an

attempt to show that a British isolate of BHV2 could be

recovered from the nervous system of the acute stage of
infection and following a period of latency.

MATERIALS AND METHODS
Virus and virus isolation
The strain of BHV2 used in this experiment was isolated in
Scotland from cows with mammillitis (Martin et al., 1964).

Swabs for virus isolation were taken directly into virus
transport medium and BEK cell cultures were inoculated with
minimal delay. When required, skin lesions were removed
sugically, under local anaesthesia, and were used to prepare
explant cultures, co-cultrues and suspensions for recovery of
virus. Tissue for co-cultures and suspensions were added to BEK
cell cultures. Samples taken at necropsy were prepared
similarly.

Isolates of virus were shown to be BHV2 by neutralisation
with specific antiserum.

Cell cultures
Secondary cultures of bovine embryonic kidney (BEK) cells
were used for the growth, titration and isolation of virus.

Eagles' medium containing 2% heat-inactivated horse serum
and antibiotics was used for BEK cell cultures and for explant
cultures Eagles' medium containing 10% foetal bovine serum and
antibiotics was used.

Neutralization tests
(a) Estimation of antibodies to BHV2 in sera from experimental
   calves.

Sera were inactivated by heating at $56^{O}C$ for 30 m and
serial twofold dilutions prepared. To each dilution was added
an equal volume of a suspension of BHV2 containing an estimated
100 $TCID_{50}$ per ml. Serum virus mixtures were incubated at room
temperature for 60 m. BEK cell cultures were inoculated and
examined for cytopathic changes after 6 days incubation at
$37^{O}C$. A virus titration was carried out concurrently to ensure
that the virus titre did not deviate markedly from expected.

(b)   Typing of virus isolates by neutralization with specific
      antiserum.

Serial ten-fold dilutions of virus isolates were prepared
in PBS containing 2% heat-inactivated horse serum. An equal
volume of a 1/10 dilution of antiserum to BHV2 with a known
titre of 1/22 against 100 $TCID_{50}$ was added to each dilution of
virus. Virus-antiserum mixtures were reacted at room
temperature for 60 m and then inoculated into BEK cell
cultures. Tests were read after 6 days incubation at $37^{\circ}C$. A
control titration of each isolate was reacted with a 1/10
dilution of heat-inactivated horse serum. In calculating the
titre of antibody, the actual dilution of serum before the
addition of virus was used.

Animals

Male Jersey calves, between 5 and 20 weeks of age, were
used. The serum from each calf was shown to be free from
antibodies to BHV2 and BHV1 prior to inoculation.

Methods of infection

Five calves were infected by intravenous (iv) injection of
1 ml of BHV2 containing between $10^{6.2}$ and $10^{6.7}$ $TCID_{50}$ of
virus. One calf was killed on each of days 7, 9 and 12
post-inoculation (pi). The two remaining calves were given a
further three iv injections of BHV2 at monthly intervals
followed 12 months later by a course of corticosteroid.

Corticosteroid treatment

The two calves which were given corticosteroid received it
16 months after primary infection. The course consisted of the
intravenous injection of 2 mg/kg dexamethasome ("Dexadreson",
Intervet Lab., Ltd.) daily for 5 days.

Histology

Biopsy samples of skin nodules and samples of tissues
taken at necropsy were fixed in Baker's calcium-formol,
dehydrated in alcohols and embedded in paraffin wax. Sections,

6 µm thick, were cut and stained with haematoxylin and eosin
and with toluidine blue for examination by light microscopy.

RESULTS

A slight febrile reaction was detected in all calves
following the injection of BHV2. Temperatures ranged from
40.1°C to 41.3°C between days 4 and 9 pi. One calf, killed on
day 7 pi, had only one detectable skin nodule at, or very close
to, the site of iv injection of virus. Each calf killed on day
9 and 12 pi had ulcerative lesions on the chin, dental pad and
lip. Several palpable plaques of thickened skin, with a
generalised distribution were detected on both of these calves.
One also had ulcers around the prepuce (Fig. 1) and on the
scrotum as described previously (Martin and Scott, 1979). The
remaining two calves reacted similarly after infection and the
areas of thickened skin were easily detectable by palpation
when the calves were examined at the time of each monthly
injection of BHV2. The skin lesions persisted over the next 12
months (Fig. 2) and appeared neither to progress or regress
although they did become painless and less sensitive to touch.
Two days after completion of the corticosteroid course however
both calves were slightly dull and several raised plaques of
skin on one calf were painful on palpation. By day 3 the
temperature of this calf was 39.7°C and the lesions were still
sensitive and painful. At this time the calf was killed. The
raised plaques in the skin of the remaining calf became neither
excessively sensitive nor painful during or after
corticosteroid administration. This calf was killed five days
after the last corticosteroid injection.

During the acute phase of infection BHV2 was isolated from
swabs of both the mouth and lip lesions from the 4 calves
sampled. Swabs were not taken from the calf killed on day 7 pi
as no lesions had developed in the mouth or on the lips.
However BHV2 was recovered from 5/14 tissues taken from this
calf at necropsy. These included nerve tissue and one
detectable skin nodule (Table 1). At day 9 pi BHV2 was
recovered from 2/15 samples including the cutaneous nerve

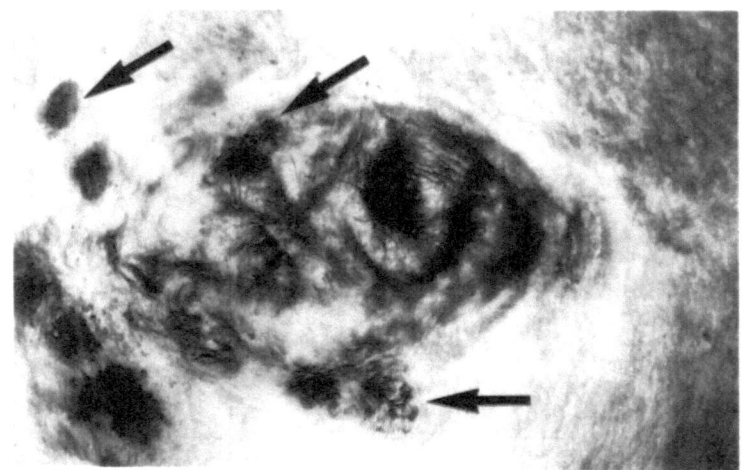

Fig. 1   Lesions (arrowed) around prepuce of calf, day
          12 pi.

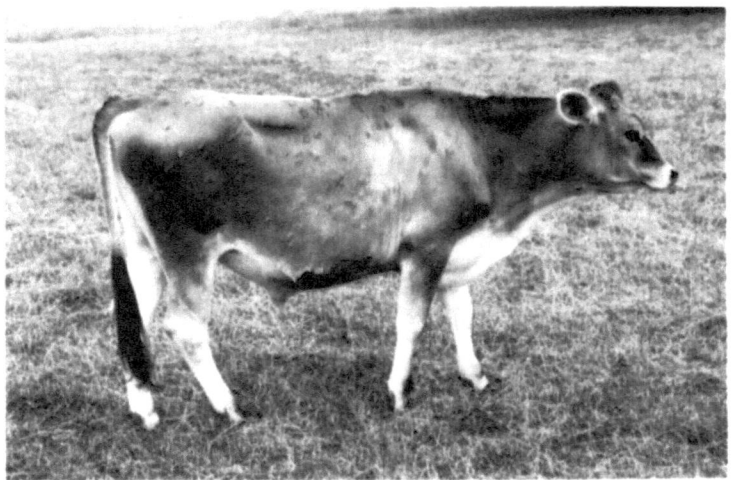

Fig. 2   Calf showing peristent skin lesions 1 year after
          infection.

supplying the lateral thoracic skin where one of the thickened
plaques was sited (Table 1). By day 12 pi BHV 2 was recovered
only from skin nodules and not from any nerve tissue.

    No virus was isolated from any of three biopsy samples
taken from either calf before corticosteroid administration.
Following corticosteroid treatment however, BHV2 was recovered

TABLE 1   Recovery of BHV2 from experimentally infected calves

Tissue	Days post inoculation		
	7	9	12
Anterior cervical ganglia	$+^b$		-
Cerebellum	$+^a$		-
Fore brain	$+^{a,b,c}$		-
Temporal cortex, thalamus	+		ND
Skin	$+^{a,b}$	$+^a$	$+^{a,c}$
Cutaneous nerve of lateral thorax	ND	$+^c$	-

+ - BHV2 isolated   a - suspensions
- - no virus isolated   b   co-cultrues
ND - not done   c - explants
Other tissues examined were:- Mesenteric lymph node,
retropharyngeal L.N. pre-cranial L.N. mesenteric ganglia,
posterior cervical ganglia, trigeminal ganglia, spinal
cord, hind brain, CSF, spleen, testis.

from 2/2 skin lesions of the calf killed on day 3 and from 1/2
skin lesions of the calf killed on day 5. BHV2 was not
recovered from the other tissues examined which were:-
Trigeminal ganglia, hind brain, mid brain, fore brain, spinal
cord, cerebellum, anterior cervical ganglia, sympathetic nerve,
maxillary nerve, cutaneous nerves to lesion (3), posterior
cervical ganglia and sub mandibular nerve.

No antibodies to BHV2 were detected in pre-inoculation
serum from any calf and no serological conversion was
demonstrated in the serum from the calves killed on days 7 and
9 pi. Antibodies to BHV2 were detected only in undiluted serum
from the calf killed on day 12 pi. In the remaining two calves
antibody titres were 1/13 and 1/22 by day 18 pi and continued
to rise until 12 weeks after the last injection of virus. Both
animals then had a neutralizing titre of 1/27 and this was
maintained for a further 8 weeks. The titres then dropped to
1/5 and 1/19 pre-corticosteroid administration and when finally

bled 3 days post- corticosteroid were not significantly
different at 1/4 and 1/18 respectively (Fig. 3).

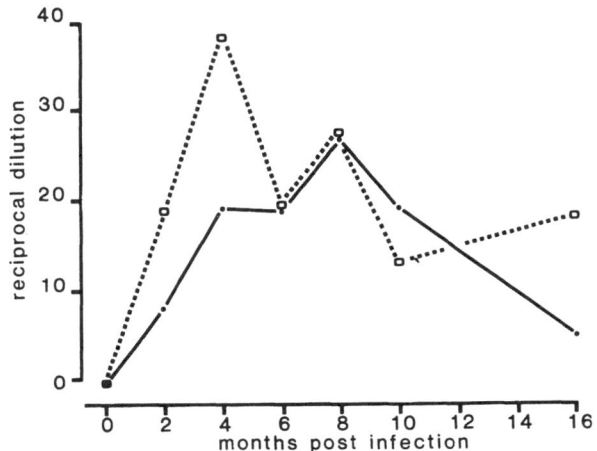

Fig. 3   Serum antibody levels to BHV2 in experimental
calves

•_____•_____• Calf killed on day 3 post corticosteroid
administration

=······=······= Calf killed on day 5 post corticosteroid
administration.

Histology (a) Skin biopsy samples. Samples taken from residual
lesions on both calves prior to corticosteroid administration
showed similar features. The loose connective tissue of the
subcutis was replaced by a thick (0.5 cm) layer of collagen
fibres arranged in bundles in criss-cross fashion and extending
into the deep layers of the corium. Mild perivascular
accumulations of mononuclear cells were also present in the
corium. These accumulations consisted of lymphocytes, mast
cells and most prominently, eosinophils. The epidermis appeared
normal.

(b) Necropsy samples.   No lesions were detected in the
tissues of the central or peripheral nervous systems. Skin
lesions ranged from thickening of the stratum germinativum with
ballooning of cells, to ulceration with necrosis of the
epidermis and infiltration of the corium and subcutis with a
mixed population of inflammatory cells among which eosinophils
were either absent or rare.

DISCUSSION

This experiment has shown that the Scottish strain of BHV2 can be isolated from the nervous system of cattle in agreement with the findings of Castrucci et al. (1982). Additionally the latent characteristic of this strain of BHV2 demonstrated by Martin and Scott (1979) is confirmed.

Thickened lesions of collagen deposited in the sub-cutis persisted in two calves for 10 months after the final experimental injection of BHV2. Histological examination of biopsy samples of these lesions revealed a cellular infiltration suggestive of a current antigenic stimulus but attempts to isolate virus from these samples were unsuccessful. Furthermore the antibody status to BHV2 of these calves did not show any rise in titre which might have indicated spontaneous reactivation of BHV2. It therefore remains unclear why these lesions not only peristed but showed little or no regression. Previous observations have indicated that skin lesions do regress and are only faintly discernible several months post infection (Cilli and Castrucci, 1976; Martin and Scott, 1978).

The calf which was given corticosteroid and which had a serum neutralizing titre to BHV2 of 1/4, showed clinical manifestations of recrudescence in skin lesions. BHV2 was recovered from both lesions excised from the skin at necropsy. The other calf which had a serum neutralizing titre of 1/18 showed barely detectable signs of recrudescence and BHV2 was recovered from only 1/2 lesions sampled. In the latter calf the antibody titre of 1/18 was apparently insufficiently high to eliminate completely the virus but may have been sufficiently high to limit recrudescence.

Castrucci et al., (1982) re-isolated BHV2 on day 6 post-corticosteroid administration from the nervous system of only 1/7 calves experimentally infected with BHV2. The other calves were killed later and BHV2 recovered only from nasal swabs. Although 2 of the calves in the experiment described here were killed on days 3 and 5 post-corticosteroid, virus could not be isolated from any of the nerve tissue sampled and it is suggested that BHV2 is present in the nervous system only for a limited time following reactivation of the virus.

Our results favour the hypothesis that the skin is an important site for BHV2 latency. Although we failed to confirm latency in the nervous system we concur with the view held by Castrucci et al., (1982) that the nervous system also may be an important site of BHV2 latency.

Acknowledgement

The authors acknowledge the assistance given by the stockmen, Mr. B. Mitchell and Mr. J. Williams for performing the biopsies and Mr. E. Brown for expert technical assistance.

REFERENCES

Castrucci, G., Rampichini, L., Frigeri, F., Ranucci, S. and Cilli, V. 1977. Preliminary studies on the diffusion of bovid herpesvirus 2 in experimentally infected calves. Folia Veterinaria Latina, 7, 243-251.

Castrucci, G., Ferrari, M., Frigeri, F., Ranucci, S., Cilli, V., Tesei, B. and Rampichini, L. 1982. Reactivation in calves of bovid herpesvirus 2 latent infection. Arch. Virol., 72, 75-81.

Cilli, V. and Castrucci, G. 1976. Infection of cattle with bovid herpes virus 2. Folia Veterinary Latina, 6, 1-44.

Gibbs, E.P.J. and Rweyemamu, M.M. 1977. Bovine herpesviruses. Part II. Bovine herpesviruses 2 and 3. Vet. Bull., 47, 411-424.

Martin, W.B., Martin, B. and Lauder, I.M. 1964. Ulceration of cows teats caused by a virus. Vet. Rec., 76, 15-16.

Martin, W.B., Martin, B., Hay, D. and Lauder, I.M. 1966. Bovine ulcerative mammillitis caused by a herpesvirus. Vet. Rec., 78, 494-497.

Martin, W.B., Wells, P.W., Lauder, I.M. and Martin, B. 1975. Features of the epidemiology of bovine mammillitis in Britain. 20th World Vet. Congress (Thessaloniki), 2, 1307-1311.

Martin, W.B. and Scott, F.M.M. 1979. Latent infection of cattle with bovid herpesvirus 2. Arch. Virol., 60, 5158.

CAPRINE HERPESVIRUS I INFECTION OF YOUNG LAMBS

F.M.M. Scott, J.M. Sharp, K.W. Angus

Moredun Research Institute, 408 Gilmerton Road,
Edinburgh, EH17 7JH

ABSTRACT

   Specific pathogen free lambs were inoculated by several
routes with the Scottish isolate of Caprine herpesvirus I. All
but one of the lambs developed interstitial changes in the
lungs and virus was recovered from the respiratory tract of
8/17 lambs. Five weeks after primary infection 3 lambs were
injected intravenously with corticosteroid and subsequently
virus was recovered from all 3 lambs.

INTRODUCTION

   Jaagsiekte or sheep pulmonary adenomatosis (SPA) is a
disease of sheep which results in the development of an
adenocarcinoma in the lungs. The aetiology of the disease is
not fully understood but studies on affected lungs have
implicated by association a herpesvirus and a retrovirus as
possible causative organisms. The experiments described here
are concerned only with the herpesvirus.

   The sheep herpesvirus was first isolated in 1969 (Mackay,
J.M.K.) from adenomatous lung tissue and has never been
isolated from any other material. The experimental inoculation
of sheep with this virus has consistently failed to establish a
causative role for the herpesvirus in the production of
pulmonary adenomatosis (Martin et al., 1980). In these
experiments attention had been concentrated mainly on the long
term effects of the virus in the sheep with the result that
little is known about the acute stage of primary infection.
Consequently the experiments described here were designed first
to examine the effects on the lamb at the acute stage of
infection and to determine from which tissues virus could be
recovered and secondly to examine the possibility of latency
resulting from primary experimental infection.

MATERIALS AND METHODS

Animals

   Specific pathogen free (SPF) lambs were inoculated at one

day of age and kept in isolation for the duration of the experiment.

Virus

The herpesvirus used, tentatively classified as Caprine Herpesvirus 1 (Roizman et al., 1981) was isolated in Scotland from a sheep affected with pulmonary adenomatosis (Mackay, 1969). The strain of this virus is known as sheep pulmonary adenomatosis herpesvirus (SPAHV). The 14th passage of SPAHV in sheep alveolar macrophage (SAM) cells was stored at -70°C until required. Virus titrations were made at the time of inoculation.

Experimental design

Acute experiment   Ten SPF lambs were each inoculated with SPAHV by several routes viz: 2 ml intravenously (IV), 5 ml intratracheally (IT), 2 ml intranasally (IN), 0.5 ml intradermally (ID), 0.5 ml intravaginally or intrapreputially and 0.2 ml instilled into one eye. The total dose for each lamb was $10^{8.9}$ $TCID_{50}$. Two lambs were killed on each of days 1, 2, 4, 6 and 11 post inoculation (pi).

Cell Cultures and Virus Isolation Procedures

SAM cell cultures grown on coverslips in Eagles medium containing 10% heat inactivated adult bovine serum were used for all *in vitro* virus studies.

Samples of leucocytes obtained from peripheral blood for virus isolation were taken before inoculation and daily for the duration of the experiment. Each sample was passaged twice in SAM cell cultures. Tissues taken at necropsy were co-cultured with SAM cells and explanted in plasma clots. Co-cultures were monitored regularly for evidence of virus and medium from explants was transferred to SAM cell cultures to check for virus infectivity. At necropsy samples of tissues were taken from each lamb from adrenal, bronchial, mediastinal and mesenteric lymph nodes, conjunctiva, kidney, liver, lung, nasal mucosa, ovary or testicle, skin, spleen, sub-mandibular salivary gland, thymus, thyroid, tonsil, tracheal mucosa, vagina or prepuce, fore-brain, cerebrum, cerebellum and superior cervical ganglion. Isolates of virus were shown to be SPAHV by neutralization with specific antiserum.

Histology   Portions of each tissue were fixed in Bakers calcium-formol and in Carnoys fixative, processed to paraffin wax, sectioned at 5 m and stained with Mayers haematoxylin and eosin.

Latency experiment   Eight lambs were inoculated by the following routes: 2 ml IV, 6 ml IM and 2 ml IN. Each lamb received a total of $10^{8.2}$ TCID$_{50}$ of SPAHV. Two lambs were killed on each of days 3 and 6 pi. One lamb died on day 25 pi of an unrelated abomasitis. The remaining lambs were given a 5 day course of corticosteroid starting on day 34 pi. One lamb was killed on each of days 1, 3 and 6 following the final corticosteroid injection.

Virus isolation   Blood for virus isolation was taken before inoculation and daily up to day 6 pi. Additionally blood for virus isolation was taken from the three surviving lambs from day 34 pi until the end of the experiment (day 44 pi). Nasal swabs were taken daily and also on the four days preceding corticosteroid administration.

        Tissues taken at necropsy and cultured for virus isolation comprised adrenal, brain (pool of fore-brain, cerebrum, cerebellum), liver, lung, spleen, sub-mandibular salivary gland, tracheal mucosa, trigeminal ganglion.

Histology   Samples of each tissue were taken for histological examination as before and portions of lung and adrenal gland only were fixed in 3% gluteraldehyde (pH 7.4) and processed for electron microscopy.

RESULTS
Acute experiment
        No lamb showed any clinical symptoms or had a febrile reaction following injection of SPAHV. Virus isolation
        The tissues from which virus was isolated are summarised in Table 1. SPAHV was recovered from leucocytes of 5/10 lambs but never after day 3 pi. Other isolates of SPAHV were made

from the respiratory tract on 4 occasions, spleen on 3 occasions, adrenal twice and once from each of the salivary gland, skin and bronchial lymph nodes. Virus was isolated from at least one tissue from 7/10 lambs 4 of which were killed on days 1 and 2 pi.

TABLE 1   Acute experiment. PAHV isolations from 10 lambs

Tissue	Day killed p.i.									
	1	1	2	2	4	4	6	6	11	11
Adrenal	-	-	-	+	-	-	-	-	+	-
Bronchial LN	-	-	-	+	-	-	-	-	-	-
Lung	-	+	-	-	-	+	-	-	-	-
Salivary Gland	-	+	-	-	-	-	-	-	-	-
Skin	-	-	-	+	-	-	-	-	-	-
Spleen	-	+	+	-	-	-	-	+	-	-
Tracheal mucosa	+	+	-	-	-	-	-	-	-	-
Leucocytes (day pi)	+(1)	+(1)	+(2)	-	-	-	+(1,3)	-	+(1,3)	-

+   -   SPAHV isolated
-    -   No virus isolated

Pathology

For the purpose of this paper only a limited pathological description of the lungs will be given. A full pathological description of lungs and other tissues will be given elsewhere (Scott et al., in preparation).

The only macroscopic pathology noted was in the lungs of both lambs killed on day 6 pi. This consisted of focal areas of deep red consolidation affecting parts of the apical and cardiac lobes (Fig. 1).

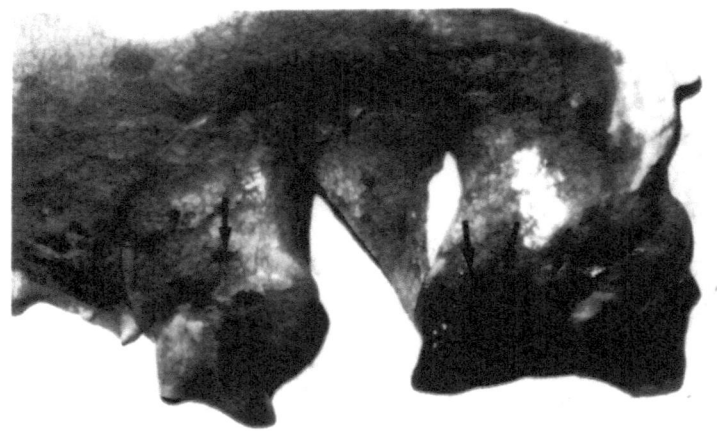

Fig. 1   Lung of lamb showing experimentally produced consolidative lesions.

Histological examination showed changes in the lungs of 9/10 lambs. On day 2 pi an interstitial reaction with focal areas of collapse and exudation of macrophages and neutrophils was present. This reaction progressed and was most severe on day 6 pi when there was consolidative pneumonia and mononuclear infiltration of alveolar walls. Other features were lymphoid cuffing of arterioles and exudation of alveolar macrophages. By day 11 pi the reaction was confined to an interstitial mononuclear cell infiltration and areas of slight collapse were all that remained.

Latency experiment

As in the acute experiment no lamb developed overt clinical illness and no pyrexia was recorded. However adventitious lung sounds were heard in 4 lambs on days 2 and 3 pi.

Virus isolation: acute stage

The results of the virus isolations are summarised in Table 2. SPAHV was recovered from the blood of 1 lamb only on day 6 pi. Virus was recovered also from nasal swabs from each of 2 lambs on one occasion. Virus isolations were made also from respiratory tract tissue, alveolar macrophages and spleen

TABLE 2   Latency experiment - acute phase SPAHV isolations
           from lambs

Tissue	Day p.i.			
	3	3	6	6
Adrenal	−	+	−	−
Liver	+	+	−	−
Lung	+	+	−	−
Tracheal musoca	+	+	+	+
Spleen	+	+	+	+
Salivary gland	−	−	−	−
Brain	−	−	−	−
Trigeminal ganglion	+	−	−	−
Alveolar macrophages	+	+	+	+
Leucocytes (day pi)	−	−	−	+(6)
Nasal swabs (day pi)	−	−	+(5)	+(4)

+   −   SPAHV isolated
−   −   No virus isolated

of both lambs killed on each of days 3 and 6 pi. Other isolates
were from liver and trigeminal ganglion of one lamb killed on
day 3 pi and from the liver of the other.

Pathology

Patchy, discoloured areas were observed in the apical and
cardiac lobes of the lungs of both lambs killed on day 3 pi.
The lungs of both lambs killed on day 6 pi were similarly
affected but in addition one had a small dark red area of
consolidation about 3 x 2 cms in the right apical lobe. The
other tissues showed no gross pathological features.

The microscopical changes observed in the lungs of both
lambs killed on day 3 and 6 pi were similar to those seen in
the acute experiment. One lamb (day 6 pi) had more advanced
lesions with a focal proliferative interstitial pneumonia and
areas of collapse and consolidation. Electron microscopical
studies revealed virus like particles, morphologically
resembling herpesvirus, in an alveolar macrophage (Fig. 2) of
one lamb.

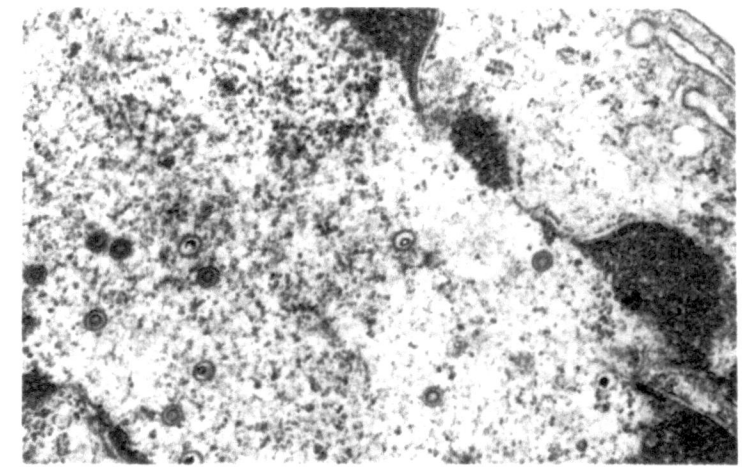

Fig. 2   Electron-micrograph of macrophage showing
intranuclear particles with herpesvirus morphology.

Virus isolation: latent stage

One lamb died of an unrelated abomasitis on day 25 pi.
This left only 3 lambs for study at this stage. SPAHV was
isolated from a nasal swab of one lamb on day 31 pi, 3 days
prior to the start of corticosteroid administration. Virus was
also recovered from this lamb on days 36 and 39 pi, from 1
other lamb on day 39 pi and from one lamb on day 40 pi (Table
3). SPAHV was isolated from peripheral blood samples of each
lamb on one occasion following the commencement of
corticosteroid injections (Table 3).

TABLE 3   SPAHV isolations from lambs following corti-
           costeroid treatment.

		Virus isolations		
dpi	No. of lambs			
		Leucocytes	Nasel swabs	Tissues
39	1	+ 1	-3, +2, +5	None
41	1	+ 3	+5	Salivary gland
44	1	+10	+6	Tracheal mucosa
		+ day from start of corticosteroid treatment		

Isolates were made from 2 tissues only; one from salivary gland on day 41 pi and the other on day 44 pi from tracheal mucosa (Table 3).

Pathology

No gross pathological changes were observed in any of the lungs. Microscopic pathology was limited to patches of mild interstitial pneumonia and infiltration of alveolar walls with mononuclear cells and neutrophils resulting in distension. The lungs of all three lambs had similar features.

DISCUSSION

The experiments described showed that experimental injection of young lambs with SPAHV consistently resulted in infection and the production of abnormal changes in lung tissue although no overt clinical signs were observed. The lungs of one lamb were unaffected but pulmonary changes observed in the other 17 ranged from a slight interstitial reaction to focal areas of consolidation or widespread pneumonia. These lesions were histologically distinct from both those of SPA (Stamp and Nisbet, 1963) and Mycoplasma Ovipneumoniae infection (Foggie et al., 1976).

The list of tissues from which isolates of SPAHV were made indicates that the virus can infect, replicate in and be recovered mainly from the respiratory tract.
Electron-microscopic examination of lung tissue of one lamb confirmed virus replication within the lung but evidence of this was obtained only in alveolar macrophage cells. Virus was recovered from 3 lambs six weeks after primary infection but from 2 of these lambs only after they had been immunosuppressed by corticosteroids. These findings show that the virus can persist in vivo for at least 6 weeks following infection and as virus was recovered from 2/3 lambs after immunosuppression it is reasonable to suggest that this herpesvirus can become latent within the host. Although latency has not been established unequivocally the experiments described indicate that during primary infection the virus had a predilection for spleen, adrenal gland and respiratory tract tissues, including

lung, which might be target sites for virus latency.

The characteristic of latency of this herpesvirus could provide an explanation for the isolation of SPAHV only from the lungs of SPA affected sheep and never from any other disease condition or normal lungs. If the lung or pulmonary cells are target sites for virus latency, reactivation of virus from this area may result from a depression of cell-mediated immunity following the development of the tumour. Alternatively metabolic or physiological changes in adenomatous lung tissue might stimulate virus reactivation from a local or distant site of latency.

The results of these experiments have shown that SPAHV can induce a sub-clinical pneumonia and can persist in vivo for at least 6 weeks following experimental infection. In addition there is evidence which clearly suggests that this virus may become latent within the host and can be reactivated and reisolated. The relationship of this herpesvirus of sheep to SPA remains conjectural but it is unlikely that the virus has a causative role in the production of pulmonary adenomatosis.

REFERENCES

Foggie, A., Jones, G.E. and Buxton, D. 1976. The experimental infection of specific pathogen free lambs with Mycoplasma ovipneumoniae. Res. Vet. Sci., 21, 28-35.
Mackay, J.M.K. 1969. Tissue culture studies of sheep pulmonary adenomatosis (jaagsiekte). I. Direct cultures of affected lungs. J. Comp. Path., 79, 141-146.
Martin, W.B., Angus, K.W., Robinson, G.W. and Scott, F.M.M. 1979. The herpesvirus of sheep pulmonary adenomatosis. Comp. Immun. Microbiol. Infect. Dis., 2, 313-325.
Roizman, B., Carmichael, L.E., Deinhardt, F., de The, G., Nahmias, A.J., Plowright, W., Rapp, F., Sheldrick, P., Takahashi, M. and Wolf, K. 1981. Herpesviridae. Definition, Provisional Nomenclature and Taxonomy. Intervirology, 16, 201-217.
Stamp, J.T. and Nisbet, D.I. 1963. Pneumonia of sheep. J. Comp. Path., 7, 319-328.

MALIGNANT CATARRHAL FEVER VIRUS:

A LYMPHOTROPIC HERPESVIRUS OF RUMINANTS

W. Plowright

A.R.C. Institute for Research on Animal Diseases,
Compton, Newbury, Berkshire, England

ABSTRACT
    Throughout this paper it would have been possible to make
frequent reference to the characteristics of MCFV which are
similar to or different from those of primate, rabbit and avian
viruses which are now classed as Gammaherpesvirinae (Roizman et
al., 1981), or lymphoproliferative herpesviruses (Epstein-Barr
virus, H. saimiri, H. ateles, H. sylvilagus and Marek's disease
virus in particular). Such comparisons have undoubtedly been
invaluable. We have been taken to task by Hunt and Billups
(1979) for our failure to recognise MCF for what it is,
comparatively speaking. This may seem a little difficult to
accept as "African" MCFV was the first of the
lymphoproliferative herpesviruses to be recognised (1960) and
there is, unfortunately, no evidence that it induces neoplastic
transformation of any cell in any species. The similarities of
MCF to infectious mononucleosis were observed in 1953
(Plowright, 1953a,b) and rabbits have been used as an
"experimental model" for nearly 50 years. Furthermore, MCF is
still a clinicopathological and not an aetiological entity;
until an identity of causal agents is proven it is important to
recognise the possibility of differences between the
wildebeest-derived and sheep-associated diseases; Hunt and
Billups (1979) unfortunately took for pathological examination
tissues from animals which were well-documented,
sheep-associated cases (Piercy, 1954) and attributed to them a
herpesvirus aetiology. It is to be hoped that this paper will
clarify some of the issues involved.

INTRODUCTION

    Malignant catarrhal fever (MCF) is an acute, generalised
disease of cattle and domesticated buffaloes, occasionally also
of a wide range of captive and free-living ungulates (cattle,
deer and antelopes) which is usually characterised by a low
morbidity and extremely high case mortality rates (Plowright,
1968; 1981). The clinical signs of MCF include sudden high
fever, severe inflammatory and degenerative changes in the
mucosae of the upper respiratory and intestinal tracts,
ophthalmia with centripetal corneal opacity, generalised
enlargement of lymphoid and haemolymph tissues, nervous
manifestations of a meningoencephalomyelitis, including

muscular tremors and sometimes diarrhoea or dysentery,
laminitis or dermatitis. The main pathological bases of these
protean clinical manifestations are two-fold - a widespread
proliferation of lymphoid cells and an angiitis, affecting many
arteries and veins.

The disease has a world-wide but highly variable
distribution, being most frequent where cattle are in prolonged
close contact with sheep or, in Africa and in zoological
gardens, with two species of wildebeest, viz. the blue or
white-bearded form (Connochaetes taurinus) and the black
(Connochaetes gnu). It is well established, both experimentally
and in natural outbreaks, that multiple cases of MCF in herds
of cattle or deer are associated with close contact with
particular flocks of normal sheep. However, the disease in its
typical form has never been reproduced in cattle by the
inoculation of sheep tissues or secretions, except when this
species has been inoculated with wildebeest virus; similarly
the inoculation of the tissues of sick cattle into sheep has
seldom reproduced the carrier state or signs of disease but see
Straver and van Bekkum, 1979; Kalunda, 1975. Plowright (1964)
failed to infect E. African fat-tailed or merino sheep with
$10^{3.1}$ to $10^{3.3}$ TCD_{50} of cattle blood virus intravenously. Both
the wildebeest-derived and sheep-associated forms are very
seldom, if ever, transmitted from bovine to bovine; the latter
are strict "end hosts". In spite of intensive efforts in a
number of centres, particularly the USA (Colorado, Storz et
al., 1976), Australia (Snowden, 1972; Westbury and Denholm,
1982), New Zealand (Horner et al., 1975) and Britain (Selman et
al., 1978; Buxton and Reid, 1980) it has not been possible to
isolate the aetiological agent of the "sheep-associated"
disease, although successful transmission to cattle and rabbits
has frequently been reported, sometimes in series.

In Africa, however, it has long been known that the
wildebeest-derived infection is readily and consistently
transmissible to cattle by parenteral inoculation (e.g. Mettam,
1923; Daubney and Hudson, 1936) and, incidentally, to rabbits
which invariably die with a characteristic clinicopathological

syndrome (Daubney and Hudson, 1936; Piercy, 1955). The causal agent was isolated from wildebeest in 1959 and identified as a herpesvirus, strictly cell-associated *in vivo* and in early passages in cell cultures (Plowright et al., 1960). This paper is primarily based on studies with this virus, although a recent breakthrough with the sheep-associated agent holds out promise of more rapid progress (Reid et al. - to be published).

THE MAINTENANCE OF THE VIRUS OF MALIGNANT CATARRHAL FEVER IN WILDEBEEST

The regular recurrence of MCF in African cattle which graze over the same ground as wildebeest was the original stimulus for investigating these reservoir species, which do not apparently develop any signs of disease as a result of infection (Mettam, 1923; Daubney and Hudson, 1936; Plowright, 1965a; Rossiter et al., 1982). Using cattle inoculation of large quantities of blood or lymphoid tissues, collected from wildebeest, virus was recovered from animals of all ages but perhaps particularly frequently from the older ($\bar{>}$ 4 years) breeding females, three out of eight in the last month of pregnancy being positive (Plowright, 1965a). Furthermore, the virus infects a proportion of their offspring *in utero*; thus, it was isolated from a foetal spleen and from the blood of 3/7 calves estimated to have been one week old or less (Plowright, 1965a,b), as well as from the nasal secretions of a 4-day calf in captivity (Mushi and Rurangirwa, 1981b). Since the "eclipse" phase in an experimentally infected wildebeest calf was 8 days it is probable that these early recoveries were evidence of *in utero* infection.

The behaviour of the virus in a group of captive wildebeest calves strongly suggested that, following its introduction by a congenitally infected animal it spread laterally to produce viraemia in all the 8 survivors between the 4th to 15th weeks of observation. In 3 animals it was shown by cultural isolation of MCFV from blood leucocytes that viraemia persisted for at least 3, 12 and 36 weeks (Plowright, 1965b). In a free-living population in Tanganyika, however, the

prevalence of viraemia was high up to 3 months of age, when 31%
of all calves were positive, but then declined to 7% for the
second and third trimesters and 2% for the fourth. Between 13
and 18 months only one isolation was made from 44 blood samples
and no viraemia was demonstrated by the cell culture technique
in 106 animals over the age of 18 months (Plowright, 1965a).
Very few susceptible wildebeest calves have been infected
experimentally but one inoculated at about 6 months of age
developed a viraemia which was continuous from the beginning of
the second to the 14th week after inoculation, being present in
greatest quantity between days 12 and 60; subsequently, a
minimal viraemia was detected only during the 31st week. There
was no free infectivity in 6-7 ml of plasma at the time of the
greatest viraemia (Plowright, 1965b).

Hence, it was concluded that wildebeest became
infected in utero or by lateral spread up to the 4th or 5th
months of life. At first they circulated virus continuously but
later they were intermittently viraemic to 13-14 months of age;
all the infectivity was associated with circulating leucocytes.
In spite of the decreasing prevalence of viraemia it is
certain, however, that some wildebeest retain the virus into
adult life and viraemia may be particularly frequent in females
in late pregnancy. It is possible that vertical transfer takes
place during periods of low level, intermittent viraemia at
this time.

Neutralising antibody is present in all or in the great
majority of adult wildebeest (Plowright, 1967; Rossiter et al.,
1983). There were indications in an earlier survey in the
Serengeti area that free-living calves normally acquired high
titre (mean VN_{50} $10^{1.94}$) antibody through the colostrum of the
dam (see also Mushi and Rurangirwa, 1981b) and that this
declined progressively during the first 4 months of life, at a
time when active infection with the virus was spreading rapidly
through the population. Thereafter the mean titre increased to
18 months ($10^{2.29}$) and then declined in animals 2 years of age
or greater (c. $10^{1.7}$). A later survey (Rossiter et al., 1983)
showed that this secondary decline in neutralising antibody may

have begun earlier in S. Kenya. It also established that
antibodies detectable by indirect immunofluorescence (IIF) in
infected monolayer cultures with "early" antigens (Rossiter et
al., 1978), as also those reacting in complement fixation (CF)
and immunoprecipitation (IP) tests (Rossiter and Jessett, 1980;
Rossiter, 1980a,b) were significantly more frequent in calves
up to 4 months old than in older animals. In contrast, IIF
antibodies to late antigens did not change significantly with
age but low-titre IgM antibodies reacting with "late" antigens
in indirect immunoperoxidase (IIP) tests (Rossiter, 1981a) were
found only in a small (3/32) proportion of calves.

THE OCCURRENCE OF HERPESVIRUSES RESEMBLING THAT OF MALIGNANT
CATARRHAL FEVER IN OTHER WILD BOVIDAE

The techniques adopted for isolation of MCFV from
wildebeest, viz. inoculation of viable tissue suspensions or
leucocytes into permissive cell cultures (or cattle) and the
in vitro cultivation of tissues to produce monolayers, were
also adopted for the attempted recovery of viruses from related
East African species such as Coke's hartebeest
(Alcelaphus buselaphus cokei), topi (Damaliscus korrigum) and
fringe-eared oryx (Oryx beisa callotis). All of these antelopes
belong to the Subfamilies Alcelaphinae and Hippotraginae of the
Family Bovidae (Gentry, 1974), and comprise the only species
which had a significant prevalence of MCFV-neutralising antibody in their sera (Reid et al., 1975).

A herpesvirus (K30) closely related serologically and
immunologically to wildebeest-derived MCFV, was isolated from
an adult Coke's hartebeest by cultivation in vitro of
trypsinised thyroid tissue (Reid and Rowe, 1973); this virus
produced typical MCF in cattle. However, three further isolates
from hartebeest, showed only a low level of cross-reactivity
with wildebeest isolates in neutralisation tests (Reid and
Rowe, 1973) and produced delayed, atypical forms of MCF in
inoculated cattle (Reid, 1974 and unpublished).

More recently, herpesviruses were isolated in kidney and
thyroid monolayers prepared from 4/18 topi calves which were

less than 6-months old (Mushi et al., 1981c). The isolates were characterised by their ability to grow in topi cells only, particularly monolayers of embryonic lung and kidney; they cross reacted in immunofluorescence tests with antisera to wildebeest isolates. On inoculation into cattle or rabbits they did not apparently infect or protect against challenge with MCFV.

Whilst no herpesviruses could be isolated from nasal swabs and leucocytes collected from them, neutralising antibody to the WC11 strain of MCFV was found recently to be present in 50/50 sera from oryx of all ages in two "tamed" herds in Kenya. The titre of antibody declined between birth and 6 to 8 months, rising rapidly to 9 months; infection appeared to have been introduced to the herds at some time between 1977 and 1979, probably by wild oryx (Mushi and Karstad, 1981).

THE EXCRETION OF MCFV BY WILDEBEEST AND ITS TRANSMISSION TO CATTLE

In the masailands of E. Africa the seasonal occurrence of MCF in cattle, i.e. predominantly March and April in N. Tanganyika and April to July in S. Kenya, has long been associated with the wildebeest calving season, i.e. January to March in Tanzania and February to April in Kenya. Hence, the disease is commonest in cattle when the wildebeest calves are 2-3 months old. In this context we can probably now dismiss the folklore which maintains that it is wildebeest placenta or the shed haircoat of the 3-4 months old wildebeest calves which are the source of contagion. By housing suceptible bovine with viraemic wildebeest calves, Plowright (1965b) showed that MCFV was naturally transmissible between the species, the incubation period in cattle being, at maximum, 30-47 days in 4/5 cases, the remaining animal developing clinical disease after 81 days. After 3 months, as we have seen, the frequency of viraemia declines rapidly and thenceforward wildebeest-to-cattle transmission is very rare, if it occurs at all.

The probable method of interspecies transmission has been elucidated recently in E. Africa. Rweyemamu et al. (1974)

isoleted MCFV from the nasal secretions of 6/23 recently captured blue wildebeest, which were stressed at the time by confinement, abrupt changes in food and sometimes by betamethasone; 2 of 3 calves and 4/19 adult females were positive. Isolates were also obtained, at death, from the tonsil and thyroid tissue of pregnant females. Surprisingly, only one of 168 blood samples from 66 animals yielded MCFV. Nasal secretions from a 2-weeks old calf were positive at capture and this animal was later found to excrete MCFV in a form not deposited by low-speed centrifugation. Incidentally, betamethasone treatment (40 mg daily for 7 days) of 8 seropositive wildebeest cows was followed, 7-9 days after first inoculation, by pustular vulvovaginitis, from which lesions in 7/8 animals IBR/IPV virus was isolated (Karstad et al., 1973); only one cow yielded MCFV in nasal secretions, 13 days after treatment began.

MCFV does not appear to be shed in the urine (Plowright, 1965b; Mushi, 1980a) or saliva (Mushiet al., 1980a) of viraemic wildebeest calves. It is, however, excreted in nasal and ocular secretions of free-living animals up to 3 months old, particularly by those in the 6-8 weeks age group. The infectivity is both cell-free and sufficiently stable in a moist environment to make it probable that transmission between young, susceptible wildebeest and from wildebeest to cattle is mediated by these materials; about 90% of cell-free preparations of virus, on filter paper at $22^{o}C$, survived at least 30 days at 100% RH. The mean titre of ocular and nasal secretions was $10^{2.25}$ and $10^{2.5}$ TCD_{50}/ml respectively, with a maximum exceeding $10^{3.2}$ TCD_{50}/ml. The source of the excreted virus was probably the mucosa covering the turbinate bones (2/12 calves positive) and the cornea (1/3 animals positive). Although 6/12 calves were excretors only 2 of them were shown to be simultaneously viraemic, whilst suspensions of spleen, tonsil, mandibular lymph node, lung, lacrimal and salivary gland tissue were all negative on inoculation into permissive cell cultures (Mushi et al., 1980a,b).

All the calves in the above study had neutralising

antibody in their serum at 3 months and thereafter IgA antibody was also present in the nasal secretions. The nasal secretions of calves >3m old had a mean neutralising titre of $10^{1.9}$ (Mushi and Rurangirwa, 1981b; Rurangirwa et al., 1981; Mushi et al., 1981a,b). This antibody presumably accounted for the cessation of recoveries of infectious virus and hence the inability of the older animals to transmit the infection to cattle. Rossiter (1980b) reported that he had found IIF antibody (L) in the ocular and nasal secretions of 7/15 wildebeest calves. Explant cultures of turbinate mucosa and cornea from free-living wildebeest calves yielded MCFV from 2 or 3 of every 5 animals examined at monthly intervals up to and including 4 months of age (Mushi et al., 1981b). It was suggested that the corneal epithelium constituted an immunologically privileged site for virus replication, from which progeny virus passed down the nasolacrimal duct to the nasal cavity (Mushi and Rurangirwa, 1981b).

So far as the natural route of virus entry to the body is concerned, it is clear that cell-free virulent MCFV, or incidentally infected cell suspensions, can infect cattle by the intranasal, aerosol or endotracheal routes (Plowright, 1968; Kalunda et al., 1981) and these methods of administration are also successful in rabbits (Mushi and Rurangirwa, 1981a). Virus excreted by wildebeest is therefore presumed to be acquired by cattle through the respiratory tract.

It was shown by Kalunda et al. (1981) that 32/53 (60%) nasal swabs, taken in early clinical stages of the disease in cattle, contained MCF infectivity demonstrable by inoculation of cell cultures and with a mean titre of $10^{1.5}$ TCD_{50}/ml. Such materials were also infectious by inoculation of cattle. Saliva (8/10 samples) from sick animals also yielded MCFV but ocular, vulval and rectal swabs were negative, as also were urinary deposits. Nevertheless, Kalunda et al. (1981) confirmed the many previous observations on failure of the wildebeest-derived disease to spread by close contact amongst cattle even on prolonged exposure (see Plowright, 1981); an apparent exception to this was recorded by Daubney and Hudson, 1936. The failure to spread amongst cattle by "natural" routes is presumably due to the absence of, or inadequate amounts of, stable cell-free infectivity in the excretions of sick cattle. There was no infectivity in large volumes (10-25 ml) of low-speed supernatants from lymph node suspensions or cell-free plasma (60-100 ml) from cattle with the acute disease, even though these were inoculated with "adapted" virus of up to 20 bovine passages (Plowright, 1964). It seems reasonable to suppose that the infectivity in cattle secretions represents infected lymphocytes (vide infra), which are still viable but die rapidly in the environment and become non-infectious.

A somewhat unexpected route of transmission in cattle was observed at the laboratory, where efforts to demonstrate congenital transmission during acute infections and in convalescent or recovered animals had hitherto failed. A cow (no. 8946) was experimentally infected and developed a viraemia which was demonstrable continuously between 9 and 16 days after inoculation and intermittently to the 15th week. This animal developed no clinical signs of MCF but resisted challenge at 13 weeks without developing viraemia and was added to a milking herd. She produced 6 calves over the period to 80 months after first inoculation and at least 4 of these were infected with MCF; only one was clinically affected at birth and another, the sixth, did not develop viraemia until the 37th day of life, with clinical signs delayed to day 120. The cow was never viraemic at the time of calving and MCFV was not recovered from tissue suspensions collected when she was killed at 84 months after infection (Plowright et al., 1972).

This incident was remarkable in proving persistent and repeated transplacental MCFV infection in cattle, which lasted until the end of the 6th year following clinically inapparent infection. It illustrated the dangers of drawing rapid conclusions about the safety of "attenuated" viruses or inapparent infections in animals protected from clinical disease by inactivated vaccines.

THE DEVELOPMENT OF MCF IN CATTLE AND RABBITS

A.   The Viraemia

The mean incubation period of "African" MCF in cattle is prolonged, even following parenteral administration of 10^3 ID_{50} to E. African grade cattle (19.5 $\pm$ SD of 3.7 days; range 11-34 days, n = 311; Plowright, 1964, 1968). Kalunda et al. (1981) have confirmed this for N. American cattle (22.3 $\pm$ SD of 6.6 days, range 14-46 days, n = 47) but, after giving 0.25 - 1.0 litres of blood, in Holland, an average of 10.6 days (range 7-16) was seen by Straver and van Bekkum (1979). There is a small minority of animals in which clinical signs are delayed even further, to about 9 or 10 weeks after inoculation. In rabbits the incubation period was about 13 $\pm$ 3 days, range 9-24 days in Kenya (Plowright, 1964), or about 16 days in Britain (Wilks and Rossiter, 1978; Rossiter et al., 1977), 14 days in Holland (Straver and van Bekkum, 1979) and 17 days in the USA (Kalunda, 1975). The variations probably reflect modifications in the material and route of passage, associated with differences in dose of infectious virus. The end of the incubation period is commonly regarded as the onset of pyrexia but occasionally animals develop indefinite clinical signs, such as enlargement of lymph nodes or ocular and nasal congestion and dicharges, 1 to 4 days prior to the onset of pyrexia (Daubney and Hudson, 1936; Plowright, 1964).

In cattle a viraemia, detectable by inoculation of buffy coat cells into permissive cell cultures (bovine thyroid monolayers), was detected 9 to 17 days after intravenous inoculation of infected blood, on average 7 days (range 3-15 days) before the onset of pyrexia (Plowright, 1968). Delays of up to 10 days and 2-7 days respectively, between the onset of viraemia and clinical signs, have been recorded by Rweyemamu et al. (1976) and Kalunda et al. (1981).

The viraemia increases in titre during the late incubation period and has commonly reached near-peak levels ($\bar{>}10^{2.0}$ TCD_{50}/ml) by the time of first pyrexia, though in some animals this occurs 3-4 days previously; there were indications that highest individual and mean levels ($10^{2.6}$ TCD_{50}/ml may occur

about the 3rd to 7th days of fever. There is no terminal
decline in fatal cases but, in the majority of the very few
survivors, viraemia has declined but remained consistently
demonstrable in cell cultures up to 50 days after onset. By
subinoculation of blood (5 ml) into cattle persistence could be
shown for 3-6 months (Plowright, 1964). According to Kalunda et
al. (1981) the titre of circulating infectivity in recovered
cattle declined and became undetectable in 45 ml samples of
blood "2-3 weeks after the disappearance of the clinical
syndrome"; this requires confirmation using a more sensitive
detection system.

Little information is available for cattle on the tissues
which are primary sites of replication and which eventually
seed infected cells into the blood. Early experiments showed
that the viraemia was largely associated with "mononuclear"
cell fractions devoid of neutrophils and eosinophils, whilst
erythrocyte and platelet-rich fractions were virus free
(Plowright, 1964). As the lymph nodes, thymus and, to a less
extent, the spleen and bone marrow, often contain more
infectivity (per gramme) than blood, with lymph nodes sometimes
attaining titres of $\bar{>}10^5$ TCD_{50}/g, and because the lymphocyte
has now been shown to be the only cell expressing viral
antigens in vivo, it is probable that the tissues named are the
source of infected circulating leucocytes.

B.   The sites of virus replication

It is generally accepted that no cytological or
electron-micrographical evidence of a herpesvirus infection can
be found in the tissues of either cattle or rabbits reacting to
infection with wildebeest-derived strains of MCFV (Plowright et
al., 1960; Plowright, 1968; Rossiter et al., 1977; Edington et
al., 1979; Kalunda et al., 1981). More recently attempts to
demonstrate viral antigens, by immunofluorescence, in a wide
range of tissues, particularly in those such as lymph nodes,
spleen and bone marrow, which were harvested at intervals
following infection, were completely unsuccessful (Rossiter et
al., 1977; Edington et al., 1979). Straver and van Bekkum
(1979) similarly failed to detect viral antigens in the tissues

of 15 affected steers and 13 rabbits, or in calves incubating
the disease (3 and 7 days after infection). However, Rossiter
(1980a) found a very few isolated cells with cytoplasmic and
nuclear fluorescence in lymph node, spleen and thymic tissue
from 3 of 6 rabbits and both of two calves reacting to MCFV
infection; a focus of fluorescent cells was also seen in the
lamina propria of the caecal tonsil of one rabbit killed 3 days
after infection but not in other animals killed at earlier or
later times. The same author (Rossiter, 1980a) observed that
rabbits given repeated inoculations of
glutaraldehyde-inactivated suspensions of infected rabbit lymph
nodes, with Freund's complete adjuvant, failed to develop any
antibody detectable in IIF tests; he therefore concluded that
any MCFV antigens in reacting rabbits are present in very low
concentration.

The site of primary replication of MCFV in rabbits was
investigated in a preliminary manner by subinoculation into
rabbits of pooled lymphoid tissue suspensions and macrophages,
collected at short intervals after intraperitoneal infection.
Infectivity was present at 2 and 4, but not at 6 and 8 days
after inoculation (Edington et al., 1979). Following
intravenous inoculation of infected lymph node cells virus was
recovered from the spleen of 2/3 rabbits at 4 days but not at
days 2 and 6; both spleen and peripheral lymph nodes were all
infectious at day 8 and subsequently. Indirect
immunofluorescence showed small numbers of antigen-bearing
mononuclear cells, 10-12μ in diameter in the spleen, lymph
nodes and thymus at 4 days, and in the spleen of all animals at
6 days; it was concluded that the spleen played a dominant role
in early virus replication in the rabbit (Edington and Patel,
1981). The fluorescing cells were located primarily in the red
pulp of the spleen, in the paracortical areas of lymph nodes
and in both cortex and medulla of the thymus (Patel and
Edington, 1980; Edington and Patel, 1981). These locations,
with the exception of the thymus, were also those in which
lymphoblastic infiltration first occurred, accompanied by focal
lymphocyte necrosis. They suggested a primary and predominant

involvement of T cells (Edington et al., 1979).

By preparing smears of freshly dispersed cells of lymph node, spleen and thymus tissue, harvested from rabbits with pyrexia, it was found by indirect immunofluorescence that only 1 to 4 cells in 10^6 were antigen-bearing at explantation; however, if surviving cell suspensions were maintained in vitro, in RPMI 1640 medium with 20% foetal bovine serum, then the numbers of positive cells increased 50-1000 fold after 48-72 hours. This process was inhibited (>99%) by either cytosine arabinoside (ara-C) or by iododeoxyuridine (IUDR), which did not permit even the production of "early" antigens (c.f. Rossiter et al., 1978). Bone marrow preparations usually contained no fluorescing cells. Suspensions from lymph nodes explanted from rabbits on the second or third days of pyrexia contained. 40-100 fold more antigen-expressing cells than those harvested on the first day of fever. The fluorescence was both cytoplasmic and intranuclear, the former diffuse, the latter sometimes particulate. A membrane antigen was later demonstrable by an $F(ab)_2$ antivirus preparation in viable explanted lymphocytes; the reaction was not due to heterophil antibodies. Infectivity was entirely associated with intact cells, the titre being directly comparable to the number of fluorescing cells, from the time of explantation up to 48 hours later; thereafter, cell death caused an increasing divergence of the figures, with more cells positive by fluorescence than infectivity. Herpes-like virions in small numbers were seen in the nucleus and cytoplasm of 0.1 to 0.3% of cultured cells; some virions were "empty", others possessed a core, but few were enveloped (Patel and Edington, 1980).

The cells with virus antigens or virions were thought to be "medium-sized lymphocytes", with a diameter of 11 ± 0.6 μm, whilst the lymphoblastoid cells which are so prominent in the lymphoreticular tissues (Edington et al., 1979) were not virus-positive. The latter were 10-14 μm in diameter with a large vesicular nucleus, an often reticulated nucleolus and high cytoplasm/nucleus ratio; they possessed a sparse endoplasmic reticulum and but few mitochondria. The lymphocytes had a low cytoplasm/nucleus ratio but their B or T lineage has not been ascertained.

When cell suspensions from infected bovine tissues (lymph nodes, spleen, thymus) were examined, the results were, broadly speaking, the same as for rabbits, except that infectivity at the time of explantation (mean 1100 infectious centres per 10^6 cells) was much higher relative to the rate of specific fluorescence ($\bar{<}2$ in 10^6 cells). The proportion of cells expressing antigen rose, usually by 24 hours, to $300-3000/10^6$ but infectivity hardly changed (Patel and Edington, 1981). The cells supporting virus replication, as in the rabbit, were differentiated medium lymphocytes, 11-13 μm in diameter. It was suggested that the difference between the species might be explained by the lytic effect of bovine complement on any infected lymphocytes which express viral antigens on their cell surface. This activity was not seen with rabbit complement and the inference was that all, or a large proportion of, infected cells in bovine cultures were latently infected at explant (Patel and Edington, 1982a).

All attempts to establish transformed lines of rabbit lymphoblasts from infected tissues have so far failed (Edington et al., 1979; Rossiter, 1980a; Plowright - unpublished). It is possible that glass or plastic-adherent cells, either peritoneal or peripheral blood macrophages can also support virus replication in the rabbit, since infectivity was continuously present in them from the third day after intravenous inoculation (Mushi and Rurangirwa, 1981a). Infectivity of low titre was also demonstrable in plastic-adherent cells, fractionated from bovine lymph node suspensions (Plowright - unpublished). In all these experiments, however, there was a possibility that the virus was simply ingested rather than replicating in the macrophages.

IMMUNITY TO WILDEBEEST-DERIVED MCFV
A.   Resistance to challenge with virulent virus
The very few cattle which survive inoculation with virulent MCFV are probably immune for life, whether they suffer

from a clinically severe, mild or inapparent infection; all wildebeest strains are immunologically homogenous. Thus, Plowright (1964, 1968) found that 15/16 cattle which were infected with one isolate (W1) resisted a first challenge at 2-12 months with the same or 5 different isolates; the exception was an animal viraemic at the time of challenge and, therefore, possibly a delayed reactor. Four of these animals were challenged 7-8 times over a period of 4 years and then later at various times up to 8 years after initial infection but failed to react. Of 9 cattle recovered from infection with 5 further isolates, 8 survived challenge, the other animal having suffered from concurrent infection with the protozoan parasite, Anaplasma marginale, which was found to increase survival rate significantly (16.3% v. 3.4% in one series) (Plowright, 1964). No rabbit has ever been recorded as surviving the disease due to MCFV.

· B.   The Development of antibodies in cattle and rabbits

Resistance to challenge inoculation is accompanied by the presence of neutralising antibody in the serum; the VN_{50} titre does not usually exceed $10^{0.8}$ (1:6) in long-term survivors, but rises to $10^{1.8}$ after challenge. It is, however, unlikely that the neutralising antibody is directly associated with resistance. Thus, it was found that moderate to high levels of neutralising antibody were induced by formalin-inactivated virus, with Freund's incomplete adjuvant, but the "vaccinated" cattle all reacted to parenteral challenge, even using cell-free virulent virus, propagated in cell cultures as an inoculum. These animals usually exhibited a rapid serological response, beginning 2-4 weeks after inoculation and before clinical reactions were observed; titres reached very high levels -$10^{2.0}$ to $\geq 10^{3.4}$ (Plowright et al., 1975). Culture virus concentrated and inactivated with formalin or AEI and combined with Freund's complete adjuvant for administration to rabbits induced high-titre neutralising antibody which was not affected by challenge with cell-free virulent virus; these animals nevertheless succumbed to challenge with infected lymph node cell suspensions after showing 4-fold increases in neutralising antibody (Edington and Plowright, 1980). An accelerated or "anamnestic" response was recorded in cattle challenged after being given "attenuated" live hartebeest virus by Reid and Rowe (1973); there was apparently some protection against cell-associated homologous virus but not against virulent wildebeest virus.

The lack of protection afforded by neutralising antibody is also manifested by the rapid dissemination of virus through freeliving populations of wildebeest calves, which nevertheless usually possess high levels of passive antibody (Plowright, 1967; Rossiter et al., 1983). Furthermore, the appearance of disease in rabbits was not influenced by the circulation of neutralising antibody, usually on the day preceding pyrexia and increasing during the course of the disease (Rossiter et al., 1977). In cattle, however, neutralising antibody develops later in survivor cattle (Plowright, 1968) but it has been detected recently in 6/13 natural, acute cases (Rossiter et al., 1980).

Apart from tests for neutralising antibody, which was the first to be investigated, a battery of other tests has been used recently to study immune reactions in cattle and rabbits. Antibodies reacting in IIF tests, using productively infected cultured cells as antigen, appeared in both species 5-7 days before the onset of pyrexia and increased continuously to death; sometimes antibody was detectable as early as 4-6 days after intraperitoneal infection in rabbits (Rossiter et al., 1977). The use in IIF tests of monolayers treated with Ara-C to produce only "early" antigens, showed that there were two of the latter, one diffuse and found throughout the cell (DEA), the other being particulate and intranuclear (PEA). Antibody to the former was found only in hyperimmunised animals, whilst activity against the PEA appeared in calves 2-3 days after that against "late" antigens and its titre was 4-8 fold lower; reacting rabbits produced very little antibody to PEA (Rossiter et al., 1978). Hence a response to early antigens in the abnormal host (cattle) appears to be induced only by active infection and to be transitory, as in the natural host (wildebeest - Rossiter et al., 1982).

Rossiter (1981a) compared the IIF and IIP (immunoperoxidase) techniques for assay of antibodies in experimentally and naturally infected cattle. All of 23 of the latter were positive by the IIP method, whereas there were 4 failures with IIF. The sensitivity of the IIP technique was approximately 8 times greater than that of IIF. All of 5 rabbits inoculated intra-peritoneally developed IIP antibodies 2-6 days before the onset of pyrexia; both IgG and IgM appeared early but the former increased at least 4 times and the IgM titre <2 fold in the course of the disease. Hence IgG predominated during the late disease (Rossiter, 1982).

Rossiter and Jessett (1980) developed a CF test, using a PEG-concentrated sonicate of infected cultured cells as antigen; CF antibodies developed in the course of infection in cattle and rabbits but required, as in wildebeest, the presence of normal calf serum (NCS) as a supplement; the time relationships were about the same as for IIF antibody. Hamdy et al. (1980) found CF antibodies by a complement-dilution method 3 weeks after inoculation of 32/44 cattle with a wildebeest isolate and, by inference, up to 1 week before clinical signs.

ID tests detected precipitating antibodies in 3/9 reacting rabbits but not in 14 experimental cattle; the CIEP technique gave many non-specific positive reactions with bovine sera (Rossiter, 1980b).

C. Cell-mediated immunity in MCF

As there was no correlation between the production of neutralising antibody and resistance to challenge attempts have been made to define the probably more important function of cell-mediated reactions. It was found in early experiments (Wilks and Rossiter, 1978) that transformation of whole-blood leucocytes by non-specific B or T-cell mitogens (antiglobulin and PHA) fell very quickly in rabbits from the end of the incubation period to death; there was no specific sensitisation to viral antigens in this system, and sensitisation to tuberculin (PPD) was suppressed. Purified lymphocyte fractions, which had been washed repeatedly, were however transformed both by mitogens and viral antigens and the anomaly was attributed to a suppressive factor present in the serum of reacting animals, possibly an antigen-antibody complex.

The significance of the above-mentioned data was questioned by Russell (1980) who found that only a proportion of reacting rabbits and no diseased calf showed reduced responses to PHA; in fact, using whole blood cultures, responses may have been enhanced in cattle and unstimulated blood and lymph node cultures from many reacting rabbits incorporated significantly more label than normals. Some sera from reacting rabbits did, however, have a suppressive effect, on some normal lymphocytes, whereas bovine sera did not.

Few observations have been recorded on delayed hypersensitivity to antigens of MCFV but Rossiter (1980a) reported a strong dermal reaction in rabbits given viral antigens in one experiment.

THE PATHOGENESIS OF THE PRINCIPAL LESIONS OF MCF IN CATTLE AND RABBITS

There are many features of the pathology of MCF which remain to be elucidated. They are discussed below: -

(A) The primary site of virus penetration

As already noted, no cytolytic cycle of infection has been demonstrated in any tissue of any host species, whether natural (wildebeest) or unusual (cattle and rabbits). If, as seems possible, the natural method of infection is by cell-free virus in the upper respiratory tract, then primary lesions in epithelia with productive infection would be expected but may be very difficult to locate, as in EB virus infection of man. The early appearance of antibodies, particularly IIF and IIP, is also evidence of such an early productive cycle.

(B) The necrosis of lymphocytes

Lymphocytes, which are known to be infected _in vivo_, undergo necrosis in the follicles of the lymph nodes of rabbits as early as 2-4 days after infection; there is concurrent congestion and haemorrhage but again no cytological or electronmicroscopical evidence of a herpesvirus infection. With the onset of the clinical reaction there is an extensive secondary episode of necrosis of lymphocytes in the paracortical areas of lymph nodes and cortex of the thymus (Edington et al., 1979). A more extensive follicular necrosis with macrophage reaction in lymph nodes has also been reported in African MCF (Plowright, 1953b) and with the SA form (Liggitt et al., 1978). The cause of this necrosis of lymphocytes has not been established.

(C)   The lymphoblastoid cells

Infiltrations of lymphoblastoid cells, which are not virus-infected and which continue to show mitoses in the areas invaded, appear not only in the lymphoid tissue but also in parenchymatous organs and subepithelial situations, where they are associated with superficial degenerative and sometimes necrotic lesions. In the rabbit these cells flood into the circulation in the terminal phases of the disease, where they often produce an absolute lymphocytosis, reaching 50,000 cu mm and resembling that of infectious mononucleosis of man. A relative but not an absolute lymphocytosis occurs in cattle (Plowright, 1953a, 1964).

Rossiter (1980a) partially characterised the "large mononuclear" cells in the lymphoid tissues of reacting rabbits. He found that they were non-phagocytic, did not adhere to plastic and probably incorporated more ^{3}H-thymidine in culture than did cells from normal animals. Many of the large atypical cells had "null" characteristics, i.e. they showed neither rosetting with sheep erythrocytes or surface immunoglobulin. A majority of those atypical cells which could be classified were found to be of T lineage (6:1 in blood and lymph nodes, 3:1 in spleen).

(D)   The vascular lesions

Perhaps the most contentious issue is the origin of the

vascular lesions which are virtually pathognomonic for this
infection. They are characterised by fibrinoid degeneration and
necrosis of the medial elements of blood vessel walls,
especially medium-sized arteries. Perivascular and intramural
infiltration of lymphocytes, lymphoblastoid cells and
macrophages is often accompanied by degeneration and oedema of
collagen fibres and by endothelial swelling, proliferation and
detachment. Thrombosis occurs but is relatively rare. It has
been suggested that these lesions, with others, occur at the
end of a long incubation period and prepatent viraemia, because
the host has become "hypersensitive to viral or viral-induced
antigens" (Plowright, 1968). Later workers hypothesised that
the disease was associated with an immune-complex formation
involving "membrane" antigens and antibodies to them (Rweyemamu
et al., 1976). Selman et al. (1974) noted similarities of the
lesions of the sheep-associated disease to a type III or IV
immune reaction (Gell and Coombes, 1968). Liggitt et al.
(1978), working with sheep-associated cases, proposed an
auto-allergic response as the basis of the vascular lesions,
whilst Liggitt and DeMartini (1980a,b) noted resemblances to
graft rejection and contact sensitivity.

Attempts to prove that the vascular lesions in cattle or
rabbits do contain immune complexes, have met with irregular
success. Thus, Rossiter (1980b) and Mushi and Rurangirwa
(1981c) found no IgG or C' in blood vessel walls and glomeruli;
the latter authors recorded a fall in serum C3 levels from the
onset of viraemia in cattle, increasing in rapidity later, but
CH_{50} levels were unchanged. There were incidentally no
significant changes in total serum IgG_1, IgG_2 and IgM, whereas
large increases might have been expected if the lesions were
really of immune complex type. Liggitt and DeMartini (1980a,b)
similarly failed to demonstrate complexes in sheep-associated
cases. Patel and Edington (1982b) described immune complexes
with immunoglobulin, C3 and conglutinin (Cg) in the glomeruli,
occasionally in the arteries, of cattle with the terminal
disease; there was also a depletion of circulating lytic
complement and conglutinin. No viral antigens were stained in

the deposits by the IIF technique and no specific activity could be demonstrated in eluates from kidney tissue. Patel and Edington (198b2) suggested that extensive binding of Cg may have masked the C3 deposits sought by other workers.

THE POSSIBLE RELATIONSHIP OF WILDEBEEST-DERIVED MCF TO THE SHEEP-ASSOCIATED DISEASE

Apart from one American report which will need verification (Hamdy et al., 1978) there has been no recent claim to have identified the agent, derived probably from sheep, which commonly causes MCF outside Africa. This paper described a virus which was isolated from a bovine case in an outbreak in Minnesota and from an inoculated steer. The virus was related immunologically to wildebeest strains and, whilst it became attenuated very rapidly for cattle, still protected if inoculated repeatedly against challenge with "African" virus. It is surprising that no attempt was made to detect antibodies to the "new" virus in the sheep which were regarded as its possible source, or to explain convincingly the very rapid attenuation, which has never been observed elsewhere with wildebeest isolates.

A recent finding more suggestive of a close relationship between the wildebeest-derived virus and the sheep-associated form of MCF was that of Rossiter (1981b). He detected IIF(L) antibodies to the "African" virus in the sera of 162/167 sheep, derived from 10 flocks in Britain, Austria, Australia and Kenya. The titre distribution resembled that in wildebeest; some high-titred sera also had antibody to the particulate early (PEA) antigen. The highest mean titre was encountered in a flock of Australian sheep known to have given rise to the disease in cattle (Snowden, 1972). Antibody was also detected in some colostrum-deprived and gnotobiotic lambs, thus suggesting that in utero transmission of the virus may have occurred. The antibody was absorbed selectively from sera by cells infected with wildebeest virus and blocked by rabbit antiserum to MCFV, not by normal rabbit serum.

A most interesting recent development is the establishment

by Reid and coworkers (1982) of a line of rabbit lymphocytes
from an animal infected with an agent derived from
sheep-associated MCF in deer (Buxton and Reid, 1980; Reid et
al., 1979). These cells required a feeder layer and possessed T
lymphocyte surface markers but no immunoglobulin; they
possessed large, dense intracytoplasmic granules and
non-specific esterase; they were also cytotoxic to cell lines
and primary cell cultures. As few as 100 of the cells
reproduced MCF in rabbits, an activity which was destroyed by
anti-T cell serum and complement, and it was suggested that
they were large granular lymphocytes or "NK" cells, exhibiting
functional disturbances caused by infection with the MCF agent
and comparable to similar lines from marmosets infected with
Herpesvirus saimiri and H. ateles (Johnson and Jondal, 1981).

In conclusion, whilst there is yet no direct evidence that
sheep-associated MCF is caused by a herpesvirus, there is
strong serological evidence that a herpesvirus related to the
wildebeest-derived isolates is extremely widespread in sheep
and, incidentally, this agent is not apparently the virus
isolated by Mackay and colleagues (Martin et al., 1979) from
cases of pulmonary adenomatosis (jaagsiekte). It is also now
undisputed that the clinico-pathological manifestations of MCF
are indistinguishable, whether caused by viruses from
wildebeest or, putatively, sheep and occasionally other
reservoir hosts. The behaviour of the sheep agent differs in
that no permissive cell culture has yet been found for it, in
spite of intense efforts. However the recent establishment of
an infected rabbit cell line, by Reid et al. (1982), not only
offers a better hope of identifying the causal agent but also
of explaining a pathogenesis unique for a naturally occurring
acute disease caused by a lymphoproliferative herpesvirus.

REFERENCES

Buxton, D. and Reid, H.W. 1980. Transmission of malignant
    catarrhal fever to rabbits. Vet. Rec., 106, 243-245.
Daubney, R. and Hudson, J.R. 1936. Transmission experiments
    with bovine malignant catarrh. J. comp. Path., 49, 63-89.
Edington, N. and Patel, J. 1981. The location of primary
    replication of the herpesvirus of bovine malignant

catarrhal fever in rabbits. Vet. Microbiol., 6, 107-112.
Edington, N., Patel, J., Russell, P.H. and Plowright, W. 1979.
The nature of the acute lymphoid proliferation in rabbits
infected with the herpes virus of bovine malignant
catarrhal fever. Europ. J. Cancer, 15, 1515-1522.
Edington, N. and Plowright, W. 1980. The protection of rabbits
against the herpesvirus of malignant catarrhal fever by
inactivated vaccines. Res. vet. Sci., 28, 384-386.
Gell, P.G.H. and Coombes, R.R.A. 1968. Clinical Aspects of
Immunology. Blackwell Scientific Publications, Oxford.
Gentry, A.W. 1974. In "Mammal Evolution in Africa" (Ed. V.J.
Maglio). (Princeton University Press, N.J., USA).
Hamdy, F.M., Dardiri, A.H. and Ferris, D.H. 1980. Complement
fixation test for diagnosis of malignant catarrhal fever.
Proc. 87th Annu. Mtg. U.S. anim. Hlth. Assoc. San Diego.
pp. 329-338.
Hamdy, F.M., Dardiri, A.H., Mebus, C., Pierson, R.E. and
Johnson, D. 1978. Etiology of malignant catarrhal fever
outbreak in Minnesota. 82nd annu. Mtg. US anim. Hlth.
Assoc., Buffalo, N.Y. pp. 248-267.
Horner, G.W., Oliver, R.J. and Hunter, R.C. 1975. An epizootic
of malignant catarrhal fever. 2. Laboratory investigations.
N.Z. vet. J., 23, 35-38.
Hunt, R.D. and Billups, L.H. 1979. Wildebeestassociated
malignant catarrhal fever in Africa: a neoplastic disease
of cattle caused by an oncogenic herpesvirus. Comp. Immun.
Microbiol. inf. Dis. 2, 275-283.
Johnson, D.R. and Jondal, M. 1981. Herpesvirus-transformed
cytoxic Tcell lines. Nature, 291, 81-83.
Kalunda, M. 1975. African malignant catarrhal fever virus;
its biologic properties and the response of American
cattle. PhD Thesis, Cornell University, N.Y., USA.
Kalunda, M., Dardiri, A.H. and Lee, K.M. 1981. Malignant
catarrhal fever. I. Response of American cattle to
malignant catarrhal fever virus isolated in Kenya.
Canad. J. comp. Med., 45, 70-76.
Karstad, L.S., Drevemo, S., Otema, J.C. and Jessett, D.M. 1973.
Vulvovaginitis in wildebeest caused by the virus of
infectious bovine rhinotracheitis. J. Wildl. Dis., 10,
392-396.
Liggitt, H.D., DeMartini, J.C., McChesney, A.E., Pierson, R.E.
and Storz, J. 1978. Experimental transmission of malignant catarrhal fever in cattle: gross and histopathologic
changes. Amer. J. vet. Res., 39, 1249-1257.
Liggitt, H.C. and DeMartini, J.C. 1980a. The pathomorphology
of malignant catarrhal fever. I. Generalised lymphoid
vasculitis. Vet. Pathol., 17, 59-73.
Liggitt, H.D. and DeMartini, J.C. 1980b. The pathomorphology
of malignant catarrhal fever. II. Multisystemic epithelial
lesions. Vet. Pathol., 17, 74-84.
Martin, W.B., Angus, K.W., Robinson, G.W. and Scott, F.M. 1979.
The herpesvirus of sheep pulmonary adenomatosis. Comp.
Immun. Microbiol. inf. Dis., 2, 313-325.
Mettam, R.W.M. 1923. Snotsiekte in cattle. 9th and 10th Reps.
Director vet. Educ. Res., Union of S. Africa. 395-432.
Mushi, E.Z. and Karstad, L. 1981. Prevalence of virus neutral-

ising antibodies to malignant catarrhal fever virus in
oryx (Oryx beisa callotis). J. Wildl. Dis., 17, 467-470.

Mushi, E.Z., Jessett, D.M., Rurangirwa, F.R., Rossiter, P.B.
and Karstad, L. 1981a. Neutralising antibodies to malignant catarrhal fever herpesvirus in wildebeest nasal
secretions. Trop. anim. Hlth. Prod., 13, 55-56.

Mushi, E.Z., Karstad, L. and Jessett, D.M. 1980a. Isolation
of bovine malignant catarrhal fever virus from ocular and
nasal secretions of wildebeest calves. Res. vet. Sci.,
29, 168-171.

Mushi, E.Z., Rossiter, P.B., Karstad, L. and Jessett, D.M.
1980b. The demonstration of cell-free malignant catarrhal
fever herpesvirus in wildebeest nasal secretions.
J. Hyg. (Camb.), 85, 175-179.

Mushi, E.Z., Rossiter, P.B. and Jessett, D. 1981c. Isolation
and characterisation of a herpesvirus from the topi
(Damaliscus korrigum Ogilby). J. comp. Path., 91, 63-68.

Mushi, E.Z. and Rurangirwa, F.R. 1981a. Malignant catarrhal
fever virus infectivity in rabbit macrophages and monocytes. Vet. Res. Commun., 5, 51-56.

Mushi, E.Z. and Rurangirwa, F.R. 1981b. Epidemiology of malignant catarrhal fever; a review. Vet. Res. Comm., 5, 127-
142.

Mushi, E.Z. and Rurangirwa, F.R. 1981c. Immunoglobulins,
haemolytic complement and serum C3 in cattle infected with
malignant catarrhal fever herpesvirus. Vet. Res. Comm.,
5, 57-62.

Mushi, E.Z., Rurangirwa, F.R. and Karstad, L. 1981b. Shedding
of malignant catarrhal fever virus by wildebeest calves.
Vet. Microbiol., 6, 281-286.

Patel, J.R. and Edington, N. 1980. The detection of the herpesvirus of bovine malignant catarrhal fever in rabbit
lymphocytes in vivo and in vitro. J. gen. Virol., 48,
437-444.

Patel, J.R. and Edington, N. (1981). The detection and behaviour of the herpesvirus of malinant catarrhal fever
in bovine lymphocytes. Arch. Virol., 68, 321-326.

Patel, J.R. and Edington, N. 1982a. The effect of antibody and
complement on the suppression of herpesvirus of bovine
malignant catarrhal fever in cultured rabbit lymphocytes.
Vet. Microbiol. in press.

Patel, J.R. and Edington, N. 1982b. Immune complexes associated
with infection of cattle by the herpesvirus of malignant
catarrhal fever. Vet. Microbiol. submitted.

Piercy, S.E. (1954). Studies in bovine malignant catarrh
V The role of sheep in the transmission of the disease.
Brit. vet. J., 110, 508-516.

Piercy, S.E. 1955. Studies in bovine malignant catarrh.
VI. Adaptation to rabbits. Brit. vet. J., 111, 484-491.

Plowright, W. 1953a. The blood leucocytes in infectious malignant catarrh of the ox and rabbit. J. comp.. Path., 63,
318-334.

Plowright, W. 1953b. The pathology of infectious bovine malignant catarrh in cattle and rabbits. XVth Internat. vet.
Congr., Stockholm. Proc. I. 323-328.

Plowright, W. 1964. Studies on malignant catarrhal fever in

cattle. DVSc Thesis, University of Pretoria, South Africa.
Plowright, W. 1965a. Malignant catarrhal fever in East Africa.
I. Behaviour of the virus in free-living populations of
blue wildebeest (Gorgon taurinus taurinus, Burchell).
Res. vet. Sci., 6, 56-68.
Plowright, W. 1965b. Malignant catarrhal fever in East Africa.
II. Observations on wildebeest calves at the laboratory
and contact transmission of the infection to cattle.
Res. vet. Sci., 6, 69-83.
Plowright, W. 1967. Malignant catarrhal fever in East Africa.
III. Neutralising antibody in freeliving wildebeest.
Res. vet. Sci., 8, 129-136.
Plowright, W. 1968. Malignant catarrhal fever. J. Amer. vet.
med. Assoc., 152, 795-804.
Plowright, W. 1981. Herpesviruses of wild ungulates, including
malignant catarrhal fever virus; In: Infectious Diseases
of Wild Mammals, 2nd Edition. (Eds. Davis, J.W., Karstad,
L.H. and Trainer, D.O.) (Iowa State University Press,
Ames, Iowa, USA). pp. 126-146.
Plowright, W., Ferris, R.D. and Scott, G.R. 1960. Blue wildebeest and the aetiological agent of bovine malignant
catarrhal fever. Nature Lond., 188, 1167-1169.
Plowright, W., Herniman, K.A.J., Jessett, D.M., Kalunda, M. and
Rampton, C.S. 1975. Immunisation of cattle against the
herpesvirus of malignant catarrhal fever: failure of inactivated culture vaccines with adjuvant. Res. vet. Sci.,
19, 159-166.
Plowright, W., Kalunda, M., Jessett, D.M. and Herniman, K.A.J.
1972. Congenital infection of cattle with the herpesvirus
causing malignant catarrhal fever. Res. vet. Sci., 13,
37-45.
Reid, H.W. 1974. Comparative aspects of herpesviruses isolated
from alcelaphine antelopes in East Africa. Trans. roy.
Soc. trop. Med. Hyg., 68, 276 (Summary only).
Reid, H.W., Plowright, W. and Rowe, L.W. 1975. Neutralising
antibody to herpesviruses derived from wildebeest and
hartebeest in wild animals in East Africa. Res. vet. Sci.,
18, 269-273.
Reid, H.W. and Rowe, L. 1973. The attenuation of a herpesvirus
(malignant catarrhal fever virus) isolated from hartebeest
(Alcelaphus buselaphus cokei Gunther). Res. vet. Sci., 15,
144-146.
Reid, H.W., Buxton, D., Corrigal, W., Hunter, A.R., McMartin,
D.A. and Rushton, R. 1979. An outbreak of malignant
catarrhal fever in red deer (Cervus elaphus). Vet. Rec.,
104, 120-123.
Reid, H.W., Buxton, D., Pow, I., Finalyson, J. and Berrie, E.L.
1982. A cytotoxic T-lymphocyte line propagated from a
rabbit infected with sheep-associated malignant catarrhal
fever. Res. vet. Sci. in press.
Roizman, B., Carmichael, L.E., Deinhardt, F., de Thé, G.,
Nahmias, J., Plowright, W., Rapp, F., Sheldrick, P.,
Takahashi, M., Wolf, K. 1981. Herpesviridae. Definition,
provisional nomenclature, and taxonomy. Intervirology, 16,
201-217.
Rossiter, P.B. 1980a. Serological and immunological

investigations in malignant catarrhal fever. Ph. D. Thesis, University of London.

Rossiter, P.B. 1980b. Antigens and antibodies of malignant catarrhal fever herpesvirus detected by immunodiffusion and counterimmunoelectrophoresis. Vet. Microbiol., 5, 205-213.

Rossiter, P.B. 1981a. Immunoperoxidase and immunofluorescence techniques for detecting antibodies to malignant catarrhal fever virus in infected cattle. Trop. anim. Hlth. Prod., 13, 189-192.

Rossiter, P.B. 1981. Antibodies to malignant catarrhal fever virus in sheep sera. J. comp. Path., 91, 303-311.

Rossiter, P.B. 1982. Immunoglobulin response of rabbits infected with malignant catarrhal fever virus. Res. vet. Sci., 33, 120-122.

Rossiter, P.B. and Jessett, D.M. 1980. A complement fixation test for antigens of and antibodies to malignant catarrhal fever virus. Res. vet. Sci., 28, 228-233.

Rossiter, P.B., Jessett, D.M. and Mushi, E.Z. 1980. Antibodies to malignant catarrhal fever virus antigens in the sera of normal and naturally infected cattle in Kenya. Res. vet. Sci., 29, 235-239.

Rossiter, P.B., Jessett, D.M., Mushi, E.Z. and Karstad, L. 1982. Antibodies in carrier wildebeest to the lymphoproliferative herpesvirus of malignant catarrhal fever. Comp. Immunol. Microbiol. inf. Dis. 6, 39-43.

Rossiter, P.B., Mushi, E.Z. and Plowright, W. 1977. The development of antibodies in rabbits and cattle infected experimentally with an African strain of malignant catarrhal fever virus. Vet. Microbiol., 2, 57-66.

Rossiter, P.B., Mushi, E.Z. and Plowright, W. 1978. Antibody response in cattle and rabbits to early antigens of malignant catarrhal fever in cultured cells. Res. vet. Sci., 25, 207-210.

Russell, P.H. 1980. The in vitro response to phytohaemagglutinin during malignant catarrhal fever of cattle and rabbits. Res. vet. Sci., 28, 39-43.

Rweyemamu, M.M., Karstad, L., Mushi, E.Z., Otema, J.C., Jessett, D.M., Rowe, L., Drevemo, S. and Grootenhuis, J.G. 1974. Malignant catarrhal fever virus in nasal secretions of wildebeest: a probable mechanism for virus trans mission. J. Wildl. Dis., 10, 478-487.

Rweyemamu, M.M., Mushi, E.Z., Rowe, L. and Karstad, L. 1976. Persistent infection of cattle with the herpesvirus of malignant catarrhal fever and observations on the pathogenesis of the disease. Brit. vet. J., 132, 393-400.

Selman, I.E., Wiseman, A., Murray, M. and Wright, N.G. (1974). A clinicopathological study of bovine malignant catarrhal fever in Great Britain. Vet. Rec., 94, 483-490.

Selman, I.E., Wiseman, A., Wright, N.G. and Murray, M. 1978. Transmission studies with bovine malignant catarrhal fever. Vet. Rec., 102, 252-257.

Snowden, W.A. 1972. Bovine malignant catarrh. Annu. Rep. Anim. Hlth., CSIRO., Australia. p. 16.

Storz, J., Okuna, N., McChesney, A.E. and Pierson, R.E. 1976.

Virologic studies on cattle with naturallyoccurring and experimentally induced malignant catarrhal fever. Amer. J. vet. Res., 37, 875-878.

Straver, P.J. and van Bekkum, J.G. 1979. Isolation of malignant catarrhal fever virus from a European bison (Bos bonasus) in a zoological garden. Res. vet. Sci., 26, 165-171.

Westbury, H.A. and Denholm, L.J. 1982. Malignant catarrhal fever in farmed Rusa deer (Cervus timorensis). 2) Animal transmission and virological studies. Aust. vet. J., 58, 88-92.

Wilks, C.R. and Rossiter, P.B. 1978. An immunosuppressive factor in serum of rabbits lethally infected with the herpesvirus of bovine malignant catarrhal fever. J. inf. Dis., 137, 403-409.

STUDIES OF PERSISTENT AND LATENT EQUID HERPESVIRUS 1
AND HERPESVIRUS 3 INFECTIONS IN THE PIRBRIGHT
PONY HERD

R. Burrows, D. Goodridge
Animal Virus Research Institute, Pirbright,
Surrey GU24 ONF, U.K.

ABSTRACT

The Pirbright pony herd is a closed herd and has no
contact with other horses. Nasopharyngeal swabs and blood
samples are collected at frequent intervals. Equine
herpesvirus 1 was isolated from several animals following
stress situations, and serological evidence of periodic EHV-1
and EHV-3 activity was obtained from many animals. Attempts
to demonstrate virus reactivation following corticosteroid
treatment or the presence of latent virus in trigeminal
ganglia were unsuccessful.

INTRODUCTION

Three herpesviruses are known to infect horses: equid
herpesvirus 1 (EHV-1) which is associated with
rhinopneumonitis and abortion (Doll and Bryans, 1963) and,
occasionally, paresis (Saxegard, 1966); equid herpesvirus 2
(EHV-2) which may or may not be associated with disease; and
equid herpesvirus 3 (EHV-3), the cause of coital exanthema
(Girard et al., 1968), a venereal disease characterised by
herpetic lesions on the external genitalia. Persistent
infections with EHV-2 in which virus can be recovered
intermittently from the nasopharynx and the white cell
fraction of the blood are well documented but persistent
latent infections with EHV-1 and EHV-3 have been less easy to
demonstrate, although Erasmus (1966) isolated EHV-1 on at
least five occasions from groups of horses three to ten days
after injecting them with live attenuated African horse
sickness viruses.

This report presents some evidence for the reactivation
of latent EHV-1 and EHV-3 infections in ponies maintained in
isolation from other horses at the Animal Virus Research
Institute, Pirbright.

MATERIALS AND METHODS

The Pirbright herd of pure and crossbred Welsh mountain ponies was established between 1967 and 1971 to provide animals with a known history for studies of the abortifacient properties of EHV-1 strains and respiratory tract viruses of horses. Apart from the introduction of new stallions in 1974 and 1977, the herd has been self-contained since October 1971. The ponies have no contact with other horses and, unless mixed for experimental or breeding purposes, are kept in separate groups according to age and sex. Most of the ponies are kept outdoors during the summer and housed during the winter. Eight separate grazing areas, ten covered courts and one isolation unit with bathing and changing facilities are available. The numbers of ponies in the herd between 1972 and 1982 ranged from 49 to 85, with a yearly average of 61. Five to 19 foals were produced each year (average 11) and one to 21 ponies (average 11) were discarded. Past and present ponies in the herd total 197.

Ponies used for experimental purposes were housed in an isolation unit and were not returned to their original group for at least six weeks. Some details of natural and experimental infections in the herd have been recorded (Burrows and Goodridge, 1973, 1975, 1978, 1979). Before and between experiments, all ponies were inspected daily and, if signs of respiratory or other disease were seen, appropriate samples were taken and screened for virus in equine foetal kidney cell cultures. Blood samples were taken at frequent intervals and the sera stored at -20°C. Neutralising antibody titres were determined by plaque reduction rests (Burrows, 1966), using equine foetal kidney or rabbit kidney cell line (RK-13) cell cultures and complement fixing antibody titres by an overnight microtest (Thomson et al., 1976).

RESULTS AND DISCUSSION

Equid herpesvirus 1

(a) Virus recovery

Virus may be isolated from the naso-pharynx of most horses for periods of eight to 10 days after infection or re-infection and from some horses for up to 14 days (Burrows and Goodridge, 1975). Virus may also be recovered from the white cell fraction of the blood for similar periods in most subtype 1 infections but not usually in subtype 2 infections (Burrows and Goodridge, 1973 and unpublished results).

No systematic attempt was made to isolate virus from ponies between experiments but virus was isolated from swabs taken for control purposes from a four-year-old mare a few days after her foal had been weaned and from a five-year-old gelding newly housed for experiment. Virus was also recovered, along with rhinovirus 1436/71, from the pharyngeal tissues of a four-year-old gelding killed in the terminal stages of Grass Sickness and from five colts a few days after castration. No clinical signs of respiratory disease were displayed by these animals and seven of the eight ponies subsequently developed increases in EHV-1 antibody.

An attempt to produce a reactivation of latent EHV-1 in ponies by treatment with synthetic corticosteroid was unsuccessful, although the treatment did result in the appearance and transmission of rhinovirus 1436/71 within the group (Table 1).

TABLE 1   Rhinovirus 2 activity in a group of ponies following treatment with synthetic corticosteroids*

Pony	\multicolumn{12}{c}{Days after treatment commenced}
	0	2	4	6	8	10	12	15	22	27	42	50
95	-†	-	-	-	-	-	-	-	-	-	-	-
96	-	-	-	-	-	-	-	-	-	-	-	-
97	-	-	-	-	-	-	-	-	-	0.7	-	2.5
99	-	-	-	-	-	-	-	2.5	3.0	2.5	2.1	2.7
105	-	-	-	-	-	-	-	-	2.0	0.7	2.6	3.2
106	-	-	-	-	-	2.1	1.8	3.1	1.7	0.7	-	2.6
111	-	-	-	-	-	-	-	-	-	-	-	-
114	-	-	-	-	-	-	-	-	-	-	-	-
122	-	-	-	1.5	1.5	-	1.3	-	-	-	-	3.1

*Flumethasone: 2.5 mg i/v day 0, 1, 2 and 3, and 3.75 mg day 5

†$\log_{10}$ pfu/nasopharyngeal swab.   - = <0.7

All ponies had been exposed three and six months earlier to EHV-1 (R/2290 - subtype 2).

Similarly, attempts to demonstrate EHV-1 in the trigeminal ganglia and other tissues at various times after infection with both subtypes of the virus have so far proved unsuccessful (Table 2).

TABLE 2   Attempts to demonstrate latent EHV-1 in tissues taken post-mortem

Pony	Age (years)	Sex	Period since last experimental infection	Sub-type	Tissues examined	Method
105	3	M			Trigeminal ganglia, guttural pouch	Organ culture and co-culti- tivation on equine foetal kidney cells. Cultures maintained for 6 weeks and sampled weekly
111	2	M				
122	2	M	15 months	2		
114	2	M				
108	2	M		1		
62	8	F	6 months	2		
68	8	F				
121	2	F	No previous			
91	4	F	experimental	-		
88	4	F	infection			
102	3	F	10 months	2		
149	$1^1/2$	M				
148	"	M	3 months	2		
142	"	M				
141	$1^1/2$	M				
143	"	M	7 months	1	Trigeminal ganglia, tonsil, pharyngeal and/or mandibular lymph nodes	Organ culture and co-culti- equine foetal lung cells. Cultures maintained for 3 weeks and sampled at 3-day intervals
150	"	M	3 months	2		
144	"	M				
131	$2^1/2$	M				
136	"	M	7 months	1		
138	"	M	2 months	2		
130	"	M				
129	"	M	6 weeks	2		
133	"	M				

(b)   Serological studies

The reactivation of a latent infection could be expected to be accompanied by virus shedding, with the possibility of infection or re-infection of contact animals. Serological screening of groups of ponies held in complete or relative

isolation has confirmed that such infections do occur. In
October 1969 15 newly purchased pony colt foals developed
rhinopneumonitis and virus was recovered from most animals
during the clinical stages of disease. Five of these colts
were placed in an animal room in the centre of the laboratory
area and held there for seven months. Serological studies
(Fig.1) confirmed that the group suffered a second infection
10 weeks after the initial infection and a third infection
three months later. Some coughing occurred during the second
infection but no virus was recovered from naso-pharyngeal
swabs taken at that time. The third infection was not
accompanied by clinical signs and was only identified in
retrospect. These results indicate that at least one of these
ponies was latently infected and was able to initiate
infections in companion animals.

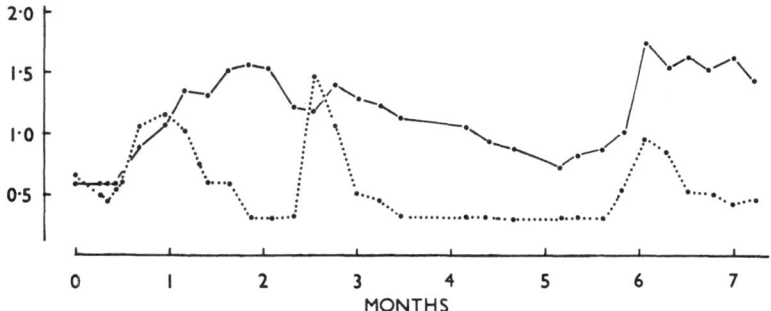

Fig.1   Geometric mean antibody titres ($\log_{10}$
reciprocal) of five 6-month-old pony foals held in
isolation. EHV-1 H-45 (subtype 2). o————o,
neutralising;   o······o, CF.

The results of similar retrospective serological studies
of our breeding mares are given in Fig.2, which presents
their geometric mean antibody titres for a three-year period.
Most animals developed significant increases in neutralising
antibody during the summers of 1976 and 1977, indicating that
some re-infections were occurring within the group at that
time.

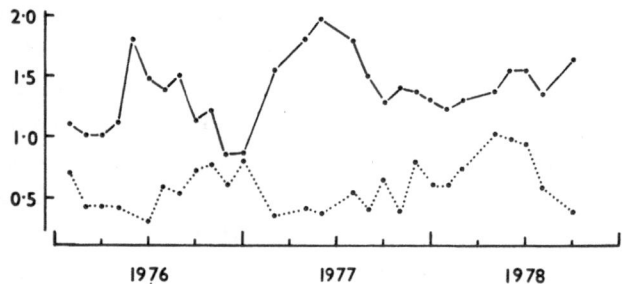

Fig.2   Geometric mean antibody titres ($\log_{10}$ reciprocal) of breeding mares. EHV-1 RAC-H (subtype 1). Mean of nine mares in 1976, 23 mares in 1977 and 22 mares in 1978.

The findings for individual mares are summarised in Table 3, which shows that 21 of the 23 mares experienced from one to three periodic increases in neutralising antibody during the periods of study. The period of study for each mare commenced at least nine months after the last experimental exposure to EHV-1. Seventeen of the 23 mares had been exposed to EHV-1 strains on one to seven occasions (average 2.8) by intranasal, intramuscular or intra-uterine injection but no virulent field strain of virus had been used in the group since April 1975 (five mares). In 1976 and 1977 many of these serological indications of either recrudescences of infection or of re-infection occurred during the late spring and early summer and they occurred in both in-foal mares and barren mares. In an earlier study of EHV-3 infection in the pony herd (see later), similar significant rises in neutralising antibody were identified in several animals at the same time of the year and it may be significant that 12 cases of Grass Sickness occurred in the herd during the early summers of 1974 and 1977. It is of interest to speculate whether subclinical cases of this disease occurred in these and other years and provided the stress factor which reactivated latent herpesvirus infections.

TABLE 3   Diagnostic increases in neutralising antibody (EHV-1, RAC-H subtype 1) in a group of breeding mares

Number of mares	Period of study (months)	Number of significant antibody rises			
		None	One	Two	Three
9	33	0	2	3	4
10	24	2	2	5	1
2	21	0	1	1	0
2	14	0	1	1	0

Mean age in January 1976:   6.4 years (3 to 12)

Mean interval between
antibody rises: 13.25 months (7 to 22)

Reports of respiratory disease occurring after influenza vaccination have been received from time to time and the possibility that influenza vaccination might impose some stress on the animal which might lead to the reactivation of latent EHV-1 was examined by looking for increases in CF activity (EHV-1) in sera. Suitable collections of sera were available from our 1971/74 study of the efficacy of four commercial vaccines (Burrows et al., 1977), the 1979/80 comparison of 10 inactivated influenza viruses (Burrows and Denyer, 1982) and the 1976/77 field trial of a prospective vaccine in trekking ponies in Wales and Scotland (Burrows and Goodridge, 1979). The results confirm that increases in EHV-1 CF antibody do occur in some animals during the two weeks after vaccination but, in the only group in which controls were available, no differences were seen between the responses of control and vaccinated animal (Table 4).

Equid herpesvirus 2

Most foals in the pony herd acquire infection during the suckling period and virus may be isolated intermittently from nasopharyngeal swabs for long periods. Twelve foals born in 1976 were sampled frequently before and after weaning at five months. Virus was isolated from 18/81 swabs (11 foals infected) collected before weaning and from 35/92 swabs (all foals infected) collected during the four months after weaning.

TABLE 4   Numbers of ponies with three-fold or greater increases in EHV-1 (H-45 subtype 2) CF antibody titre during the 14 days following vaccination with commercial or experimental inactivated influenza-virus vaccines

Study	Number of ponies	Number of ponies with increases following			
		First primary	Second primary	First annual	Second annual
Pirbright 1971/74	32	2	5	7	6
Pirbright 1979/80	20	1	2	3	-
Field trial 1976/77	94	13	5	17	-
Controls	22	5	1	4	-

Equid herpesvirus 3

Clinical lesions associated with EHV-3 infection were first seen in the pony herd in June 1975, although routine testing of sera in 1972 had disclosed that subclinical infections had occurred since 1971. The acquisition and transmission of infection during the breeding seasons 1971 to 1975 are summarised in Table 5.

The serological findings indicate that in 1971 a young "virgin" stallion, B/68, was infected by mare 12/66 which had joined the herd in October 1970. This mare developed an increase in EHV-3 neutralising antibody before being mated and subsequently the stallion and two of eight other mares mated developed antibody. In 1972 stallion B/68 infected five of ten susceptible mares but whether the stallion or mare 17/65 was the initial source of virus that year is not known.

Stallion A/64 was infected in 1972 by mare 13/65. In

TABLE 5   Acquisition and transmission of EHV-3
infection during the breeding season

Stallion	Season	Mated	With antibody before mating	Developing antibody after mating
	1967 to 1971	4 to 11	2 (*2 and 4)	0
	1972	5	2 (12 and 13)	0
A/64	1973	7†	0	4
	1974	6†	0	3
	1975	8	3	2
	1971	9	1 (12)	2 (13 and 17)
	1972	11	1 (17)	5
B/68	1973	8	4	2
	1974	6	4	2
	1975	7	7	-

(Number of mares spans Mated / With antibody before mating / Developing antibody after mating)

Note: Stallion A first developed antibody July 1972,
infected by Mare 13
Stallion B, virgin stallion in 1971, developed
antibody June 1971, infected by Mare 12

* Identity of infected mares
† Virgin fillies

1973 and 1974 he was used only to mate with virgin fillies
and in both years transmission of infection occurred.

The neutralising antibody titres of mare 12/66 which had
been infected before entering the pony herd and the two mares
(13/65 and 17/65) infected in 1971 were measured over a
period of 20 months (Fig.3). Titres dropped to below 0.6 (log
reciprocal) some 15 to 20 weeks after infection or
recrudescence of infection and remained at this level for
variable periods ranging from one to six months before
increasing to titres of 1.7 to 2.0.

Similar findings were obtained for mares infected in
1974 and 1975 (Fig.3). Attempts to correlate these secondary
increases in neutralising antibody with episodes of virus
growth and excretion were made by examining vaginal and nasal
swabs periodically from week 50 to week 95 from mares 61/71
to 68/71. Virus was recovered from vaginal swabs of mare
61/71 on five occasions from week 54 to week 59 during the
primary infection (virus amounts ranged from $10^{0.7}$ to $10^{2.7}$

316

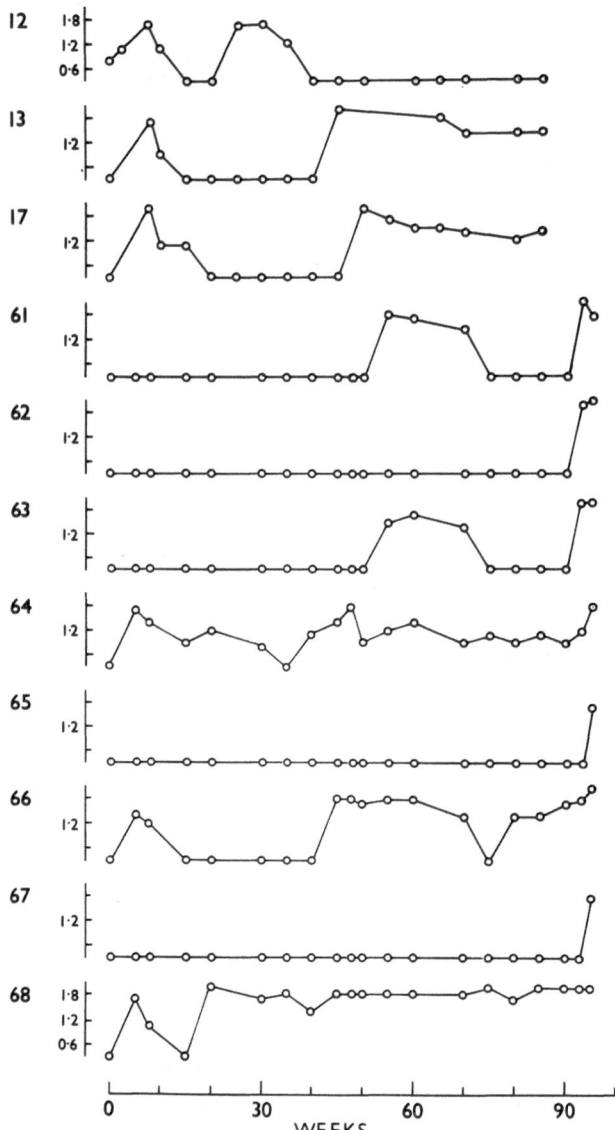

Fig.3   EHV-3 neutralising antibody titres (log$_{10}$ reciprocal) of selected mares.
Periods: Mares 12, 13 and 17 - May 1971 to Jan. 1973
          Mares 61 to 68   - May 1974 to March 1976
Stallion B/68 running with mares 12, 13 and 17 from weeks 0 to 5 in 1971 and mare 17 from weeks 52 to 58 in 1972.

Fig. 3 (continued)

Stallion A/64 running with mares 12 and 13 from weeks 52
to 58 in 1972, with virgin mares 63 to 68 from weeks 0
to 5 in 1974, and virgin mares 61 and 62 and mares 63 to
68 from weeks 52 to 58 in 1975.

pfu/swab) and again from two samples taken during week 90
(mean titre $10^{3.1}$ pfu/swab). Clinical signs of coital
exanthema in form of a single lesion at the same site on the
vulva were evident on both occasions. The neutralising
antibody titres of mares 61/71 and 63/71 increased from <0.6
to 2.0 between weeks 90 and 93. Primary infections also
occurred in mares 62/71, 65/71 and 67/71 at this time, but
virus was not recovered from swabs and no clinical signs of
disease were seen. Precautions had been taken to avoid
transmission of infection during sampling procedures but some
grooming and tail trimming had been carried out during week
90.
    These studies of natural EHV-3 infection in the breeding
herd provide some information relevant to the epizootiology
of the disease and an explanation of its sporadic appearance
in breeding establishments. Infection was introduced in
October 1970, yet no obvious clinical signs of the disease
were seen until June 1975. The stallions and mares ran as
groups for six weeks each season and the mares were inspected
daily for evidence of recent coitus. During these years both
stallions and eighteen mares acquires infection and
unequivocal evidence was obtained of the long-term
persistence of virus in both the stallion and the mare. The
virological and serological results indicated that, some
months after a primary infection, neutralising antibody
levels decreased to pre-infection levels and then increased
again after a variable peroid. Virus was not recovered from
samples taken from the vagina or the nose during periods when
primary subclinical infections took place, as a result of
either coitus or cross-infection, or when secondary increases
in antibody occurred. However, small amounts of virus were
obviously produced at these times, as transmission of

infection to susceptible animals took place. Some
experimental evidence that large amounts of virus are
required to produce clinical disease and that smaller amounts
produce subclinical infections was reported by Bryans and
Allen (1973). Virus was recovered for a period of five weeks
from one mare which displayed a single lesion and again from
a lesion which appeared in the same area some eight months
later. Cross-infection to three susceptible mares occurred on
this latter occasion but whether the virus was transmitted by
grooming activities, flies (Gibbs et al., 1972) or inhalation
(Bryans and Allen, 1973) is not known.

ACKNOWLEDGEMENTS

This study was supported in part by the Horserace
Betting Levy Board. It is a pleasure to thank Mrs. Mary
O'Sullivan for technical assistance, Mr. G. Hutchings for his
attempts to demonstrate virus in tissues collected after
death (Table 2) and Mr. A. Tiffin and Mr. N.B. Collins for
their care of the pony herd.

REFERENCES

Bryans, J.T. and Allen, G.P. 1973. In vitro and in vivo
    studies of equine coital exanthema. Proc. 3rd Int. Conf.
    Equine Infectious Diseases, Paris, 1972 (Ed. J.T. Bryans
    and H. Gerber). (Karger, Basel). pp.322-366.
Burrows, R. 1968. Rhinopneumonitis virus neutralising
    antibody levels of British Thoroughbred mares. Proc. 1st
    Int. Conf. Equine Infectious Diseases, Stresa, 1966 (Ed.
    J.T. Bryans). (Grayson Foundation, Lexington, Kentucky),
    pp.122-130.
Burrows, R. and Denyer, M. 1982. Antigenic properties of some
    equine influenza viruses. Arch. Virol., 73, 15-24.
Burrows, R. and Goodridge, D. 1973. In vivo and in vitro
    studies of equine rhinopneumonitis virus strains. Proc.
    3rd Int. Conf. Equine Infectious Diseases, Paris, 1972.
    (Ed. J.T. Bryans and H. Gerber). (Karger, Basel).
    pp.306-321.
Burrows, R. and Goodridge, D. 1975. Experimental studies on
    equine herpesvirus type 1 infections. J. Reprod. Fert.
    Suppl., 23, 611-615.
Burrows, R. and Goodridge, D. 1978. Observations of
    picornavirus, adenovirus and equine herpesvirus
    infection in the Pirbright pony herd. Proc. 4th Int.
    Conf. Equine Infectious Diseases, Lyon, France, 1976.
    (Ed. J.T. Bryans and H. Gerber). (Veterinary

Publications Inc., Princeton, New Jersey). pp.155-164.

Burrows, R. and Goodridge, D. 1979. Equid herpesvirus 1 (EHV-1): Some observations on the epizootiology of infection and on the innocuity testing of live virus vaccines. Proc. 24th Ann. Conf. Amer. Assoc. Equine Pract., St. Louis, Missouri, 1978. pp.17-28.

Burrows, R., Spooner, P.R. and Goodridge, D. 1977. A three-year evaluation of four commercial equine influenza vaccines in ponies maintained in isolation. Develop. biol. Standard., 39, 341-346.

Doll, E.R. and Bryans, J.T. 1963. Epizootiology of Equine Viral Rhinopneumonitis. J. Am. vet. med. Ass., 142, 31-37.

Erasmus, B.J. 1968. The activation of herpes virus infections of the respiratory tract in horses by immunisation against Horsesickness. Proc. 1st. Int. Conf. Equine Infectious Diseases, Stresa, 1966. (Ed. J.T. Bryans). (Grayson Foundation, Lexington, Kentucky). pp.117-121.

Gibbs, E.P.J., Roberts, M.C. and Morris, J.M. 1972. Equine coital exanthema in the United Kingdom. Equine Vet. J., 4, 74-80.

Girard, A., Greig, A.S. and Mitchell, D. 1968. A virus associated with vulvitis and balanitis in the horse - a preliminary report. Canad. J. comp. Med., 32, 603-604.

Saxegard, F. 1966. Isolation and identification of equine rhinopneumonitis virus (equine abortion virus) from cases of abortion and paralysis. Nord. Vet. Med., 18, 504-512.

Thomson, G.R., Mumford, J.A., Campbell, A., Griffiths, L. and Clapham, P. 1976. Serological detection of equid herpesvirus 1 infections of the respiratory tract. Equine Vet. J., 8, 58-65.

CHARACTERIZATION OF THE FELINE HERPESVIRUS GENOME
AND MOLECULAR EPIDEMIOLOGY OF ISOLATES FROM
NATURAL OUTBREAKS AND LATENT INFECTIONS

Sigrid-C. Herrmann, Rosalind M. Gaskell*,

B. Ehlers, H. Ludwig

Institut für Virologie der FU Berlin,
im Robert Koch Institut,
Nordufer 20, 1000 Berlin 65
*Department of Veterinary Medicine,
Langford House, University of Bristol,
Bristol U.K.

ABSTRACT

Felid herpesvirus type 1 (FHV 1), the cause of severe respiratory diseases in Felidae, has a DNA of low GC content and of an approximate molecular weight of 80×10^6 Daltons. Various isolates from different countries and different clinical outbreaks or originating from latent infections showed a considerably homogeneity in their genomes when restriction enzyme analysis was applied. These results are discussed in comparison with other viruses of the herpes group, which have an obvious DNA heterogeneity. One speculative conclusion would be that the FHV 1 genome has a unique structure.

INTRODUCTION

One of the major clinical problems in diseases of Felidae is associated with respiratory tract infections. The great majority of these cases are caused by one of two viruses; felid herpesvirus I (FHV I) and feline calicivirus. Both viruses are found worldwide (Gaskell and Wardley, 1978). Our report deals with FHV I, which is a typical member of the herpesvirus group attributed to sub family alphaherpesvirinae (Roizman et al., 1981). It is known to undergo latency (Povey, 1979). Its biological properties, virus host cell relationship, antigenic properties and characteristics of its carrier state have been studied in some detail and will be intensively discussed at this meeting (Gaskell and Povey, 1977, 1979; Povey, 1979; Gaskell and Goddard, 1982 this issue). One of the outstanding features of FHV I is its restrictedness in vivo and in vitro to Felidae and feline cells. This narrow host range together with other biological

properties bears some resemblence to Varicella-zoster virus
(VZV). Different FHV I isolates examined by conventional,
serological cross neutralisation techniques appear to be
uniform and in general are of uniform pathogenicity.
Nevertheless strains of modified virulence do exist having
been developed for use in vaccines (Slater and York, 1976;
Davis and Beckenhauer, 1976; Bittle and Rubic, 1975). No
relationship has been observed to the other feline herpesvirus
(FHV 2, felid cytomegalovirus) or any other member of the
herpesvirus group (Povey, 1979).

In this report the first detailed studies on the genome of
FHV I isolates are presented. The viruses originated from
Europe or Northern America and were obtained from cats showing
both typical and atypical signs of infection with FHV I.
Attention was also given to re-isolates from persistently
infected cats in order to determine if the virus altered
during latency and passage in the host. Our results present
surprising uniformity in FHV I genomes which is quite in
contrast to data obtained with bovine herpesviruses and
pseudorabiesviruses also reported in this issue (Pauli et al.,
1982; Ludwig, 1982; Herrmann et al., 1982).

MATERIALS AND METHODS
VIRUSES

Wildtype isolates from clinical cases of FHV 1 infections
(feline viral rhinotracheitis) in Bristol or Berlin, a
laboratory strain (B927) used for experimental infections,
isolates recovered from the trigeminal ganglia of latently
infected cats and an attenuated vaccine strain originating
from Northern America, are summarized in Table 1.

CELLS

Viruses were grown in Crandell feline kidney (CRFK) cells
or in a permanent cat cell line (kindly provided by N. Hirano,
Iwate University, Morioka, Japan) under standard conditions.

DNA ISOLATION AND RESTRICTION ENZYME ANALYSIS

Viral DNA was either isolated from cell-free supernatant
or from infected cells utilizing known techniques (Darai et

TABLE 1: Biological data of FHV-I isolates used in DNA restriction analyses

No	Source*	Place Date of isolation	Reference	Titre TCID$_{50}$ per ml	Passage[+] No.	Purification	DNA - analyses
1	Case B 927	Bristol 1972 UK	Gaskell, Povey (1979 b)	$10^{5.6}$	P9	P1-P4 3x terminal dilution	Reference DNA pattern
2	as above			$10^{6.1}$	P20	as above	as reference (1)
3	Isolate from TG** explant from cat expt. infected with P4 B927 11 months before.	Bristol 1973 UK	Gaskell, Povey (1979 a)	$10^{6.9}$	P4	none	as ref. (1)
4	Isolate from cat naturally infected 21 months before & re-exceting after cortico-steroid	Bristol 1974 UK		$10^{6.9}$	P4	none	Change in DNA patterns of Pst I, EcoR I, Kpn I comp. to ref. (1)
5	Case GB: na-tural infec-tion in ex-perimental cat	Bristol 1980 UK		$10^{6.9}$	P7	P1-P4 3x terminal	Slight difference from reference (1), seems similar to (6)
6	Isolate from TG** explant from expt.cat naturally inf. as (5) one year before	Bristol 1981 UK		$10^{5.6}$	P6	none	seems similar to (5)

continue TABLE 1

7	Case J31	Bristol	1979	$10^{7.1}$	P3	none	Slight difference from ref.(1)
8	"	"	"	$10^{6.9}$	P7	Plaque purified 3x	Slight difference from ref.(1) and earlier passage (7)
9	Case G547	"	1977	$10^{5.9}$	P3	none	Slight difference from ref.(1)
10	Case J593	"	1979	$10^{6.1}$	P3	none	"
11	Case FU:Isolate from natural case with evidence of generalized FHV-I infection plus some nervous signs. Virus recovered from respiratory, abdominal tissues and also brain	"	1973	$10^{6.6}$	P4	none	Slight difference from ref.(1)
12	Case H1254: isolate from case of skin ulceration	"	1978 Flecknell et al. (1976)	$10^{6.3}$	P4	none	Slight difference from ref.(1)
13	Temperature-sensitive strain of FHV I	USA	? Slater & York (1976)	$10^{5.6}$	more than P 200	none	Slight difference from ref.(1)

continue TABLE 1

14 Case V I 12/30 Berlin	1981	$10^{4.8}$	P3	none	Slight difference from ref.(1)
15 Case V I 12/35	" 1981	$10^{5.4}$	P3	none	Slight difference ref.(1)
16 Case Jens Isolate from lachrymal fluid	" 1981	$10^{6.5}$	P3	none	Slight difference from ref.(1)

Footnotes:

* unless stated otherwise =
  (i) oro-pharyngeal swab isolate, and
  (ii) from case with typical upper respiratory signs of FHV 1 infection

** trigeminal ganglion

+ isolates 1-12 passaged in secondary feline embryo cells or a diploid cell line (courtesy Prof. O. Jarrett)

TABLE 2: Molecular weights of FHV - I DNA-fragments obtained by restriction enzyme cleavage

Hind III Fragment	MWx10^6	Eco RI Fragment	MWx10^-6	Bam HI Fragment	MWx10^-6	Bst EII Fragment	MWx10^-6	Kpn I Fragment	MWx10^-6	Pst I Fragment	MWx10^-6
1	19,2	1	8,5	1	9,7	T-1	19,5	1	15	1	19,5
2/3	9,7	2	7,0	2	8,8	2/3	6,5/6,4	2	11,5	2	14,6
4	8	3	6,3	3	6,3	4	5,3	3	9,0	3	9,6
5	4	4	5,75	4	5,6	5/6	4,7/4,6	4	6,3	4	7,9
6	3,5	5	5,1-4,8	5	5,0	7/8	4,0/3,9	6/7	5,2	5	6,5
7	3,1	6	4,6	6	4,3	9	2,7-2,6	8	4,25	6	6
8	2,6	7	4,3	7	4,1-4,0	T-10	2,5-2,3	9/10	3,7-3,9	7	5,25
9	2,4	8/9	4	8/9	3,3/3,2	11	2,0	11	3,2	8	4,6
10	2,3	10	3,4-3,15	T-10	3,0-2,9	12	1,9	12	2,4	9	4,15
11	2,25	11	3,2	11/12	2,4	13	1,8	13	2,0	10	2,6
12	2,1	12	3,0	13	2,05	14	1,6	14/15	1,75/1,6	11	2,5
13/14	1,85/1,8	13	2,8-2,65	14	1,9	15	1,4	16	1,3	12	2,3
15	1,5	14/15	2,4/2,2	15	1,7-1,6	16	1,3	17	1,2	13	1,7
16	1,2	16	2,15	16	1,45	17	1,2	18	0,9		
17	1,05	17/18	1,85	17	1,35	18	1,0				
		19	1,65	18	1,3	19	0,9				
		20	1,55	19	1,2	20	0,8				
		21	1,5	20	1,1						
		22	1,35	21	1,0						
		23	1,15	22-25	2,4						
		24	0,9								
tot.	76,25	tot.	84,85	tot.	73,55	tot.	73,9	tot.	78,7	tot.	87,2

(mean values of 4-6 agarose slab gels 0,8-1%)

T = terminal fragment

al., 1975; Pignatti et al., 1979) and digested with different
restriction enzymes under conditions recommended by the
supplier (BRL). The resulting DNA fragments were separated on
0.8-1% agarose gels at 110 V for 3 hours (horizontal gels) or
35 V for 18 hours (vertical gels). These slab gels were
stained with ethidium bromide and photographed with a Polaroid
Land camera.

RESULTS
    An insufficient yield of FHV 1 DNA from virus particles of
the cell-free supernatant motivated us to establish the growth
conditions and virus production using B927 as reference strain
in CRFK cells. As shown in Fig. 1, FHV 1 remained relatively
strongly cell associated with titres of two logs higher
compared to virus released in the supernatant. This explains
the low DNA yield in preliminary experiments when DNA
isolation was performed from concentrated supernatant
preparations. In all consecutive experiments DNA isolation
followed the procedure of Pignatti et al. (1979), which had
already proven to be advantageous in VZV DNA extraction
(Gilden et al.., 1982). Such partially purified DNAs analysed
by preparative CsCl equilibrium centrifugation (Ludwig, 1972)
had buoyant densities of 1.7o8-1.710 g/cm³ (Fig. 2). CRFK cell
DNA (e = 1.698 g/cm³) and pseudorabies (PsR) virus DNA (e =
1.731 g/cm³) served as markers. The GC-content of FHV 1 DNA
was calculated to be approximately 50 Mol %, which is close to
that of cell DNA and corresponds well to a value of 46%
reported by Plummer et al. (1969). It is also close to the
value of 46% obtained for VZV DNA (Ludwig et al., 1972).
    The total amount of DNA received from one infected cell
batch (1 Roux bottle) was approximately 20 µg. This was
sufficient to perform all the following experiments. A total
of 6 different enzymes (Hind III, Eco R I, Bam H I, Bst E II,
Kpn I, and Pst I) was used for cleavage of 16 FHV 1 DNAs. The
results are given in Table 2. The molecular weight calculated
from the sum of the fragments was estimated to be
approximately 80x10^6 Daltons. This result was calculated

328

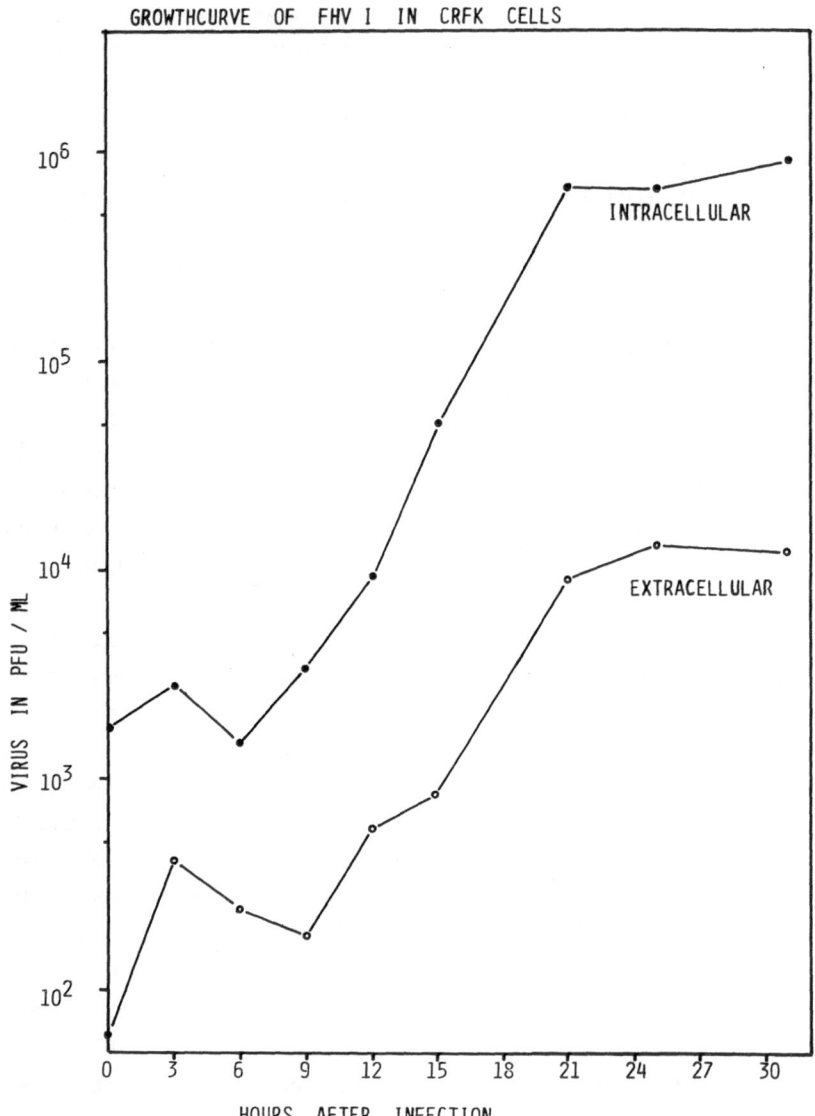

Fig. 1   CRFK cells were inoculated with FHV 1 stockvirus
B297 (1 PFU/cell). After adsorption for 1 hour (0) samples
of supernatant and cells were collected at the indicated
times and frozen at -70°C until the titre in plaque assay
was determined.

independently from six agarose gels and is a mean value from
all enzymes applicated, using the Bam H I fragments of PsR

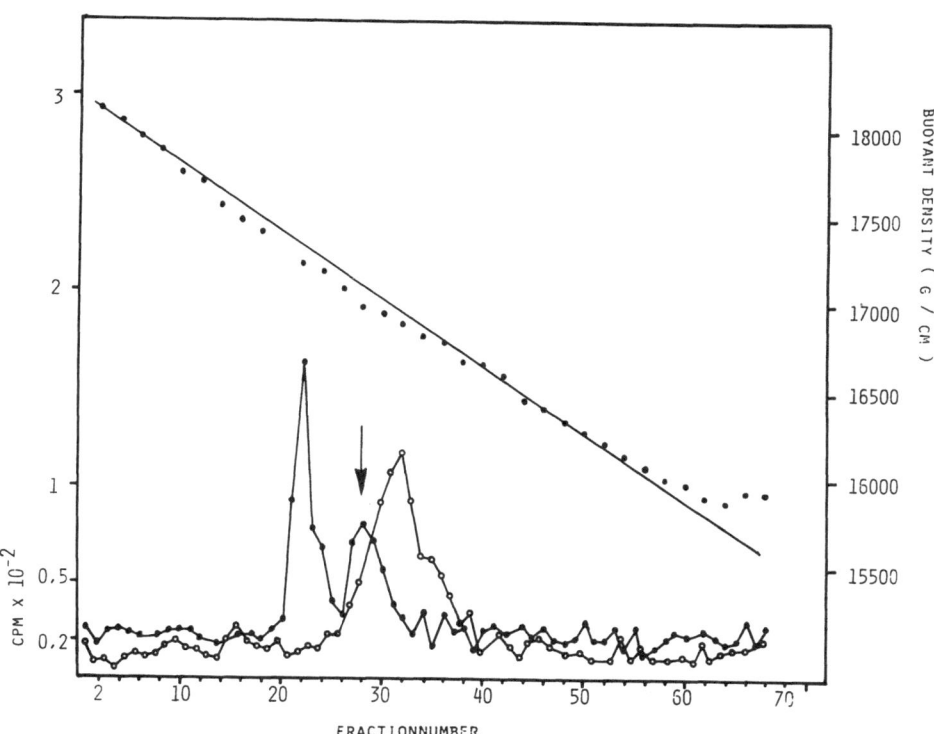

Fig. 2   CRFK cells, infected with FHV 1 stockvirus B927
and mink lung cells, infected with PsR virus were labelled
4 hrs. p.i. with ³H-Thymidine. Simultaneous mock-infected
CRFK cells were lysed, treated as described previously
(Ludwig, 1972) and centrifuged to equlibrium in CsCl
gradients. The arrow indicates FHV 1 DNA, PsR- and CRFK
cell DNA were used as internal markers.

virus DNA (Rixon and Ben-Porat, 1979) as molecular weight
markers. The molecular weight of FHV 1 DNA is unusual low for
a herpesvirus DNA. However, our estimates seemed to be in the
correct range because in simultaneous electrophoresis on the
same slab gel the mobility of the intact PSR virus DNA (MW =
92×10^6 Daltons) was considerably lower than that of the felid
herpes virus, pointing to a molecular weight difference of
$10 - 15 \times 10^6$ Daltons. Further investigations are on the point
of being accomplished since molecular weight estimates from

DNA cleavage patterns may be erroneous (Hayward et al., 1975).

In restriction enzyme analysis of the DNAs of 16 FHV 1 isolates no obvious differences in the cleavage patterns were observed when 5 of the above mentioned enzymes were used (Fig. 3 and 4). Only with Eco RI were two types of cleavage patterns

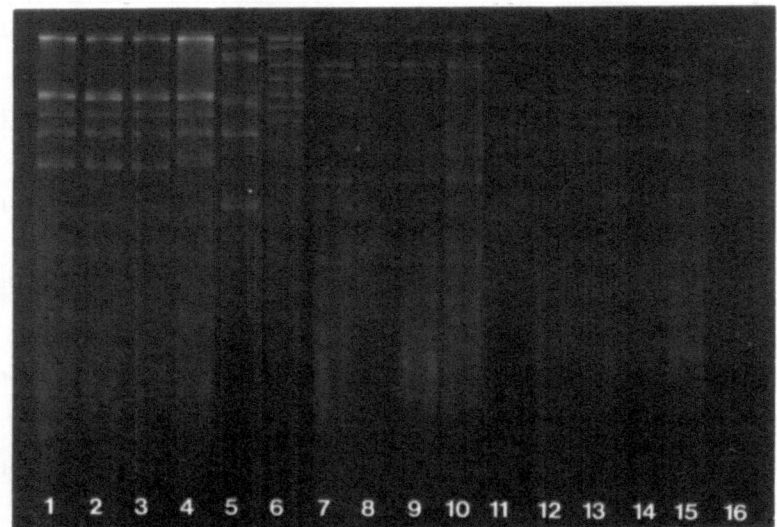

Fig. 3   DNA cleavage patterns of FHV 1 isolates after digestion with different restriction endonucleases: Lanes 1-4 FHV 1 DNAs Bst E II digested; Lanes 5 and 11 PsR virus DNA Bam H I digested (serving as molecular weight markers); Lane 6 FHV 1 DNA Pst I digested; Lanes 7-10 FHV 1 DNAs Hind III digested; Lanes 12-15 FHV 1 DNAs Bam H I digested; Lane 16 FHV 1 DNA Kpn I digested. The DNA fragments were separated by electrophoresis on a 0.8% agarose gel at 40 V for 18 hours, stained with ethidiumbromide (1µg/1) and photographed under UV transillumination with a Polaroid Land camera.

observed, but these showed only minor differences (Fig. 5). With all the other enzymes only slight shifts in the electrophoretic mobility of one or two fragments were evident (Fig.3 and 4, further data not shown). One of these fragments seemed to represent an end fragment as found by exonuclease treatment in preliminary experiments using Bst E II or Bam H I enzymes.

Isolates 2 and 3 represent re-isolates of the standard stock virus B927 (isolate 1, Table 1) and all have identical or nearly identical DNA patterns. Isolate 2 was passaged

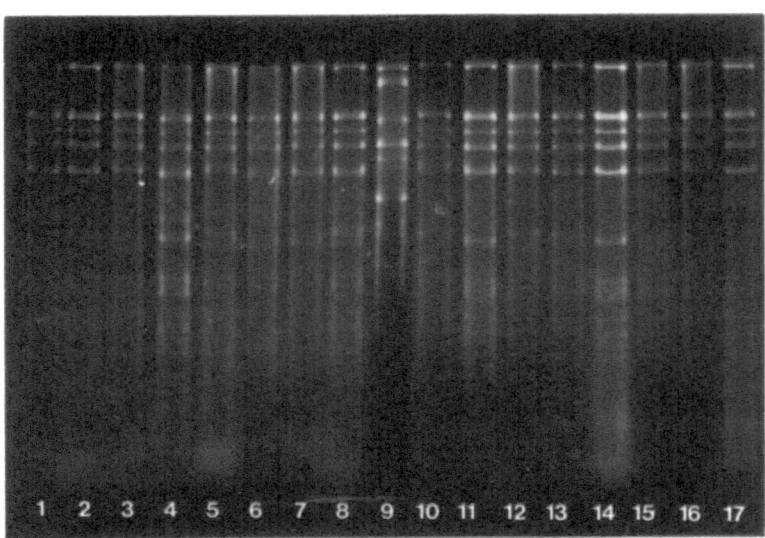

Fig. 4   DNA cleavage patterns of FHV 1 isolates after digestion with Bst E II: Lanes 1-8 FHV 1 isolates 1,3,4,2,7,8,11 and 12 (see Table 1); Lane 9 PsR virus DNA Bam H I digested (molecular weight marker); Lanes 10-17 FHV 1 isolates 9,10,5,6,13,14,15, and 16 (see Table 1). Conditions for separation and visualization were as indicated in Fig. 3.

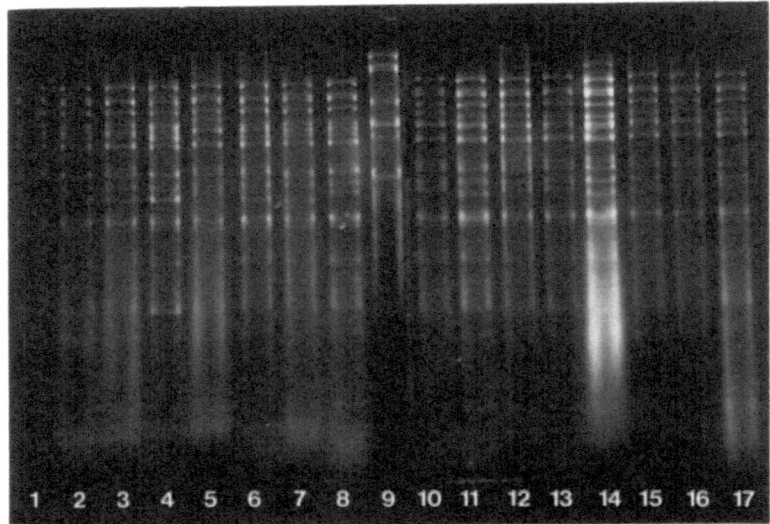

Fig. 5   DNA cleavage patterns of FHV 1 isolates after digestion with Eco R I. Arrangement of samples and conditions as in Fig. 4.

11xmore _in vitro_ than isolate 1; isolate 3 was present in a latently infected cat for 11 months before re-isolation from its trigeminal ganglia. Two other isolates, numbers 5 and 6 also have identical or very similiar DNA cleavage patterns. They derive from the same outbreak (Table 1), but isolate 6 was present in a latently infected cat for 1 year before re-isolation from its trigeminal ganglia. Isolates 7 and 8, however, which are representatives of the same virus strain, but differ only in a threefold plaque purification procedure, do not show a similiar DNA pattern (Fig. 4 and 5). They exhibit the same slight shifts in mobility of some fragments as all the other unrelated isolates. However, looking at the overall cleavage pattern, no major differences were visible between isolates from different countries, different clinical entities or from latently infected cats. It is of further interest that the attenuated strain from Northern America, which is used as vaccine shows no obvious changes in the DNA pattern compared to the wild-type European strains.

DISCUSSION

The characterization of the FHV 1 genome revealed that this virus has a low DNA GC content (approximately 50 Mol %), similiar to that of VZV DNA (46%). If the molecular weight of FHV 1 DNA (about $80x10^6$ Daltons) could be confirmed by other techniques, this would also agree with the size of VZV DNA (Dumas and Geelen, 1981). FHV 1 also shares other similiarities with this human herpesvirus, like cell association and narrow host range. Analysis of FHV 1 points to a relatively uniform structure of the genome. Whether this correlates with the relatively uniform pathogenicity of the virus and its restriction of infection only to members of the Felidae, remains to be investigated further. The comparison of a variety of strains points to a unique genomic situation in FHV 1, since in some other herpesvirus groups, like herpes simplex virus, herpesvirussaimiri and equine herpesvirus, considerably more heterogeneity has been found, when enzymes were used which cleaved approximately the same number of fragments (Lansdale et al., 1980; Desrosiers and Falk, 1982; Studdert et al., 1982). There are other herpesvirus groups which exhibit less variability in their genomes compared to the former e.g. bovine herpesviruses and pseudorabies viruses (Engels et al., 1981; Herrmann et al., 1982 this issue), but they are still more heterogeneous than FHV 1. Nevertheless one group seems to behave similiarly to FHV 1: the VZV genome; but there is only a limited amount of information on this as yet (Martin et al., 1982; Richards et al., 1979).

There is no evidence in the present study that the FHV 1 genome alters during a period of latency in the host. Both re-isolates obtained from the trigeminal ganglion explant cultures 11 and 12 months after the initial infection appeared to be virtually identical to the original infecting virus. A similiar situation has been shown for HSV in man (Lansdale et al., 1980; Buchman et al., 1980). As in HSV 1 (Buchman et al., 1980) the reference strain B927 (isolate 1) did not appear to alter on in vitro passage. However, another isolate (7) showed a visible change (8) in DNA pattern after a threefold plaque purification procedure. This may be because of heterogeneity in the original virus population.

Isolates from a variety of clinical cases, some with unusual manifestations of FHV 1 infection, were all very similar, though some slight differences both from each other and from reference strain B927 (1) were observed. However, these differences were not as marked as in some other herpesvirus infections (e.g. bovine herpesvirus 1) where differences in pathogenicity of isolates may be correlated with restriction enzyme cleavage patterns (Engels et al., 1981; Pauli et al., 1982 this issue). This is perhaps not surprising in that strains with particular tropisms do not appear to be common in FHV 1 infection, and an unusual clinical manifestation may represent a difference in the host's response rather than in the virus. It is also noteworthy that an attenuated vaccine strain (13) did not differ markedly from wild-type isolates, as compared to the quite different situation with some other herpesviruses

(Studdert et al., 1981; Herrmann et al., 1982 this issue; Martin et al., 1982).

Isolates from the three different geographical locations of Berlin, Bristol, U.K., and the U.S.A. also appeared to be very similar, showing only slight differences from each other and from the reference strain B927 (1).

In conclusion, the most outstanding finding with FHV 1 compared to other herpesviruses was the marked stability of the viral genome. The virus is known to persist as a latent infection in cat. It periodically produces severe outbreaks of disease, and is worldwide in distribution. Therefore theoritically it has the same opportunities for recombination as HSV and other herpesviruses, and these show a considerably higher genome heterogeneity. This suggests that the FHV 1 genome may have a unique structure.

REFERENCES
Bittle, J.L. and Rubic, W.J. 1975. Immunogenic and protective effects of the F2 strain of feline viral rhinotracheitis virus. Am. J. vet. Res., 21, 547-550.
Buchman, T.G., Roizman, B. and Nahmias, A.J. 1979. Demonstration of exogenous genital reinfection with herpes simplex type 2 by restriction endonuclease fingerprinting of viral DNA. J. of Inf. Diseases, 140, 295-304.
Buchman, T.G., Simpsom, T., Nosol, C., Roizman, B. and Nahmias, A.J. 1980. The structure of herpes simplex virus DNA and its application to molecular epidemiology. Ann. of the New York Acad. of Sci., 354, 279-290.
Darai, G., Lorentz, A., Kammer, K., and Munk, K. 1975. The fate of herpes simplex virus type 2 DNA during abortive infection at 42°C of human embryonic lung cells. Virology, 68, 92-104.
Davis, E.V. and Beckenhauer, W.H. 1976. Studies on the safety and efficacy of an intranasal feline rhinotracheitis-calici virus vaccine. Vet. Med. small Anim. Clin., 71, 1405-1410.
Desrosiers, R.C. and Falk, L.A. 1982. Herpesvirus saimiri strain variability. J. of Virol., 43, 352-356.
Dumas, A. and Geelen, J.L.M.C. 1981. Restriction enzyme maps of the two orientations of the varicella zoster virus. In "International Workshop on Herpesviruses" (Eds. A.S. Kaplan, M.La Placa, F. Rapp and B. Roizman) (Esculapio Publ. Co., Bologna, Italy). p.31.
Engels, M., Steck, F. and Wyler, R. 1981. Comparison of the genomes of IBR- and IPV virus strains by means of restriction enzyme analysis. Arch. Virol., 67, 169-174.
Flecknell, P.A., Orr, C.M., Wright, A.T., Gaskell, R.M. and Kelly, D.F. 1979. Skin ulceration associated with herpes

virus infection in cat. Vet. Rec. <u>104</u>, 313-315.

Gaskell, R.M.. and Povey, R.C. 1977. Experimental induction of feline viral rhinotracheitis virus re-excretion in FVR-recovered cats. Vet. Rec., <u>100</u>, 128-133.

Gaskell, R.M. and Wardley, R.C. 1978. Feline viral respiratory disease: A review with particular reference to its epizootiology and control. J. Small Anim. Pract., <u>19</u>, 1-16.

Gaskell, R.M. and Povey, R.C. 1979a. Feline viral rhinotracheitis: Sites of virus replication and persistence in acutely and persistently infected cats. Res. in Vet. Sci., <u>27</u>, 167-174.

Gaskell, R.M. and Povey, R.C. 1979b. The dose response of cats to experimental infection with feline viral rhinotracheitis virus. J. comp. Path., <u>89</u>, 179-191.

Gaskell, R.M.. and Goddard, L.E. 1982. The epizootiology of feline viral rhinotracheitis with particular reference to the nature and role of the carrier state. CEC Symposium on "Latency of Herpesviruses", Tübingen, Sept. 21-23 (this issue).

Gilden, D.H., Shtram, Y., Friedmann, A., Wellish, M., Devlin, M., Cohen, A., Fraser, N. and Becker, Y. 1982. Extraction of cell associated varicella zoster virus DNA with Triton X-100 NaCl. J. of virol. Meth., <u>4</u>, 263-275.

Hayward, G.S., Frenkel, N. and Roizman, B. 1975. Anatomy of herpes simplex DNA: Strain differences and heterogeneity in the locations of restriction endonuclease cleavage sites. Proc. Nat. Acad. Sci. USA, <u>72</u>, 1768-1772.

Herrmann, S.-C., Heppner, B. and Ludwig, H. 1982. Pseudorabies viruses from clinical outbreaks and latent infections grouped into four major genome types. CEC Symposium on "Latency of Herpesviruses", Tübingen, Sept. 21-23 (this issue).

Lonsdale, D.M., Brown, S.M., Lang, J., Subak-Sharpe, J.H., Koprowski, H. and Warren, K.G. 1980. Variations in herpes simplex virus isolated from human ganglia and a study of clonal variation in HSV 1. Ann. of the New York Acad. Sci., <u>354</u>, 291-308.

Ludwig, H. 1972. Untersuchungen am genetischen Material von Herpesviren. Microbiol. Immunol., <u>157</u>, 186-211.

Ludwig, H., Haines, H., Biswal, N. and Benyesh-Melnik, M. 1972. The characterization of varicella zoster DNA. J. gen. Virol., <u>14</u>, 111-114.

Ludwig, H., 1982. Latent reactivable bovine herpesviruses, their role and characterization. CEC Symposium on "Latency of Herpesviruses", Tübingen, Sept. 21.-23 (this issue).

Martin, J.H., Dohner, D.E., Wellinghoff, W.J. and Gelb, L.D. 1982. Restriction endonuclease analysis of varicella zoster vaccine virus and wilt-type DNAs. J. med. Virol., <u>9</u>, 69-76.

Pauli, G., Gregersen, J.-P., Storz, J. and Ludwig, H. 1982. Biology and molecular biology of latent bovine herpesvirus type 1, (BHV 1). CEC Symposium on "Latency of Herpesviruses", Tübingen, Sept. 21-23 (this issue).

Pignatti, P., Cassai, E., Meneguzzi, G., Chenciner, N. and Milanesi, G. 1979. Herpes simplex virus DNA isolation from infected cells with a novel procedure. Virology, <u>93</u>, 260-264.

Plummer, G., Goodheart, C.R., Henson, D., Bowling, C.P. 1969. A comparative study of the DNA density and behaviour in tissue cultures of fourteen different herpesviruses. Virology, <u>39</u>, 134-137.

Povey, R.C. 1979. A review of feline viral rhinotracheitis (feline herpesvirus 1 infection). Comp. Immun. Microbiol., <u>2</u>, 373-387.

Richards, J., Hyman, R.W. and Rapp, F. 1979. Analysis of the DNAs from several varicelly zoster virus isolates. J. of Virol., <u>32</u>, 812-821.

Rixon, F.J. and Ben-Porat, T. 1979. Structural evolution of the DNA of pseudorabies- defective viral particles. Virology, <u>97</u>, 151-163.

Roizman, B., Carmichael, L.E., Deinhardt, F., De-The, G., Nahmias, A.J., Plowright, W., Rapp, F., Sheldrick, P., Takahashi, M., Wolf, K. 1981. Herpesviridae. Definition, provisional nomenclature, and taxonomy. Intervirol., <u>16</u>, 201-217.

Slater, E. and York, C. 1976. Comparative studies on parenteral and intranasal inoculation of an attenuated feline herpesvirus. Devel. biol. Stand., <u>33</u>, 410-416.

Studdert, M.J., Simpson, T. and Roizman, B 1981. Differentiation of respiratory and abortigenic isolates of equine herpesvirus 1 by restriction endonucleases. Science, <u>214</u>, 562-564.

THE EPIZOOTIOLOGY OF FELINE VIRAL RHINOTRACHEITIS
WITH PARTICULAR REFERENCE OF THE NATURE AND ROLE
OF THE CARRIER STATE

R.M. Gaskell, L.E. Goddard
University of Bristol
Department of Veterinary Medicine
Langford House, Langford Bristol

ABSTRACT

Feline viral rhinotracheitis (FVR) virus, now known as felid herpesvirus 1 (FHV-1), is a major cause of feline upper respiratory tract disease. This paper reviews briefly the present state of knowledge of this virus and the clinical syndrome it produces. The epizootiology of the disease is discussed with particular emphasis on the nature and role of the carrier state. Information is presented on the interactions between vaccination and the carrier state.

INTRODUCTION

Felid herpesvirus 1 (FHV 1) is a major respiratory pathogen of cats. It was first isolated in 1957 in the USA by Crandell and Maurer (1958) and the disease, an acute, febrile syndrome, characterised by copious ocular and nasal discharges, was called feline viral rhinotracheitis (FVR) (Crandell and Despeaux, 1959). Later work confirmed that the agent was a herpesvirus (Ditchfield and Grinyer, 1965; McEwan and Miles, 1967) and in 1973 the identification felid herpesvirus I, subfamily alphaherpesvirinae, was proposed by the International Committee on Taxonomy of Viruses (Roizman et al., 1981).

THE AGENT

The morphology, physicochemical properties, cultural and other characteristics of the virus have been reviewed in some detail by Crandell (1973) and Povey (1979). Only features of the agent relevant to its epizootiology will be presented here.

FHV-1 is a comparatively labile virus, surviving for only up to 18 hours in a moist external environment at approximately 15°C, and less than 12 hours in a similar but dry environment (Povey and Johnson, 1970). As an aerosol, it is relatively unstable at midrange and higher relative humidities (Donaldson and Ferris, 1976). The virus is susceptible to the effects of heat and acid (Miller and Crandell, 1962; Johnson, 1966) and to all common disinfectants (Scott, 1980).

Both the natural and experimental host range of FHV-1 appears to be highly restricted in contrast to some other herpesviruses such as Aujeszky's disease virus or herpes simplex virus. Despite attempts to culture it in a number of laboratory animals and cell lines from various species (reviewed by Povey, 1979), in vivo it appears only to infect members of the Felidae and in vitro, apart from one unconfirmed report of adaptation to a rabbit kidney cell line (Ditchfield and Grinyer, 1965), its replication is confined to cells of feline origin. There is one report of an abortive infection in human cells pre-treated with inactivated Sendai virus (Tegtmeyer and Enders, 1969).

All FHV 1 isolates so far examined appear to be closely related antigenically on the basis of conventional serological cross-neutralisation tests (Crandell et al., 1960; Bittle et al., 1960; Johnson and Thomas, 1966); more refined serological techniques such as neutralisation kinetics or plaque reduction assays have not been used. Recent work using restriction enzyme analysis of the viral DNA has confirmed this high degree of similarity between strains (Herman et al., 1982) which, in general, is reflected in the relatively uniform biological behaviour of isolates. Nevertheless strains of modified virulence do exist, having been produced in recent years for use in vaccines (Slater and York, 1976; Davis and Beckenhauer, 1976; Bittle and Rubic, 1975). When one of these, a ts mutant, (Slater and York, 1976) was examined it also showed a similar DNA cleavage pattern to the other isolates when the major DNA fragments were compared (Herman et al., 1982). More extensive work is needed to confirm this apparent lack of heterogeneity in FHV 1.

FHV 1 is highly infectious to susceptible cats and generally produces a reasonably uniform upper respiratory tract syndrome. The natural route of infection is almost certainly intranasal, oral or conjunctival. Experimentally, the intranasal route is most commonly used, but several other routes have also been investigated (reviewed by Povey, 1979). Because of the affinity of some other herpesviruses for both respiratory and genital tracts, some attention has been given to a possible genital tract tropism for FHV 1. Bittle and Peckham (1971) showed that vaginal instillation of virus resulted in congenitally infected kittens. Transplacental infection and abortion has been demonstrated following intravenous inoculation of virus, but although abortions also occurred following the more natural intranasal route of inoculation, no virus was recovered from aborted material (Hoover and Griesemer, 1971). Thus abortion was attributed to non-specific effects of the severe debilitating upper respiratory disease and not to the effects of the virus itself.

In the typical, respiratory experimental infection, replication of FHV 1 as assessed by (1) pathological findings together with the presence of intranuclear inclusion bodies, and (2) the occurrence of maximal virus titres in tissues, takes place predominantly in the mucosae of the nasal septum, turbinates, nasopharynx and tonsils; other tissues including conjunctivae, mandibular lymph nodes and upper trachea are also often involved (Crandell et al., 1961; Gaskell and Povey, 1979a). A viraemia has only rarely been reported (Bürki et al., 1964; Hoover at al., 1970; Gaskell and Povey, 1979a).

THE CLINICAL SYNDROME

FHV 1 produces a characteristic syndrome in susceptible cats (Crandell et al., 1961; Bürki et al., 1964; Gaskell and Povey, 1979b). The incubation period is usually 2-6 days, but may be longer. Experimentally it has been shown that increasing virus dosage (from 10^2 to 10^7 $TCID_{50}$) is significantly correlated with a shortening of the incubation period and to some extent with the severity of clinical signs (Gaskell and Povey, 1979b), but in general, the syndrome is reasonably uniform.

Early signs of the disease include depression, marked

sneezing and clear ocular and nasal discharges. There is
usually fever (39.5°C) and loss of appetite. As the disease
progresses, the discharges gradually turn muco-purulent.
Conjunctivitis, hypersalivation, and sometimes dyspnoea and
coughing may develop, and there may be a recurrence of th
pyrexia. A leucocytosis with a left shift is present throughout
the course of the disease. The majority of clinical signs has
usually resolved in 10-20 days but some animals may be left
with chronic sequelae. Mortality may be high in very young or
debilitated cats. Other signs seen less commonly include tongue
ulcers and ulcerative and interstitial keratitis (Karpas and
Routledge, 1968; Bistner et al., 1971). Generalised disease may
also occasionally occur, particularly in younger animals
(Gaskell and Wardley, 1978): other rarer manifestations such as
skin ulcers and nervous signs, have also been reviewed by
Gaskell and Wardley, together with a discussion of various
factors which on some occasions may account for variations in
the host's response.

MAINTENANCE OF THE VIRUSES IN THE POPULATION
     FHV 1 is a highly successful virus in cats. It is worldwide
in distribution (Crandell, 1973) and together with feline
calicivirus, accounts for the majority of cases of feline
respiratory disease (Kahn and Hoover, 1976; Gaskell and
Wardley, 1978). Clinically, it is the most significant of the
feline respiratory pathogens. Serological surveys prior to
vaccination demonstrated serum neutralising antibody titres in
26-70% of cats, depending on the nature of the sample
population (Studdert and Martin, 1970; Povey and Johnson, 1971;
Ellis, 1981); in general, infection is less common in isolated
household pets than in colony animals. Thus in cats, FHV 1 has
filled the respiratory ecological niche which in many species
is filled by a number of other virus families.
     FHV 1 is relatively fragile and short-lived in the external
environment. Thus outside the cat it probably only persists
long enough for indirect transmission to occur within the
closed confines of a cattery. It has no known reservoir or

alternative hosts. Therefore like many herpesviruses it must rely for its continued survival on its ability to persist in the host, such persistence being achieved firstly, by continuous horizontal spread from the acute case to susceptible cat, and secondly, by means of carriers.

The FHV 1 carrier state is characterised by a latent phase with only intermittent episodes of virus shedding (Gaskell and Povey, 1973; 1977). In the latent phase, virus is undetectable by normal sampling techniques, but during re-excretion episodes, virus is present in oro-pharyngeal secretions and the cats are infectious to other cats (Gaskell and Povey, 1982). As with other herpesvirus carrier states there is no evidence that the carrier state is self-limiting (Gaskell, 1975).

Re-excretion may occur spontaneously, but is most likely to occur following stress. Experimentally in a group of 33 FVR-recovered cats it was shown that a change of housing induced virus shedding in four (18%) of 22 individuals on six (15%) of 40 occasions; corticosteroid in 22 (69%) of 32 cats on 31 (54%) of 57 occasions; and during lactation there was a marginally increase shedding rate (40% of a group of 10 queens experienced an episode of shedding within 10 weeks post-partum) (Gaskell and Povey, 1973; 1977). Climatic stress appeared to be ineffective at inducing re-excretion. The apparently spontaneous shedding rate in the 33 cats over a mean period of 8.8 months was 0.9% on any one day. In these studies, a total of 82% of the FVR-recovered cats shed endogenous virus on at least one occasion, and 45% shed virus spontaneously or under natural "stress" conditions and could thus be considered to be epidemiologically important. Similar findings on the FHV 1 carrier state have been reported by Ellis (1981).

Experimentally a lag period occurred before onset of virus shedding from 4-11 days (mean 7.2) after corticosteroid treatment and from 4-10 days (mean 7.2) after re-housing (Gaskell and Povey, 1973; 1977). The duration of virus shedding ranged from 1-13 days (mean 6.5) after corticosteroid and 4-9 days (mean 7.2) after re-housing. In some cases (72% following corticosteroid stress, 30% following re-housing) shedding was

accompanied by recrudescence of mild clinical signs, though
occasionally signs were seen in carriers unassociated with
detectable episodes of re-excretion.

It appeared that there was a refractory period following an
episode of corticosteroid induced re-excretion during which
further administration of corticosteroid was less effective
(Gaskell and Povey, 1977). Cats which did re-excrete as a
result of treatment had last shed virus on an average of 16
weeks before, whereas cats which did not re-excrete had
experienced their last episode of virus shedding on an average
of only eight weeks before (p 0.01). Considerable variation
was apparent however, both within and between individuals.

In the field situation, surveys of clinically normal cats
have shown an apparently spontaneous shedding rate of 1-2%
(Wardley et al., 1974; Ellis, 1981); in Ellis' study only 26%
of the cats sampled had FHV 1 antibody but their shedding rate
may have been increased by having been brought to a cat refuge.
Gaskell (1975) recorded FHV 1 re-excretion in 3(4%) of 75 cats
9-12 days after entering a boarding cattery.

Possible sites of latency with particular emphasis on a
possible neural site, have been investigated by Plummer (1973)
and Gaskell and Povey (1979a). Plummer was unsuccessful in
attempts to isolate FHV 1 from the trigeminal ganglia of at
least 10 FVR-recovered cats, despite successfully isolating
herpesviruses from human and monkey trigeminal ganglia using
similar coculture techniques. Gaskell and Povey examined the
trigeminal ganglia by explant or coculture technique, and a
range of other tissues mainly by tissue homogenisation in 20
non-stressed latently infected FVR-recovered cats. None yielded
virus except the turbinates and trigeminal ganglia culture of
one cat spontaneously shedding virus at the time it died. Virus
was isolated from the ganglia at 15 days and again at 47 days
after initiation. Attempts to repeat this observation by
examining tissues from 17 cats killed sequentially and induced
to shed by corticosteroid or re-housing, yielded virus in
turbinates and in some cases other oro-pharyngeal tissues, but
not in trigeminal ganglia. Virus was recovered by coculture

from the olfactory bulbs and tracts of one of four cats
however. This is interesting in view of the proximity of these
tissues to and their association with the turbinates, and also
because pathological changes have been recorded here in the
acute stages of the disease (Hoover et al., 1970). In addition,
olfactory spread has been shown as well as spread via the
trigeminal system in experimental HSV infection in mice
(Johnson, 1964; Baringer, 1975).

The implications of this work were discussed by Gaskell and
Povey (1979a) but, in the meantime, more studies are needed to
confirm the importance of a possible neural site of latency for
FVR, possibly with the use of more sophisticated techniques
such as in situ DNA hybridisation. In addition, it may be
possible to enhance isolation of the virus from trigeminal
ganglia cultures by slightly altering the culture technique:
minor differences have been shown to influence the recovery
rate in other systems (Warren and Lewis, 1981). In our original
studies the explant method of Baringer and Swoveland (1973) was
used, but more recently we have isolated virus from the
trigeminal ganglia of one latently infected FVR-recovered cat
by a modification of the method of Harbour et al. (1981). This
work is being continued.

TRANSMISSION AND THE SIGNIFICANCE OF THE CARRIER

The major method of spread of FHV 1 is by direct cat-to-cat
contact. During the acute stage of the disease, titres of up to
$10^{6.8}$ (mean 10^4) $TCID_{50}$ of virus are shed per ml of
oropharyngeal, nasal and conjunctival secretions for a period
of 1-3 weeks; during re-excretion episodes from carriers,
levels shed are generally lower (p 0.01), up to $10^{5.8}$ (mean
$10^{3.1}$) $TCID_{50}$ per ml for 1-13 days (Gaskell, 1975).
Experimentally titres of from 10^2 - 10^7 $TCID_{50}$ inclusive have
been shown to be infective (whereas 10 $TCID_{50}$ was not),
transmission being achieved by macrodroplet instillation of the
virus onto the mucosa of the upper respiratory tract (Gaskell
and Povey, 1979b). Cats have also been infected by the aerosol
route (Bartholomew and Gillespie, 1968) but this is probably

not an important natural route for there is some evidence that
the cat does not produce an infectious aerosol of either FHV 1
or feline calicivirus during normal respiratory movements
(Wardley and Povey, 1976; Gaskell and Povey, 1982). Thus under
field conditions most infections are probably the result of
direct cat to cat contact through infectious discharges and
sneezed macrodroplets. The distance through which sneezed
droplets can be carried is not known but in relatively still
air it appears they may reach a distance of 1.2m (Povey and
Johnson, 1970).

Indirect or fomite transmission via a contaminated
environment, personnel, or feeding and cleaning utensils may
also occur and is probably an important route of transmission
where groups of cats are housed together. However, in view of
the fragility of FHV 1 ouside the cat, indirect sources of
virus are unlikely to be of long term importance in the
transmission of the disease. Other factors that influence the
survival of FHV 1 in the external environment, and hence
indirectly affect the efficacy of transmission, include
temperature, relative humidity and ventilation (Povey and
Johnson, 1970).

It is likely that under natural conditions the efficacy of
cat-to-cat transmission of the virus will depend on both the
amount of virus being shed by the infecting animal and on the
duration and intimacy of contact of the susceptible animal with
the infected secretions. Therefore it might be expected that
virus might be more readily transmitted by cats in the acute
stage of the disease where the discharges are usually more
copious and in slightly higher titre, than by shedding
carriers. Thus it has been shown that although cross-infection
from acutely infected to susceptible cats may be readily
achieved (Horváth et al., 1965; Povey and Johnson, 1967;
Bartholomew and Gillespie, 1968), under experimental
conditions, fairly intimate contact of several days duration
appears to be necessary before successful transmission may
occur from a shedding carrier to an unrelated susceptible
individual (Gaskell and Povey, 1982). Thus in cages 2m x 0.75m^2

or larger, transmission was not achieved, but in cages of
0.7m x 0.9m x 0.6m it was.

Under more natural conditions, however, it is likely that
the greatest importance of the carrier lies in its ability to
transmit the virus within the close contact of family groups,
thus enabling it to perpetuate the virus-host relationship into
the next generation. Thus we looked at the transmission of
FHV 1 virus from carrier queens to their kittens (Gaskell and
Povey, 1982). In the 10 week post-partum period, the shedding
rate from queens did appear to be marginally increased above
the spontaneous rate: four of 10 queens re-excreted virus, and
four kittens from three litters developed a contact infection.
None showed clinical signs, and were presumably infected under
cover of passive immunity. Two shed virus transiently for one
day only and did not become carriers (as evidenced by
corticostoid treatment) and two shed virus for 15 and 25 days
and were subsequently shown to have become carriers; their SN
antibody titres rising from <1 in 4 and 1 in 8 prior to
re-excretion, to 1 in 96 and 1 in 128 after. The establishment
of a latent carrier state under cover of passive immunity in
animals which then become sero-negative, has also been shown
for HSV 1 infection in mice (Sekizawa et al., 1980).

From other studies it appears that there are many cases
where carrier queens shed virus either when their own or when
other kittens is close contact are unprotected by maternal
antibody, and cases of acute disease result (Povey and Johnson,
1967; Crandell, 1971). In general, however, this is not a good
method for the virus to perpetuate itself in its host as
mortality in young kittens can be high. The findings outlined
above, however, show that on some occasions at least, the cat
has an ideal method of perpetuating a balanced virus-host
relationship which does not depend on the development of
clinical disease. This then leads to the establishment in the
next generation of the latent carrier state, so that the cycle
is complete.

VACCINATION AND THE CARRIER STATE

Since the advent of vaccination against FVR, in the UK
seven years ago, it was pertinent to determine if vaccinated
animals were protected against infection or just against the
disease, and therefore whether such vaccinated animals could
still be epidemiologically important. In a limited study using
a modified live systemic vaccine, it was shown that all four
vaccinated cats replicated field virus following challenge, and
one of these was subsequently shown to have become a latent
carrier. Virus re-isolated from this animal following
corticosteroid treatment induced FVR in a susceptible cat (Orr
et al., 1978). In similar studies with an intranasal vaccine,
it appeared that there was little or no virus replication
following challenge and no animals appeared to have become
carriers (Orr et al., 1980). Thus in the short term, at least,
and in this small group (8) of animals, this vaccine appeared
to protect cats against the development of a field virus
carrier state. More work is needed to elucidate vaccine/carrier
state interactions.

REFERENCES

Baringer, J.R. 1975. Herpes simplex virus infection of nervous
    tissue in animals and man. In "Progress in Medical
    Virology" 20 (Ed. J.L. Melnick). (S. Karger, Basel) pp.
    1-26.
Baringer, J.R. and Swoveland, P. 1973. Recovery of herpes
    simplex virus from human trigeminal ganglions. New Engl. J.
    Med. 288, 648-650.
Bartholomew, P.T. and Gillespie, J.H. 1968. Feline viruses. 1.
    Characterisation of four isolates and their effect on young
    kittens. Cornell vet. 58, 248-265.
Bistner, S.K., Carlson, J.H., Shively, J.N. and Scott, F.W.
    1971. Ocular manifestations of feline herpesvirus
    infection. J. Am. vet. med. Ass. 159, 1223-1237.
Bittle, J.L. and Peckham, J.C. 1971. Comments: genital
    infection induced by feline rhinotracheitis virus and
    effects on newborn kittens. J. Am.. vet. med. Ass. 158,
    927-928.
Bittle, J.L. and Rubic, W.J. 1975. Immunogenic and protective
    effects of the F2 strain of feline viral rhinotracheitis
    virus. Am. J. vet. Res. 36, 89-91.
Bittle, J.L., York, C.J., Newberne, J.W. and Martin, M. 1960.
    Serologic relationship of new feline cytopathogenic
    viruses. Am. J. vet. Res. 21, 547-550.
Bürki, F. Lindt, S. and Frendiger, U. 1964. Enzootischer,

virusbedingter Katzenschnupfen in einem Tierheim.
Mitteilung: Virologischer und experimenteller Teil. Zbl.
Vet.-Med. 11B, 110-118.
Crandell, R.A. 1971. Virologic and immunologic aspects of
feline viral rhinotracheitis virus. J. Am. vet. Med. Ass.
158, 922-926.
Crandell, R.A. 1973. Feline viral rhinotracheitis (FVR). Adv.
vet. Sci. comp. Med. 17, 201-224.
Crandell, R.A. and Maurer, F.D. 1958. Isolation of a feline
virus associated with intranuclear inclusion bodies. Proc.
Soc. exp. Biol. Med. 97, 487-490.
Crandell, R.A. and Despeaux, E.W. 1959. Cytopathology of feline
viral rhinotracheitis virus in tissue cultures of feline
renal cells. Proc. Soc. exp. Biol. Med. 101, 494-497.
Crandell, R.A., Ganaway, J.R., Niemann, W.H. and Maurer, F.D.
1960. Comparative study of three isolates with the original
feline viral rhinotracheitis virus. Am. J. vet. Res. 21,
504-506.
Crandell, R.A., Rehkemper, J.A., Neumann, W.H., Ganaway, J.R.
and Maurer, F.D. 1961. Experimental feline viral
rhinotracheitis. J.Am. vet. med. Ass. 138, 191-196.
Davis, E.V. and Beckenhauer, W.H. 1976. Studies on the safety
and efficacy of an intranasal feline rhinotracheitis -
calici virus vaccine. Vet. Med. small Anim. Clin. 71,
1405-1410.
Ditchfield, J. and Grinyer, I. 1965. Feline rhinotracheitis
virus: a feline herpesvirus. Virology 26, 504-506.
Donaldson, A.I. and Ferris, N.P. 1976. The survival of some
air-borne animal viruses in relation to relative humidity.
Vet. Microbiol. 1, 413-420.
Ellis, T.M. 1981. Feline respiratory virus carriers in
clinically healthy cats. Austr. vet. J. 57, 115-118.
Gaskell, R.M. 1975. Studies on feline viral rhinotracheitis
with particular reference to the carrier state. Ph.D.
Thesis, University of Bristol.
Gaskell, R.M. and Povey, R.C. 1973. Re-excretion of feline
viral rhinotracheitis virus following corticosteroid
treatment. Vet. Rec. 93, 204-205.
Gaskell, R.M. and Povey, R.C. 1977. Experimental induction of
feline viral rhinotracheitis virus re-excretion in
FVR-recovered cats. Vet. Rec. 100, 128-133.
Gaskell, R.M. and Povey, R.C. 1979a. Feline viral
rhinotracheitis: sites of virus replication and persistence
in acutely and persistently infected cats. Res. vet. Sci.
27, 167-174.
Gaskell, R.M. and Povey, R.C. 1979b. The dose response of cats
to experimental infection with feline viral rhinotracheitis
virus. J. Comp. Path. 89, 179-191.
Gaskell, R.M. and Povey, R.C. 1982. The transmission of feline
viral rhinotracheitis. Vet. Rec. in press.
Gaskell, R.M. and Wardley, R.C. 1978. Feline viral respiratory
disease: a review with particular reference to its
epizootiology and control. J. small Anim. Pract. 19, 1-16.
Harbour, D.A., Hill, T.J. and Blyth, W.A. 1981. Acute and
recurrent herpes simplex in several strains of mice. J.
gen. Virol. 55, 31-40.

Hermann, S., Gaskell, R.M., Ehlers, B. and Ludwig, H. 1982. Molecular epidemiology of latent herpesvirus felinis (This volume).

Hoover, E.A. and Griesemer, R.A. 1971. Experimental feline herpesvirus infection in the pregnant cat. Am. J. Path. 65, 173-188.

Hoover, E.A., Rohousky, M.W. and Griesemer R.A. 1970. Experimental feline viral rhinotracheitis in the germfree cat. Am. J. Path. 58, 269-282.

Horváth, Z., Bartha, A., Papp, L. and Juhász, M. 1965. On feline rhinotracheitis. Acta vet. Acad. Sci. hung. 15, 415-420.

Johnson, R.H. 1966. Feline panleucopaenia virus III. Some properties compared to a feline herpesvirus. Res. vet. Sci. 7, 112-115.

Johnson, R.H. and Thomas, R.G. 1966. Feline viral rhinotracheitis in Britain. Vet. Rec. 79, 188-190.

Johnson, R.T. 1964. The pathogenesis of herpesvirus encephalitis. I. Virus pathways to the nervous system of suckling mice demonstrated by fluorescent antibody staining. J. exp. Med. 119, 343-356.

Kahn, D.E. and Hoover, E.A. 1976. Infectious respiratory diseases of cats. Vet. Clins. N. American. 6, (3) 399-413.

Karpas, A. and Routledge, J.K. 1968. Feline herpesvirus: isolations and experimental studies. Zbl. Vet.-Med. 15, 599-606.

McEwan, P.J. and Miles, J.A.R. 1967. An electron microscope study of viruses associated with upper respiratory tract infections in cats. Proc. Univ. Otago med. Sch. 45, (2), 21-23.

Miller, G.W. and Crandell, R.A. 1962. Stability of the virus of feline viral rhinotracheitis. Am. J. vet. Res. 23, 351-353.

Orr, C.M., Gaskell, C.J. and Gaskell, R.M. 1978. Interaction of a combined feline viral rhinotracheitis - feline calicivirus vaccine and the FVR carrier state. Vet. Rec. 103, 200-202.

Orr, C.M., Gaskell, C.J. and Gaskell, R.M. 1980. Interaction of an intranasal combined feline viral rhinotracheitis, feline calicivirus vaccine and the FVR carrier state. Vet. Rec. 106, 164-166.

Plummer, G. 1973. Isolation of herpesviruses from trigeminal ganglia of man, monkeys and cats. J. infect. Dis. 128, 345-348.

Povey, R.C. 1979. A review of feline viral rhinotracheitis (feline herpesvirus 1 infection). Comp. Immun. Microbiol. infect. Dis. 2, 373-387.

Povey, R.C. and Johnson, R.H. 1967. Further observations on feline viral rhinotracheitis. Vet. Rec. 81, 686-689.

Povey, R.C. and Johnson, R.H. 1970. Observations on the epidemiology and control of viral respiratory disease in cats. J. small. Anim. Pract. 11, 485-494.

Povey, R.C. and Johnson, R.H. 1971. A survey of feline viral rhinotracheitis and feline picornavirus infection in Britain. J. small Anim. Pract. 12, 233-247.

Roizman, B., Carmichael, L.E., Deinhardt, F., de The, G., Nahmias, A.J., Plowright, W., Rapp, F., Sheldrick, P.,

Takahashi, M. and Wolf, K. 1981. Herpesviridae. Definition, provisional nomenclature, and taxonomy. Intervirol. 16, 201-217.

Sekizawa, T., Openshaw, H., Wohlenberg, C. and Notkins, A.L. 1980. Latency of herpes simplex virus in absence of neutralising antibody: model for reactivation. Science 210, 1026-1028.

Scott, F.W. 1980. Viricidal disinfectants and feline viruses. Am. J. vet. Res. 41, 410-414.

Slater, E. and York, C. 1976. Comparative studies on parenteral and intranasal inoculation of an attenuated feline herpesvirus. Devel. biol. Stand. 33, 410-416.

Studdert, M.J. and Martin, M.C. 1970. Virus diseases of the respiratory tract of cats. I. Isolation of feline rhinotracheitis virus. Austr. vet. J. 46, 99-105.

Tegtmeyer, P. and Enders, J.F. 1969. Feline herpesvirus infection in fused cultures of naturally resistant human cells. J. Virol. 3, 469-476.

Wardley, R.C., Gaskell, R.M. and Povey, R.C. 1974. Feline respiratory viruses: their prevalence in clinically healthy cats. J. small Anim. Pract. 15, 579-586.

Wardley, R.C. and Povey, R.C. 1976. Aerosol transmission of feline calici-viruses. An assessment of its epidemiological importance. Br. vet. J. 133, 504-508.

Warren, K.G. and Lewis, M.E. 1981. Rate of recovery of herpes simplex virus from human trigeminal ganglion explantation monolayers. In "International Workshop on Herpesviruses" (Eds. A.S. Kaplan, M. La Placa, F. Rapp, and B. Roizman) (Esculapio Publ. Co., Bologna, Italy). p.159.

IMMUNITY TO FELID HERPESVIRUS 1

A review and report on recent work

L.E. Goddard*, R.M. Gaskell*, C.J. Gaskell*,

R.C. Wardley**

*Department of Veterinary Medicine, University of Bristol,
Langford, Bristol, England
**Animal Virus Research Institute,
Pirbright, Woking, Surrey, England

ABSTRACT

Felid herpesvirus 1 (FHV 1) shares many epidemiological
characteristics with other alphaherpesviruses. Control of
these diseases in vivo relies on complex interactions between
components of both specific and non-specific immunity. This
paper briefly reviews anti-herpesvirus immune mechanisms in
general, and then describes current knowledge on immunity to
FHV 1. Preliminary investigations of the ability of antibody
and complement to lyse infected cells, and the use of a
lymphocyte transformation test are described.

INTRODUCTION

Felid herpesvirus 1 (FHV 1) is an alphaherpesvirus of

cats causing a severe upper respiratory disease. Its

epidemiology and carrier state have been described elsewhere

(R.M.Gaskell, this volume), and it is apparent that many

characteristics of this host/virus relationship are similar to

those of other alphaherpesviruses (such as herpes simplex

virus (HSV), bovid herpesvirus 1 (BHV1), Aujeszky's disease

virus and varicella-zoster virus (VZV)). Irrespective of

whether herpesvirus latency is a static, or a dynamic state

(Roizman, 1965), it is the shedding of infectious virus,

whether symptomatic or not, which is of clinical and

epidemiological importance. Thus once shedding, or increased

shedding, has been stimulated, it is the immune system's task

to contain the virus in a "safe" state. From this it follows

that studies of anti-herpesvirus immunity are of critical

importance in the control of these diseases.

ANTI-HERPESVIRUS IMMUNE MECHANISMS

Mechanisms of anti-herpesvirus immunity, and their

relative importance in both the acute phase of infection and

in the control of latency have been reviewed in some detail by
Rouse and Babiuk (1978), Babiuk and Rouse (1979) and Shore and
Feorino (1981). A number of non-specific immune mechanisms are
of great importance in resisting disease, especially in the
non-immune host. Different cell types may vary in their degree
of permissiveness for herpesvirus replication both within and
between individuals, and thus could influence the
establishment of disease. Macrophages have been shown to play
a crucial role in herpesvirus resistance. Their state of
permissiveness for virus replication and many functions may
vary with the age of the animal (Hirch et al., 1970; Lopez and
Dudas, 1979; Stanwick et al., 1980) and also upon infection
(Forman and Babiuk, 1982). Similarly, the polymorphonuclear
leukocyte (PMN) is emerging as an important effector. Bovine
PMN can secrete an interferon-like mediator in response to
stimulation by herpesvirus (Rouse et al., 1980) and
complement-dependent neutrophil cytotoxicity has been shown to
lyse BHV 1 infected cells (Grewal, Rouse and Babiuk, 1980).
Both PMN and macrophages can interact with the components of
the specific immune system to give greatly enhanced
anti-herpesvirus effects.

Natural killing of HSV targets has been reported (Ching
and Lopez, 1979; Kohl et al., 1981) but Campos et al., (1982)
could not demonstrate NK activity in a bovine system against
BHV 1 using peripheral blood mononuclear cells, although lung
lavage cells were reported to be successful.

Initially, specific herpesvirus immune status was
measured by serumneutralising antibody (SN Ab) titres,
although the role of this alone in controlling disease has
long been controversial (reviewed by Rouse and Babiuk, 1978).
Consequently many other components of the immune system have
been studied both in isolation and in various combinations, in
an attempt fo define the anti-herpesvirus immune response.

In the acute disease particularly, the cell-mediated
immune system (CMI) has come to be regarded as highly
important and CMI assays have been shown to become positive
earlier in the acute disease than Sn Ab (Davies and

Carmichael, 1973; Rouse and Babiuk, 1974 and 1975), although recently more sensitive techniques for antibody detection such as radioimmuno assay and Antibody-Dependent Cell-Mediated Cytotoxicity (ADCC) assay have shown earlier antibody' development (Kohl et al., 1981). Direct T cell killing has been demonstrated for HSV (Pfizenmaier et al., 1977; Eberle et al., 1981) and is subject to genetic restriction. Interferons and other lymphokines produced from sensitized T cells enhance both specific and non-specific immune mechanisms (Babiuk and Rouse, 1978).

Antibody dependent mechanisms are most likely to be of importance in the control of latent infection, where antibody (Ab) is already present. Antibody and complement-mediated lysis and ADCC, with or without facilitation by complement, have been demonstrated (Rouse et al., 1976, 1977; Shore et al., 1976), the latter operating especially at low antibody levels (as in the early stages of disease).

Attempts to correlate changes in immunological parameters with recrudescent disease have produced conflicting results (Davies and Carmichael, 1973; Rasmussen, 1974; Russell, 1974; Sørensen et al., 1980; Starr et al., 1975; Thong et al., 1975; Wilton et al., 1972). With increasing study, the interaction, at least in vitro, between all these mechanisms and especially between specific and non-specific types is becoming increasingly apparent.

IMMUNITY TO FHV 1

Several workers have studied the SN Ab response of cats after exposure to FHV 1 (Povey and Johnson, 1967; Walton, 1968; Walton and Gillespie, 1970). Results of this early work indicated that immunity in recovered cats was not necessarily associated with detectable SN Ab, and that furthermore seroconversion could occasionally occur in the absence of disease. Gaskell and Povey (1979) showed that 40% of cats were seropositive by 20 days after infection, 73% by 40 days, and that seroconversion tended to coincide with cessation of virus shedding. Two cats had undetectable titres again by 52 days, and in contrast, one cat did not seroconvert until after a corticosteroid-induced episode of FHV 1 recrudescence. Thus cats may occasionally develop latent infections in the absence of detectable SN Ab. Mean SN Ab titres in cats after primary infection were low with a mean titre of 1 in 12.4 (range 1 in 4-1 in 64). Gaskell (1975) demonstrated that, after the initial episode of recrudescence, a significant rise in SN Ab titre occurred in 19 of 23 cats. Interesting parallels exist between this situation and the rapid HSV latency mouse model of Sekizawa et al., (1981) where development of SN Ab in seronegative carriers was used to detect recrudescence. Once FHV 1 antibody levels were high, titres tended to be relatively constant in carriers even in the absence of virus shedding and subsequent recurdescences did not consistently raise the titre. SN Ab titres rarely exceeded 1 in 256 and the maximum recorded was 1 in 1024. A similar situation exists with persistent HSV infection in man (Lopez and O'Reilly, 1977).

Immune assays based on haemagglutination inhibition (Gillespie et al., 1971; Mochizuki et al., 1979a, b, c), Immunodiffusion (Tan and Miles, 1971), and complement fixation (Tan, 1970) have been described for FHV 1, but none have been used routinely for assessment of FHV 1 immune status. Wardley et al., (1976) described a preliminary investigation of the likely efficiency of Ab-complement-mediated lysis, ADCC and direct cytotoxicity in limiting the spread of FHV 1 in vitro. Four FHV recovered cats were shown to perform the first two of these functions, although only some cats on some occasions performed direct cytotoxicity. It is possible that genetic restriction between effectors of direct cytotoxicity and targets confused this situation, or that a natural killing phenomenon was involved. ADCC and Ab-complement lysis operated from about the time of infectious intracellular virus production and spread by the intra-cellular route, and thus may be important in limiting virus spread. The ADCC effector was thought to be a lymphoid cell, although macrophages could also mediate it.

The direct lymphocyte-mediated killing operated from the time of extra-cellular virus appearance, and thus was less likely to be capable of limiting virus spread.

APPLICATION OF ANTIBODY AND COMPLEMENT-MEDIATED LYSIS AND LYMPHOCYTE TRANSFORMATION ASSAYS TO A FHV 1 SYSTEM

Current work aims to extend this in vitro approach to studies of the latently infected carrier cat using assays of Ab-complement lysis, lymphocyte transformation (LT), ADCC, T cell killing in authochthonous systems and natural killing.

MATERIALS AND METHODS

A local FHV 1 isolate (GB $P_7$9 was used at the 7th passage grown in Crandell Feline Foetal Kidney Cells (Cr FK, Passages 120-150) and cultured in Eagle's MEM (Wellcome) supplemented with 4% heat-inactivated foetal calf serum, antibiotics and $NaHCO_3$. Feline complement consisted of fresh cat serum stored at -70°C, and FHV 1 antiserum was pooled (heat inactivated) serum from FHV recovered cats.

Antibody-complement lysis assay

The method of Wardley et al. (1976) was adapted, using a 2-hour incubation with previously determined optimal concentrations of feline complement (50 ml) and FHV 1 antiserum (100 ml). Briefly, confluent Cr FK monolayers about 2×10^6/dish were infected at a multiplicity of 1, and at 17 hours pi were labelled with 80 μ Ci $Na^{51}_2CrO_4$ (Amersham International Ltd.) for one hour. Targets were harvested and suspended at 2×10^5/ml in MEM. 100 μl of targets were incubated with antiserum and complement as described above. Controls included complement alone, antiserum alone and uninfected targets. At the end of incubation, 100 μl aliquots were counted for radioactive release and results expressed as % specific lysis =

$$\frac{\text{test cpm - background cpm}}{\text{total cpm - background cpm}} \times 100\%$$

Lymphocyte transformation assay

Culture medium was removed from FHV 1 infected Cr FK, and monolayers were U.V.-irradiated to inactivate infectious virus. Whole cells were resuspended at a previously determined suitable concentration of 1.2×10^5/ml in RPMI 1640 medium (Flow Laboratories), supplemented with 10% foetal calf serum, 476 mg HEPES, 2.0g $NaHCO_3$, and 300 mg L-glutamine per litre plus antibiotics. Antigen was stored at -70°C. Control antigen consisted of uninfected CrFK treated as above. Concanavalin A (Sigma No. C-2020) was used at 10 µg/well. Whole heparinized blood was diluted 1:20 in RPMI medium. 150 µl were then incubated with 50 µl of Con A (3 days), or FHV antigen (7 days) in 96 well round bottom microculture plates (Nunclon). Controls included medium only and uninfected cell antigen. Plates were pulsed with 0.5 µ Ci tritiated thymidine (Amersham International Ltd.) in 50 µl RPMI for 6 hours after the end of incubation and harvested on a Skatron automatic cell harvester. Paper discs were immersed in Scintran Cocktail T (BDH) and ß emissions counted. Stimulation ratios were calculated as SR =

$$\frac{test\ cpm}{control\ cpm}.$$

RESULTS AND CONCLUSIONS
In vitro virus - host system

Fig. 1 shows a single step growth curve for GB P_7 in CR FK cells. Infectious intracellular virus titres began to rise at 8-9 hours pi, and the extracellular release of virus commenced about 4 hours later. Spread of virus by the intracellular route, as shown by an infectious centre assay, occurred at 8-9 hours pi.

Antibody and complement-mediated lysis

Complement activity was rapidly diluted out and abolished by the heat inactivation of Factor B at 50°C, for 20 minutes (Fig. 2), indicating involvement of the alternative pathway of complement activation. Targets first became susceptible to

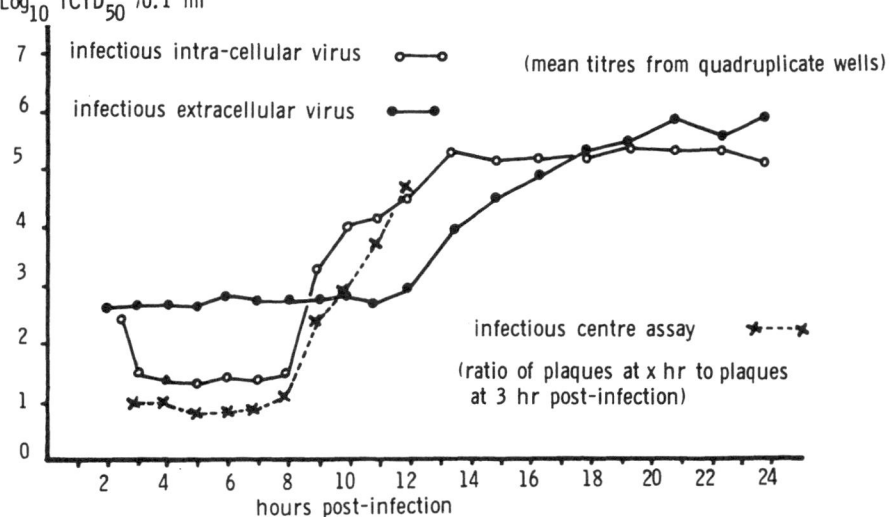

Fig. 1   One-step growth curve for GBP$_7$ isolate of FHV-1 in Crandell Foetal Kidney Cells.

lysis at 7-8 hours pi (8 hour lysis increase significant at p 0.01), (Fig. 3) which was one hour before virus spread began, and thus this mechanism could be useful in limiting FHV 1 in cats with pre-existing Ab titres. This data confirms the observations of Wardley et al. (1976).

Lymphocyte transformation

Stimulation ratois increased with time post infection of antigen, peaking at 11 hours pi, which was one hour before extracellular release of virus, and increased with the number of days of culture. The 11 hour antigen and a 7-day culture time were routinely used. Mean SR of 9 FHV 1 recovered cats were 21.7 $\pm$ 14.4 SD (range 5.3-48.7) and was concistently less than 1.5 for 9 non-FHV 1 exposed cats.

Studies in FHV recovered cats

It is intended to subject FHV 1 recovered cats (82% of which will be carriers - Gaskell and Povey, 1977) to natural stresses known to provoke recrudescence of the latent virus, and to observe these and other immune parameters sequentially.

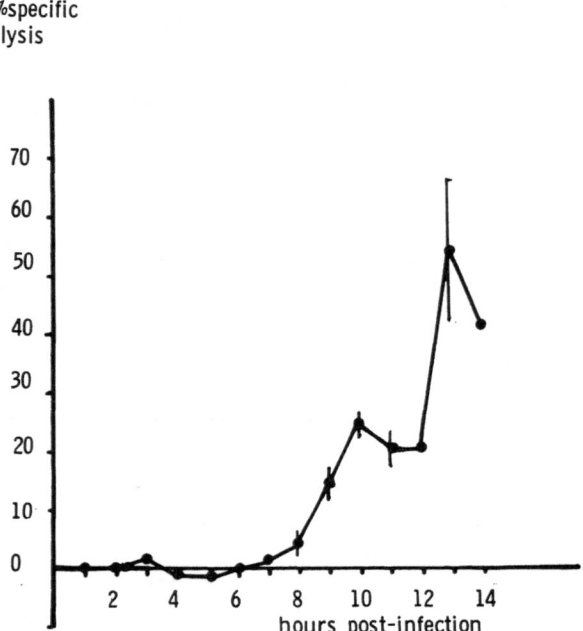

means (n=4) ± 1SD

%specific
lysis

Fig. 2   Variation of antibody complement lysis with
dilution of complement, and inactivation of complement at
50°C for 20 minutes.

One such stress is rehousing, shown to induce recrudescence of
FHV 1 in 18% of cats on 15% of occasions. (Gaskell and Povey,
1977). A group of 20 FHV-recovered cats are under study. To
date 4 cats have been rehoused in isolation, but no detectable
virus shedding occurred. No distinct changes in lymphocyte
transformation in response to Con A or FHV 1 antigen were
observed in the 7 days prior to stress, or during the
subsequent 21 days. Investigations of this and other immune
parameters in recrudescent FHV 1 infection continue.

Such sequential studies in the cat are severely limited
by its relatively small blood volume (especially for assays of
CMI activity requiring isolated leukocytes). However, the cat
provides a useful model of a herpesvirus infection in the
natural host, with a well characterized carrier state

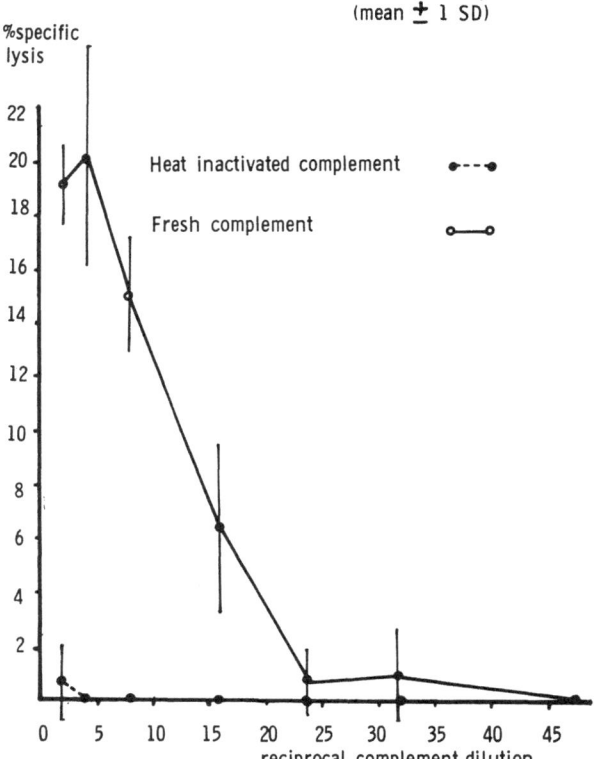

Fig. 3   Variation of antibody complement lysis with
dilution of complement, and inactivation of complement at
50°C for 20 minutes.

epidemiology, and future immunological studies should
contribute to the wider understanding of the interaction
between alphaherpesvirus and host.

REFERENCES
Babiuk, L.A. and Rouse, B.T. 1979. Immune control of
    herpesvirus latency. Can. J. Microbiol. 25, 267-274.
Babiuk, L.A. and Rouse, B.T. 1978. Interactions between
    effector cell activity and lymphokines: Implications for
    recovery from herpesvirus infections. Int. Archs. Allergy
    appl. Immun. 57, 62-73.
Campos, M., Ross, C.R. and Lawman, M.J.P. 1982. Natural
    cell-mediated cytotoxicity of bovine mononuclear cells
    against virus-infected cells. Infec. Immun. 36,
    1054-1059.
Ching, C. and Lopez, C. 1979. Natural killing of herpes
    simplex virus type 1 - Infected target cells: Normal
    Human Responses and Influence of Anti-Viral Antibody 26,

49-56.

Davies, D.H. and Carmichael, L.E. 1973. Role of cell-mediated immunity in the recovery of cattle from primary and recurrent infections with infectious bovine rhinotracheitis virus. Infec. Immun. 8, 510-518.

Eberle,R., Russell, R.G. and Rouse, B.T. 1981. Cell-mediated immunity to herpes simplex virus: Recognition of type-specific and type-common surface antigens by cytotoxic T cell populations. Infec. Immun. 34, 795-803.

Forman, A.J. and Babiuk, L.A. 1982. Effect of infectious bovine rhinotracheitis virus infection on bovine alveolar macrophage function. Infec. Immun. 35, 1041-1047.

Gaskell, R.M. 1975. Studies on feline viral rhinotracheitis with particular reference to the carrier state. PhD. Thesis. University of Bristol.

Gaskell, R.M. and Povey, R.C. 1977. Experimental Induction of feline viral rhinotracheitis virus re-excretion in FVR-recovered cats. Vet. Rec. 100, 128-133.

Gaskell, R.M. and Povey, R.C. 1979. The dose response of cats to experimental infection with feline viral rhinotracheitis virus. J. Comp. Path. 89, 179-191.

Gillespie, J.H., Judkins, A.B. and Scott, F.W. 1971. Feline viruses XII. Hemagglutination and hemadsorption tests for feline herpesvirus. Cornell Veterinarian LXI, 159-171.

Grewal, A.S., Rouse, B.T. and Babiuk, L.A. 1980. Mechanisms of recovery from viral infections: Destruction of infected cells by neutrophils and complement. J. Immunol. 124, 312-319.

Hirsch, M.S., Zisman, B. and Allison, A.C. 1970. Macrophages and age-dependent resistance to herpes simplex virus in mice. 104, 1160-1165.

Kohl,S., Lawman, M.J.P., Rouse, B.T. and Cahall, D.L. 1981. Effect of herpes simplex virus infection on murine antibody dependent cellular cytotoxicity and natural killer cytotoxicity. 31, 704-711.

Lopez, C. and Dudas, G. 1979. Replication of herpes simples virus type 1 in Macrophages from resistant and susceptible mice. Infec. Immun. 23, 432-437.

Lopes, C. and O'Reilly, R.J. 1977. Cell-mediated immune responses in recurrent herpes virus infections. 1. Lymphocyte proliferation assay. J. Immunol. 118, 895-902.

Mochizuki, M., Konishi, S. and Ogata, M. 1977. Studies on cytopathogenic virus from cats with respiratory infections. III Isolation and certain properties of feline herpes viruses. Jap. J. Vet. Sci. 39, 27-37.

Mochizuki, M., Konishi, S. and Ogata, M. 1977. Sero diagnostic aspects of feline herpesvirus infection. Jap. J. Vet. Sci. 39, 191-194.

Mochizuki, M., Konishi, S. and Ogata, M. 1977. Studies on cyto-pathogenic viruses from cats with respiratory infections. IV. Properties of hemagglutinin in feline herpesvirus suspensions and receptors on feline erythrocytes. 39, 389-395.

Pfizenmaier, K., Jung, H., Starzinski-Powitz, A., Röllinghoff, M. and Wagner, H. 1977. The role of T cells in anti herpes simples virus immunity. 1. Induction of antigen-specific cytotoxic T lymphocytes. J. Immunol. 119, 939-944.

Povey, R.C. and Johnson, R.H. 1967. Further observations on feline viral rhinotracheitis. Vet. Rec. 81, 686-689.

Rasmussen, L.E., Jordan, G.W., Stevens, D.A. and Merigan, T.C. 1974. Lymphocyte interferon production und transformation after herpes simplex infections in humans. J. Immunol. 112, 728-736.

Roizman, B. 1965. An inquiry into the mechanisms of recurrent herpes infection of man. In "Perspect. Virol. IV" (Ed. Pollard) (Harper & Row). pp. 283-304.

Rouse, B.T. and Babiuk, L.A. 1974. Host defense mechanisms against infectious bovine rhinotracheitis virus: In vitro stimulation of sensitized lymphocytes by virus antigen. Inf. Immun. 10, 681-687.

Rouse, B.T. and Babiuk, L.A. 1075. Host defense mechanisms against infectious bovine rhinotracheitis virus: II. Inhibition of viral plaque formation by immune peripheral blood lymphocytes. Cell Immun. 17, 43-56.

Rouse, B.T. and Babiuk, L.A. 1978. Mechanisms of recovery from herpesvirus infections - A Review. Can. J. Comp. Med. 42, 414-427.

Rouse, B.T., Babiuk, L.A. and Henson, P.M. 1980. Neutrophils in antiviral immunity: Inhibition of virus replication by a mediator produced by bovine neutrophils. J. Infect. Dis. 141, 223-232.

Rouse, B.T., Grewal, A.S., Babiuk, L.A., Fujimiya, Y. 1977. Enhancement of antibody-dependent cell-mediated cytotoxicity of herpes-virus infected cells by complement. Infec. Immun. 18, 660-665.

Rouse, B.T., Wardley, R.C. and Babiuk, L.A. 1976. The role of antibody dependent cytotoxicity in recovery from herpesvirus infections. Cell Immunol. 22, 182-186.

Russell, A.S. 1979. Cell-mediated immunity to herpes simplex virus in man. J. Inf. Dis. 129, 142-146.

Sekizawa, T., Openshaw, H., Wohlenberg, C. and Notkins, A.L. 1980. Latency of herpes simplex virus in absence of neutralizing antibody: Model of reactivation. Science, 210, 1026-1028.

Shore, S.L. and Feorino, P.M. 1981. Immunology of primary herpes virus infections in humans. In "The Human Herpes viruses" (Ed. A.J. Nahmias and R.F. Schinazi).

Shore, S.L., Black, C.M., Melewicz, S.M., Wood, P.A., Nahmias, A.J. 1976. Antibody-dependent cell-mediated cytotoxicity to target cells infected with type 1 and type 2 herpes simplex virus. J. Immunol. 116, 194-201.

Sørensen, O.S., Haahr, S., Moller-Larsen, A. and Wildenhoff, K. 1980. Cell-mediated and humoral immunity in herpesvirus during and after herpes zoster infections. Infec. Immun. 29, 369-375-

Stanwick, T.L., Campbel, D.E., Nahmias, A.J. 1980. Spontaneous cytotoxity mediated by human monocyte-macrophages against human fibroblasts infected with herpes simplex virus - augmentation by interferon. Cell Immunol. 53, 413-416.

362

Starr, S.E., Karatela, S.A., Shore, S.A., Duffey, A., Nahmias, A.J. 1975. Stimulation of human lymphocytes by herpes simplex virus antigens. Infec. Immun. 11, 109-112.

Tan, R.J.S. 1970. Serological comparisons of feline respiratory viruses.Jap. J. Med. Sci. Biol. 23, 419.

Tan, R.J.S. and Miles, J.A.R. 1971. Further studies on feline respiratory virus diseases. 2. Immunodiffusion tests. New Zealand. Vet. J. 19, 15.

Thong, Y.H., Vincent, M.M., Hensen, S.A., Fuccillo, D.A., Rola-Plaszczynski, M. and Bellanti, J.A. 1975. Depressed specific cell-mediated immunity to herpes simplex virus type 1 in patients with recurrent herpes labialis. Infec. Immun. 12, 76-80.

Walton, T.E. Jr. 1968. Feline herpes virus: in vivo and in vitro studies including a microbiological survey of the domestic cat (Felis domesticus). PhD. Thesis, Cornell University.

Walton, T.E. and Gillespie, J.H. 1970. Feline viruses. VII. Immunity to the feline herpescirus in kittens inoculated experimentally by the aerosol method. Cornell Veterinarian 60, 232-239.

Wardley, R.C., Rouse, B.T., Babiuk, L.A. 1976. Observations on recovery mechanisms from feline viral rhinotracheitis. Can. J. Comp. Med. 40, 257-264.

Wilton, J.M.A., Ivanyi, L. and Lehner, T. 1972. Cell-mediated immunity in herpesvirus hominis infections. B.M.J. 1, 723-726.

SESSION III

PORCINE, HERPESVIRUS (AUJESZKY'S DISEASE VIRUS)

Chairlady: Tamar Ben-Porat
Co-chairman: J.B. McFerran

LATENCY OF PSEUDORABIES VIRUS

Tamar Ben-Porat*, Anne M. Deatly*, B.C. Easterday**,
Denise Galloway***, A.S. Kaplan*, Sandy McGregor**
*Department of Microbiology
Vanderbilt University School of Medicine
Nashville, Tennessee 37232, USA
**Department of Veterinary Sciene and School of Vet.Med.
University of Wisconsin
Madison, Wisconsin 53706, USA
***Fred Hutchinson Cancer Research Center
Seattle, Washington 98104, USA

ABSTRACT
The restriction patterns of genomes of twelve different
field isolates of PrV were analyzed. All were found to differ.
In most cases, the basis of the differences in restriction
patterns was found to lie in the acquisition or deletion of
sequences which appear to be nonessential to the productive
infection of RK cells. Mutagenesis of a laboratory virus stock
also resulted in the isolation of mutants with similar
modifications in their genomes.
The difference in the restriction patterns of the
different genomes of the PrV isolates was exploited to
ascertain whether superinfection of swine which had previously
been exposed to PrV would result in colonization of the ganglia
by the superinfecting strain. Colonization of the ganglia by
the superinfecting virus strain was not observed; only the
strain used for the primary infection was recovered from the
ganglia of these animals.
Attempts to study the state of the viral genome and its
expression in the latently infected ganglia using "Southern"
and "Northern" blotting techniques, as well as in situ DNA-RNA
hybridization, were unsuccessful. No hybridization signals were
obtained with probes which should have detected one viral
nucleic acid molecule per twenty cells. However, sequence
homologies between some regions of the viral genome and some
regions of the genome of the pig cells were observed.

INTRODUCTION

Interaction of pseudorabies (Pr) virus with susceptible
cells is in most cases productive, resulting in cell death and
the production of progeny virions. However, Pr virus also
remains in a latent state in animals which have recovered from
disease and virus may be isolated for relatively long periods
of time from a number of organs of animals which have recovered
from infection (Sabo, 1969; Sabo and Rajcani, 1976; Beran et
al., 1980). After virus can neither be detected nor recovered
from most organs, it still is present in the trigeminal ganglia

(Beran et al., 1980; Rziha et al., 1981; Easterday and McGregor, unpublished results) and can be recovered by cocultivation with susceptible cells.

Attempts to induce virus shedding in swine that have recovered from experimental infection with Pr virus, using agents effective in inducing the shedding of HSV in man, were not successful at first (McFerran and Dow, 1964; Sabo and Rajcani, 1976). However, under stress (severe climatic conditions (Howarth, 1969) or after immunosuppression (Mock et al., 1980; Rziha et al., 1981) reactivation of virus in the latently infected pigs will occur. Furthermore, spontaneous shedding of Pr virus from a postparturient sow in isolation has been reported (Davies and Beran, 1980). Thus it appears that in animals which recover from infection, Pr virus enters a latent state in the trigeminal ganglia and that under certain conditions, virus may be reactivated and shed without the appearance of clinical signs. It is well established that the presence of circulating antibody does not prevent release of virus (see, for example, Sabo, 1969; Beran et al., 1980; Wittmann et al., 1980).

That Pr virus remains associated with the ganglia of latently infected pigs was corroborated by the detection of viral DNA in these tissues using cRNA-DNA hybridization (Gutekunst, 1979; Gutekunst et al., 1980). Furthermore, Rziha et al. (1981) detected approximately 5-6 genome equivalents/cell in the brain or cortex of animals 11-13 weeks after infection. Thus, the PrV genome can be detected in the ganglia of swine, however, little is known about its molecular state.

Another important question, unanswered at present, is whether colonization of the ganglia by Pr virus will be prevented in immune animals. This question relates to the efficacy of immunization against latent viruses, such as the herpesviruses, i.e., whether immunization will prevent not only disease but also the establishment of the virus in the ganglia and the consequent potential shedding of virulent virus throughout life.

Temporary shedding of virus occurs either spontaneously or after challenge of immune animals with virulent strains. Thus, when animals were vaccinated with an attenuated strain of PrV and then challenged with a virulent strain, release of virulent virus, i.e., its multiplication and dissemination, was observed despite the presence of serum antibody (Sabo, 1969; Sabo and Grunert, 1971). However, Gutekunst and Pirtle (1979) reported that upon infection of swine, which had been previously immunized with an inactivated vaccine, excretion of virus was considerably less copious and occurred for a shorter period than in nonimmune swine. The finding that replication of virulent virus occurs in immune pigs is not surprising since virus is sometimes shed by animals which have recoverdd from the disease and are therefore immune. Whether shedding of the virus after infection of immune animals is temporary or whether the virus can colonize the ganglia of animals which may sporadically shed virus thereafter remains to be ascertained. If colonization of the ganglia by superinfecting virus were inhibited in immunized pigs, long term spread of the virulent strain would not occur.

The experiments that shall be discussed relate to the following two questions:

(1) Will colonization of the ganglia occur after superinfection of swine which had previously been exposed to Pr virus?

(2) What is the state of the Pr virus genome in the ganglia of latently infected swine and are some of the viral genes expressed in these latently infected ganglia?

Because the variability of the restriction patterns of the genomes of different isolates of Pr virus forms the basis of the rationale for some of the experiments that we have performed, information dealing with the genome variability of the virus will be discussed first.

Differences in restriction enzyme patterns between genomes of different field isolates, as well as between different mutants of Pr virus

Restriction endonucleases generate fragments of DNA at distinct positions on the genome where given recognition nucleotide sequences occur. The number and sizes of the fragments generated from different populations of molecules therefore yield information about their genetic makeup. Thus, if cleavage of the DNA of two different strains of virus by a given enzyme generates fragments which differ in their number and sizes, genetic heterogeneity between the two strains exists. Genetic heterogeneity, based on differences in restriction fragmentation patterns between strains of herpes simplex virus (HSV), as well as of cytomegalovirus, is well decomented (Hayward et al., 1975; Kilpatrick et al., 1976). These differences are useful in epidemiological studies (Buchmann et al., 1979).

We have analysed the genomes of several isolates of Pr virus recovered from different epidemics of pseudorabies and have found, not surprisingly, that their restriction fragmentation patterns differed (Figs. 1 and 2). Indeed, Herrman (1981) has previously reported differences between some isolates of Pr virus. All the different field isolates we have analyzed (a total of 12) could be differentiated from one another on the basis of their restriction patterns.

The differences in migration patterns of the restriction fragments between different isolates could be due to a loss of cleavage sites (generating fusion fragments), deletions or insertion of nucleotide sequences (thereby yielding smaller or larger fragments), or translocation of sequences from one region of the genome to another (thereby also changing the sizes of the fragments).

We have analyzed the restriction digests of the DNA of different strains of Pr virus to determine the basis for the differences in migration patterns of the restriction fragments. To determine the identity of the various DNA bands, and to determine whether translocation of genes from one area of the genome to another had occurred, we hybridized nicktranslated, cloned fragments from our laboratory strain (Ka) of Pr virus to the restriction fragments generated by digestion of the DNA of different isolates fixed to nitrocellulose filters (Southern, 1975). No translocation between sequences present in a given fragment of the Ka strain to a different fragment was found in

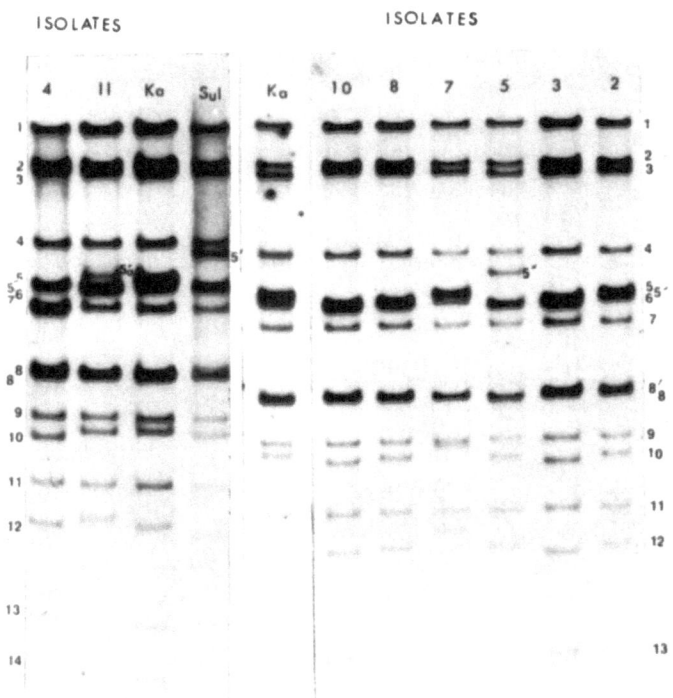

Fig. 1   Autoradiograms of ^{32}P-labeled Bam HI-digested DNA obtained trom different field isolates of PrV. Numbers indicate the different isolates. Sul: PrV (Sullivan Strain). Ka: a PrV strain obtained originally from Richard Shope and carried for the last 25 years in our laboratory.

any of the isolates that were analyzed and the total colinearity between the genes of the different strains seems to have been retained in all cases (data not shown). Furthermore, analysis of the genomes of twelve different isolates after digestion with 3 different restriction enzymes (see Fig.3) which give a total of more than 60 cleavage sites on Pr virus DNA showed that only two had lost a restriction site,i.e.,

instead of the two restriction fragments normally found, a
fusion fragment was observed.

Differences in the migration patterns of fragments
generated from most regions of the genome were observed.
However, the regions of the genome which differed most
frequently were located within the inverted repeat, as well as
near the left end of the genome. A summary of the results

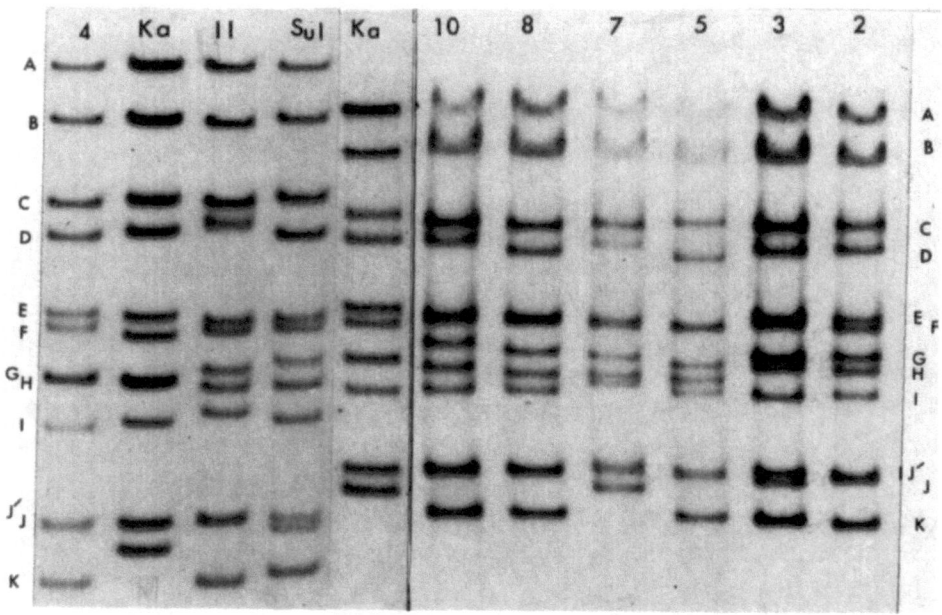

Fig. 2   Autoradiograms of ^{32}P-labeled Kpn I digests of
DNA obtained from different field isolates of PrV (see
Fig.1).

obtained with two representative Bam HI fragments (Fig.3) show
that they varied by as much as 35%. Thus, it appears that
acquisition or deletion of sequences within different regions
of the genome are the reason for the differences in sizes of
the fragments generated from different isolates and that
nonessential sequences, which can be deleted without loss of
viability, are present at various positions along the genome of
some Pr virus isolates.

A variation in the restriction patterns of the genomes of
mutants that have been isolated in our laboratory, which

genetically behave as being mutated in a single gene (Ben-Porat et al., 1982; Ihara et al., 1982) was also observed (Fig.4). Interestingly, the regions of the genome that were modified in the mutants were not necessarily near the regions in which the mutations had been located by marker rescue (Ihara et al., 1982). Such variation in the restriction patterns of the mutant genomes were observed after selection of TK⁻ mutants using exposure of the infected cells to increasing amounts of Ara-T

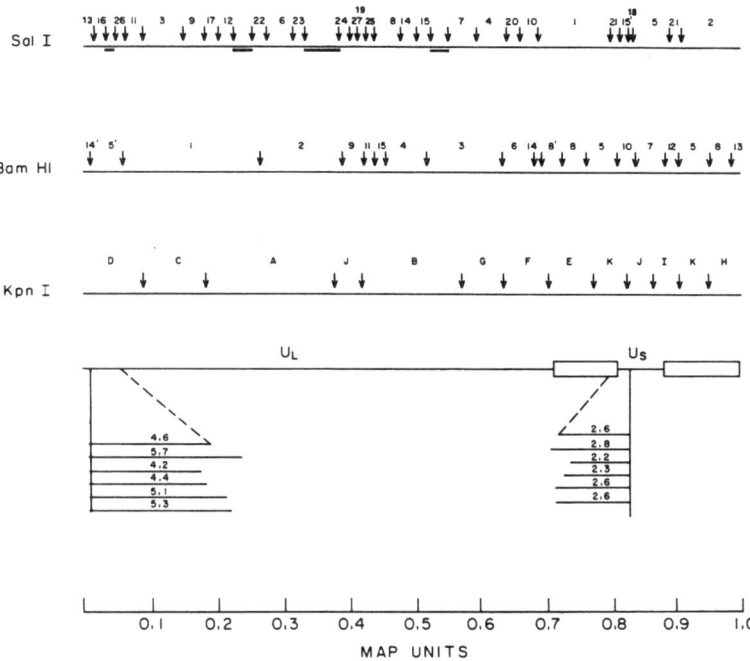

Fig. 3   Restriction maps of the DNA Ka strain. These 3 restiction endonucleases were used to analyze the different field isolates. The underlined regions on the Sal I map are composed of small fragments (smaller than 0.5x10⁶ daltons) and have not been mapped. The variation in sizes of two representative Bam HI fragments present in the restriction digests of the genomes of five of these isolates are also indicated.

(a procedure which is probably mutagenic), as well as after mutagenesis by ultraviolet light irradiation, nitrosoguanidine, and BUdR. Although, to avoid the isolation of multiple mutants, the doses of the mutagen were kept low (survival of infectious virus was 2-10%), secondary nonlethal mutants nevertheless must have been introduced into many of the genoms as indicated by the differences in the restriction patterns of the DNA of these mutants and that of the parental wild type virus. Thus, the genome of Pr virus appears to allow for a high degree of pleomorphism. After mutagenesis, changes in the restriction patterns of the DNA resulting from acquisition or deletion of sequences can arise at relatively high frequency. On the other hand, repeated plaque purification of the same isolates (data not shown), as well as passage of any given strain in animals (see below), does not change the restriction pattern of the genome.

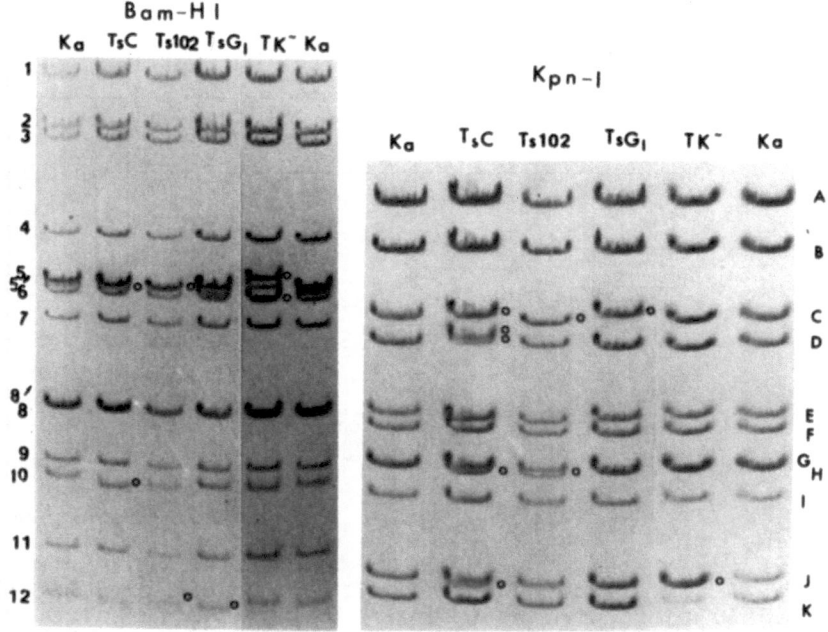

Fig 4   Variation in restriction patterns of the DNA of various mutants obtained by mutagenesis of PrV (Ka strain).

Can superinfecting virus colonize the ganglia of previously
infected animals?

To determine whether superinfecting virus colonizes the
ganglia of immune animals, we took advantage of the
availability of virus strains which differ from one another in
their DNA restriction patterns. An experiment was designed to
determine whether pigs which had survived primary infection
with one strain of Pr virus and were then superinfected with
another strain would harbor only one or both strains of virus
in their ganglia.

Weanling pigs (4-6 weeks of age), all negative for serum
neutralizing antibody against Pr virus, were exposed to the
virus (Pr Sullivan strain) by intranasal instillation of 10^5
PFU per pig. Thirty-five percent (7/20) of the pigs died within
two weeks following exposure to the virus. All surviving pigs
were bled for antibody determination 33 days after infection;
all had significant levels of antibody to Pr virus (data not
shown). At periodic intervals thereafter, some of the pigs were
killed and fragments of various tissues were cocultivated with
either rabbit kidney (RK) or swine testis (ST) cells.

At 24 weeks of age, five of the pigs which had been
exposed to PrV (Sullivan strain) and three pigs which had not
been previously exposed to PrV were bled (for serology) and
inoculated intranasally with 10^5 PFU of PrV (isolate 7). All
pigs were observed for signs of disease. The three seronegativ
pigs (622, 630, 674) had fevers 3 to 4 days after inoculation
while the pigs which had been pre-exposed to Pr virus showed no
sign of the disease. At different times the animals were killed
and fragments of various tissues were cocultivated with RK
cells.

Tables 1 and 2 summarize the results of this experiment.
Of all the tissues obtained from the latently infected or
superinfected animals, virus could be recovered from the
trigeminal ganglia only. Similarly, virus could be recovered
only from the trigeminal ganglia (and in one case from the
parotid gland) of pigs which were infected for the first time
at 24 weeks of age (Table 2). When younger pigs (4-6 weeks old)

TABLE 1 Protocol of superinfection experiment and type of virus recovered from ganglia

Pig No.	Infected with Sullivan at 4-6 weeks	Sacrificed 8 weeks later	Antibody level at 24 weeks*	Infected with Isolate 7 at 24 weeks	Time killed after super-infection with Isolate 7 (days)	Strain recovered from ganglia
743	+	+				None
799	+	+				Sullivan
128	+	-	>1280	+	6	None
600	+	-	295	+	6	Sullivan
741	+	-	200	+	30	Sullivan
745	+	-	160	+	56	Sullivan
746	+	-	>1280	+	56	Sullivan
622	-	-	Seronegative	+	6	Isolate 7
630	-	-	Seronegative	+	6	Isolate 7
674	-	-	Seronegative	+	6	Isolate 7

* Serum neutralizing antibody titer expressed as reciporcal of the serum dilution required to give 50% reduction in plaque number

were similarly inoculated, virus could be recovered from a
variety of tissues by 6 days after infection (data not shown).

PrV (Sullivan strain) can easily be distinguished from PrV
(isolate 7) by restriction endonuclease analysis (see Figs. 1
and 2). To determine whether the superinfecting strain of virus
had colonized the ganglia, the DNA of the virus population
recovered by cocultivation of the ganglia with RK cells was
analyzed by restriction endonuclease digestion (Fig. 5). Only
the virus strain used for the first infection (PrV Sullivan)
could be recovered from the ganglia of the superinfected
animals. This was true for animals which had high, as well as
lower, levels of circulating neutralizing antibodies at the
time of superinfection (see Table 2). That the superinfecting
strain (PrV-isolate 7) can colonize the ganglia is shown by the
fact that it was consistently recovered from the ganglia of
matched controls which had not been pre-exposed to PrV.

TABLE 2   Pr virus recovery after cocultivation of various
           tissues obtained from animals inoculated as
           summarized in Table 1

Pig No.	Tonsils	Submax. lymph node	Submax. salivary gland	Trigem. ganglia	Parotid gland	Brain (Temporal lobe)
743	–	–	–	–	–	–
799	–	–	–	+	–	–
128	–	–	–	–	–	–
600	–	–	–	+	–	–
741	–	ND	ND	+	ND	ND
845	–	ND	ND	+	ND	ND
746	–	ND	ND	+	ND	ND
622	ND	–	–	+	–	–
630	ND	–	–	+	–	–
674	ND	–	–	+	+	–

ND, not done.

As mentioned in the introduction, reinfection, as well as virus shedding, of immunized pigs is well documented. In the experiment described above, colonization of the ganglia by the

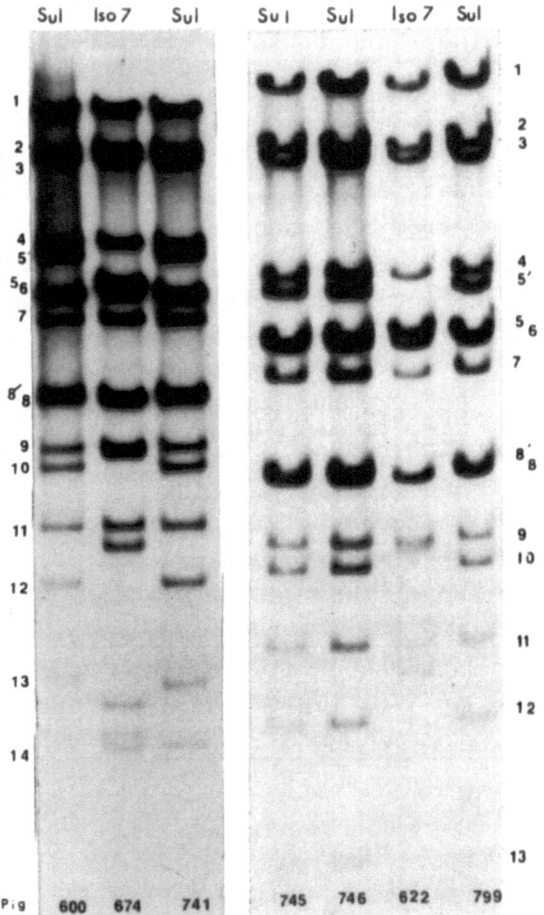

Fig. 5   Restriction patterns obtained after digestion of the DNA obtained from virions recovered by cocultivation of ganglia of swine with RK cells subjected to different protocols of infection and superinfection. The protocol of the experiment is summarized in Table 2.

superinfecting strain did not occur. However, colonization of the ganglia upon superinfection may be dependent on the general condition of the animal as well as upon its immunological status and we cannot therefore state unequivocally that it will not occur under any conditions.

Information is available indicating that colonization of
the ganglia after superinfection with HSV also does not occur.
While individuals previously infected with HSV-2 can be
reinfected by a different strain of that virus (Buchman et al.,
1979), the ganglia of a given individual all appear to be
infected with a single strain of HSV only, indicating that
colonization of the ganglia by superinfecting strains may not
occur (Lonsdale et al., 1979). Experiments with animal models
also indicate that active immunization against HSV prevents
colonization of the ganglia (Price and Schmitz, 1979;
Centifanto et al., 1982). Thus, it appears, the information
available to date indicates that colonization of the ganglia by
superinfecting strains of both HSV and PrV does not occur in
actively immunized animals.

Studies on the State and expression of the genome of PrV in latently infected ganglia

As mentioned above, PrV is latent in the sensory ganglia
of swine as is HSV in man. Before embarking on a description of
the experiments that we have performed dealing with the state
and expression of PrV in the ganglia, it is useful to summarize
the information available concerning the state and expression
of the HSV genome in latently infected ganglia, a subject of
intense study in several laboratories.

Puga et al. (1978) found low levels of viral DNA but no
detectable amounts of viral RNA (indicating that the genome may
not be transcribed) in the ganglia of mice latently infected
with HSV. On the other hand, viral thymidine kinase activity
was detected in these ganglia by Yamamoto et al. (1977).
Whether transcription had occurred but was undetected in the
latently infected ganglia or whether the thymidine kinase
activity detected was a remnant of the acute stage is unknown.
However, the presence of thymidine kinase activity in the
ganglia is interesting in view of the important role this
enzyme appears to play in the colonization of the ganglia
(Tenser et al., 1979).

That part of the viral genome may be transcribed in
latently infected ganglia was also indicated by the report that

immediate-early proteins, but not capsid proteins, were detectable in some neurons of rabbits latently infected with HSV (Green et al., 1981).

The expression of the viral genome has also been investigated using DNA-RNA in situ hybridization (Galloway et al., 1979; Tenser et al., 1981). Using this sensitive method, viral RNA was detected in the neurons of latently infected guinea pigs, as well as in human ganglia obtained at autopsy. Furthermore, using cloned restriction fragments of viral DNA as probes, it was found that transcripts complementary to some regions of the HSV genome only were detectable in the neurons (Galloway et al., 1982). Since transcripts of only some regions of the genome were found in these latently infected ganglia, it is unlikely that they reflect a slow lytic cycle resulting from inactivation of the virus.

From the evidence summarized above, it appears that some functions of the viral genome may be expressed in ganglia latently infected with HSV. However, the state of the HSV genome, as well as its expression in latently infected ganglia, is far from clear.

It has been estimated that few of the cells (0.1%) in the trigenimal ganglia of latently infected mice (one of the model systems used for the study of latency of HSV) harbor the viral genome (Walz et al., 1976). Because of the paucity of viral genomes, it is therefore difficult to study the state of the viral genome in this system. Gutekunst (1979) reported the detection of PrV DNA in latently infected ganglia of swine using conditions of hybridization which would detect this DNA only if several copies were present per cell. Furthermore, Rziha et al. (1981) found that several genome copies per cell were present in the brain and cortex of latently infected pigs. It appeared therefore that it should be possible to define the state of the Pr viral genome in the latently infected tissues of swine.

We designed a set of experiments in which DNA extracted from latently infected ganglia was digested with appropriate restriction enzymes with the aim of establishing the following:

(1) Are most of the Pr genomes in the ganglion of latently infected swine in a linear form (the form of mature genomes) or are most in the form of circles or concatemers, i.e., the form in which the genomes are expressed and replicated (Ben-Porat, 1982) and (2) are some of the viral genomes integrated into the cellular genomes?

The DNA of latently infected ganglia was extracted and digested with a restriction enzyme (Eco RI) that does not cleave PrV DNA, as well as with a restriction enzyme (Kpn I) that introduces several cuts into the viral genome. The fragmented DNA was electrophoresed, transferred to nitrocellulose paper (Southern, 1975) and hybridized to nick-translated, cloned Pr viral DNA fragments. Reconstruction experiments in which various amounts of viral and RK DNAs were mixed, similarly digested, transferred to nitrocellulose paper, and hybridized to the labeled viral DNA probes showed that the techniques used were sufficiently sensitive to detect the presence of one viral DNA molecule per 20 cells. (The probes had a specific activity of approximately $2-5 \times 10^8$ cmp/μg).

Distinct bands of DNA obtained from the ganglia of latently infected pigs hybridized to some of the probes of cloned viral DNA fragments. However, similar bands were seen when DNA from ganglia of seronegative pigs was analyzed. Furthermore, DNA extracted from uninfected cultured pig kidney cells but not rabbit kidney cells also gave hybridization signals with some cloned fragments of viral DNA. The bands of DNA which hybridized with the probes were, however, not in the position expected of viral DNA and we conclude therefore that they represent cellular DNA with sequence homology to some regions of the viral genome. Some of the clones of viral DNA did not have any detectable homology to cellular DNA. These clones also did not detectable hybridize to DNA extracted from ganglia of latently infected pigs.

Our results thus show that few of the cells in the latently infected ganglia examined (less than 1 in 20) harbored the viral genome. Because the level of viral genomes was below detection by the methods used, we could not, of course, reach any conclusions concerning the state of the viral DNA.

Viral RNA should, in principle, be detected more easily than viral DNA because many transcripts can arise from a single genome. To clarify the degree of expression of the viral genome in the latently infected ganglia, we analyzed the tissues for the presence of viral RNA. To this end, RNA was extracted from the ganglia, electrophoresed, transferred to nitrocellulose filters, essentially by the methods described by McMaster and Carmichael (1977) and Thomas (1980), and hybridized to cloned, nick-translated restriction fragments of PrV DNA.

In productively infected RK cells, approximately 50 major species of mRNA hybridizing to different restriction fragments of DNA are easily detectable at late times after infection using probes with a specific activity of $2x10^7$ cpm/μg. However, no RNA was detectable in preparations obtained from latently infected ganglia using a probe with a 10-fold higher specific activity (data not shown). Thus, if the genomes present in the latently infected ganglia are transcribed, RNA accumulation is below the level of detection we have used.

Using in situ hybridization, Galloway et al. (1979) have demonstrated the presence of viral RNA in human ganglia obtained at autopsy. This technique has the advantage of detecting viral RNA in a single cell and thus, even if very few of the cells harbor the viral genome but the cells which harbor the genome, express at least part of it, viral RNA should be detectable within these individual cells. When this technique was applied to ganglia obtained from pigs latently infected with PrV, viral transcripts were not detected, even though the conditions used were similar to those which gave positive results with human ganglia (Galloway et al., 1979).

Our results show that in ganglia of pigs which have recovered from infection with PrV (Sullivan strain) relatively few cells harbor the viral genome. Because of the paucity of viral DNA in these ganglia, our studies did not shed light on the state of the PrV genome in latently infected pig ganglia. However, the in situ hybridization technique used should have detected viral transcription (had it occurred) within the rare cell in the ganglia which harbors the genome. Since none was observed, we tentatively suggest that in PrV latently infected ganglia transcription of the viral genome does not occur.

The number of PrV genomes per latently infected ganglion in the tissues that we have analyzed is considerably lower than that found by others in similar tissues. Both Rziha et al. (1981) and Gutekunst (1979) have reported the presence of relatively high concentrations of viral DNA in the ganglia or brain tissue of pigs that have recovered from PrV infection. It is possible that the differences between our results and those previously published are due to differences in the strains of virus, the immune status of the animals, or both.

ACKNOWLEDGEMENT

This investigation was supported by Grant No. AI-10947 from the National Institutes of Health.

REFERENCES
Ben-Porat, T. 1982. Organization and replication of herpesvirus DNA. In "Organization and Replication of Viral DNA" (Ed. A.S. Kaplan). (CRC Press, Inc., Boca Raton, Fla.) pp. 147-172.
Ben-Porat, T., Hoffmann, P., Brown, L., Feldman, L. and Blankenship, M.L. 1982. Partial characterization of temperature-sensitive mutants of pseudorabies virus. Virology, in press.
Beran, G.W., Davies, E.B., Arambulo, P.V. III, Will, L.A., Hill, H.T. and Rock, D.L. 1980. Persistence of pseudorabies virus in infected swine. J. am. Vet. Med. Assoc. 176, 998-1000.
Buchman, T.G., Roizman, B. and Nahmias, H.J. 1979. Demonstration of exogenous genital reinfection with HSV-2 by restriction finger-printing of viral DNA. J. Infect. Dis. 140, 195-304.
Centifanto-Fitzgerald, Y.M., Varnell, E.D. and Kaufmann, H.E. 1982. Initial herpes simplex virus type 1 infection prevents ganglionic superinfection by other strains. Infect. Immun. 35, 1125-1132.
Davies, E.B. and Beran, G.W. 1980. Spontaneous shedding of PrV from a clinically recovered postparturient sow. J. Am. Vet. Med. Assoc. 176, 1345-1347.
Galloway, D.A., Fenoglio, C.M. and McDougall, J.K. 1982. Limited transcription of the herpes simplex virus genome when latent in human sensory ganglia. J. Virol. 41, 686-691.
Galloway, D.A., Fenoglio, C., Shevchuk, M. and McDougal, J.K. 1979. Detection of herpes simplex RNA in human sensory ganglia. Virology 95, 265-268.

382

Green, M., Courtney, R.J. and Dunkel, E.C. 1981. Detection of an immediate-early HSV-1 polypeptide in trigeminal ganglia of latently infected animals. Infect. Immun. 34, 987-992.

Gutekunst, D.A. 1979. Latent PrV infection in swine detected by RNA-DNA hybridization. Am J. Vet. Res. 40, 1568-1571.

Gutekunst, D.E. and Pirtle, E.L. 1979. Humoral and cellular immune responses in swine after vaccination with inactivated Pr virus. Am. H. Vet. Res. 40, 1343-1346.

Gutekunst, D.E., Pirtle, E.C., Miller, L.D. and Steward, W.C. 1980. Isolation of pseudorabies virus from trigeminal ganglia of a latently infected sow. Am. J. Vet. Res. 41, 1315-1316.

Hayward, G.S., Frenkel, N. and Roizman, B. 1975. Anatomy of HSV DNA; Strain differences and heterogeneity in the location of restriction endonuclease cleavage sites. Nat. Acad. Sci. USA 72, 7768-7772.

Herrmann,S. (1981). Differentiation of PrV strains. International Workshop on Herpesviruses, Bologna, Italy, p.17.

Howarth, J.A. 1969. A serologic study of pseudorabies in swine. Am. J. Vet. Med. Assoc. 154, 1583-1589.

Ihara, S., Ladin, B.F. and Ben-Porat, T. 1982. Comparison of the physical and genetic maps of pseudorabies virus shows that the genetic map is circular. Virology, in press.

Kilpatrick, B.A., Huang, E.S. and Pagano, J.S. 1976. Analysis of cytomegalovirus genomes with restriction endonucleases Hind III and Eco RI. J. Virol. 18, 1095-1105.

Lonsdale, D.M., Brown, S.M., Subak-Sharpe, J.H., Warren, K.G. and Koprowski, H. 1979. The polypeptide and the DNA restriction enzyme profiles of spontaneous isolates of herpes simplex virus type 1 from explants of human trigeminal, superior cervical and vagus ganglia. J. Gen. Virol. 43, 151-171.

McFerran, J.B. and Dow, C. 1964. The secretion of Aujeszki's disease by experimentally infected pigs. Res. Vet. Sci. 5, 405-410.

McMaster, G.K. and Carmichael, G.C. 1977. Analysis of single and double stranded nucleic acids on polyacrylamide and agarose gels using glyoxal and acridine orange. Nat. Acad. Sci. USA 74, 4835-4838.

Mock, R.E., Crandell, R.A., Mesfin, G.M. 1981. Induced latency in pseudorabies vaccinated pigs. Can. J. Comp. Med. 45, 56-59.

Price, R. and Schmitz, J. 1979. Route of infection, systemic host resistance, and integrity of ganglionic axions influence acute and latant herpes simplex virus infection of the superior cervical ganglion. Infec. Immun. 23, 373-383.

Puga, A., Rosenthal, J.D., Openshaw, H. and Notkins, A.L. 1978. Herpes simplex virus DNA and mRNA sequences in acutely and chronically infected trigeminal ganglia of mice. Virology 89, 102-111.

Rziha, H.J., Döller, P.C. and Wittmann, G. 1981. Detection of pseudorabies and viral DNA in organ tissue of latently infected pigs. International Workshop on Herpesviruses, Bologna, Italy, p.147.

Sabo, A. 1969. Persistence of perorally administered virulent Pr virus in the organisms of nonimmune and immune pigs. Acta Virol. 13, 229-235.

Sabo, A. and Grunert, S. 1971. Persistence of virulent pseudorabies virus in herds of vaccinated and nonvaccinated pigs. Acta Virol. 15, 87-94.

Sabo, A. and Rajcani, J. 1976. Latent pseudorabies virus infection in pigs. Acta Virol. 20, 208-214.

Southern, E.M. 1975. Detection of specific sequences among DNA fragments separated by gel electrophoresis. J. Mol. Biol. 98, 503-517.

Tenser, R.B., Dawson, M., Ressel, S.J. and Dunstan, M.E. 1981. Detection of herpes simplex virus mRNA in latently infected trigeminal ganglion neurons by in situ hybridization. Ann. Neurol. 11, 285-291.

Tenser, R.B., Miller, R.L. and Rapp, F. 1979. Trigeminal ganglion infection by thymidine kinase negative mutants of herpes simplex virus. Science 205, 915-917.

Thomas, P.S. 1980. Hybridization of denatured RNA and small DNA fragments to nitrocellulose filters. Nat. Acad. Sci. 77, 5201-5205.

Walz, M.A., Yamamoto, H. and Notkins, A.L. 1976. Immunological response restricts the number of cells in sensory ganglia infected with herpes simplex virus. Nature (London) 264, 554-556.

Wittmann, G., Jakubik, J. and Ahl, R. 1980. Multiplication and distribution of Aujeszky's disease (PrV) in vaccinated and nonvaccinated pigs after intranasal infection. Arch. Virol. 66, 227-240.

Yamamoto, H., Walz, M.A. and Notkins, A.L. 1977. Viral-specific thymidine kinase in sensory ganglia of mice infected with HSV. Virology 76, 866-869.

RESTRICTION ENDONUCLEASE PATTERNS OF THE GENOME OF
AUJESZKY'S DISEASE VIRUS ISOLATED FROM LATENTLY INFECTED PIGS

A.L.J. Gielkens

Central Veterinary Institute, Department of Virology
39, Houtribweg, 8221 RA Lelystad, The Netherlands

ABSTRACT
    Latency of the virulent Northern Ireland Aujeszky three
(NIA-3) strain of Aujeszky's disease virus (ADV) was
established in seronegative pigs, vaccinated pigs and pigs with
high maternal antibody. The latent virus was reactivated by in
vivo and in vitro methods (Van Oirschot, these proceedings).
    The present study was conducted to determine whether the
viruses isolated after primary infection and reactivation were
identical based on DNA restriction profiles.
    Four months after infection of maternal immune pigs with
NIA-3, virus was reactivated by corticosteroid treatment. Virus
recovered from oropharyngeal fluid (OPF) samples was grown in
pig kidney cells and infected cell DNA was analysed with the
restriction endonuclease Bam HI in combination with Southern
blot hybridization (Gielkens and Berns, 1982). The DNA fragment
patterns of viruses isolated from swabs after primary infection
and corticosteroid treatment were shown to be parental-like.
However, they both revealed an additional Bam HI DNA fragment
of approximately 3 kb, not present in the parental NIA-3 virus
stock. Virus isolated from cultured ganglionic tissue of these
pigs showed the same pattern. We are presently characterizing
the 3 kb DNA fragment to determine whether it originates from
defective genomes.
    By analysis of DNA of virus isolated from ganglionic and
tonsillar tissue of several seronegative pigs infected with
NIA-3 1-2 months previously, it was shown that the restriction
profiles were identical to that of NIA-3 isolated shortly after
primary infection (NIA-3 pi).
    In OPF of pigs intranasally vaccinated with Bartha's K
strain virus can be detected for several days after
vaccination. The DNA-fragment patterns of these isolates were
shown to be Bartha-like. After challenge of these pigs with
NIA-3 some virus containing OPF samples were grown in pig
kidney cells and infected cell DNA was analysed. The bam HI
restriction profiles obtained were indistinguishable from that
of NIA-3 pi. Ten weeks after challenge the pigs were treated
with corticosteroids and sentinel pigs were introduced (Van
Oirschot, these proceedings). Again, virus isolated from the
reactivated pigs and the sentinel pigs could not be
distinguished from the NIA-3 pi isolates. No evidence was
obtained for simultaneous excretion of the avirulent Bartha's K
strain.
    In conclusion, by restriction endonuclease analysis of ADV
reactivated from latently infected pigs, it was shown that the
state of the viral genome during establishment and maintenance
of the latent phase presumably does not result in structural
changes in the viral DNA.

REFERENCES
Gielkens, A.L.J. and Berns, A.J.M. 1982. Differentiation of
    Aujesky's disease virus strains by restriction endonuclease
    analysis of the viral DNA's. In "Ausjeszky's Disease" (Ed.
    G. Wittmann and S.A. Hall). Curr. Top. Vet. Med. Anim.
    Sci., 17, 3-13. Martinus Nijhoff Publishers.

PSEUDORABIES VIRUSES FROM CLINICAL OUTBREAKS AND LATENT INFECTIONS GROUPED INTO FOUR MAJOR GENOME TYPES

Sigrid-C. Herrmann, Bernhard Heppner and Hanns Ludwig
Institut für Virologie der Freien Universität Berlin,
im Robert Koch-Institut, Nordufer 20, 1000 Berlin 65,
Germany

ABSTRACT
About 150 isolates of pseudorabies virus were collected worldwide from fatally infected piglets, cattle and carnivores. Their DNAs were analysed by restriction enzmye cleavage and compared with the published physical map of a standard strain. In addition, four vaccine strains were included in the investigation. Four main genome groups were evident, clustering in distinct geographic areas (Northern Europe, Middle Europe and Thailand). Isolates within these genome groups can additionally be subdivided according to epizootiological relatedness. Nucleotide sequence homology of the DNAs derived from the different groups was ascertained by hybridization. The DNA patterns of the four vaccine strains are slightly different from those of wildtype strains and there is evidence that two of the vaccine strains have a deletion in the short unique region of the genome.

INTRODUCTION

Two taxonomically distinct viruses have been isolated from pigs: suid herpesvirus 1, better known as pseudorabies (PsR) virus, and suid herpesvirus 2, pig cytomegalovirus. According to clinical specificity and genome structure, they are classified as members of the alphaherpesvirinae (PsR virus) or betaherpesvirinae (pig cytomegalovirus), respectively (Roizman et al., 1981).

As the causative agent of Aujesky's Disease, PsR virus is of economic importance throughout the world (Aujeszky, 1902). Besides young pigs, a variety of carnivores and other animals are fatally infected, whereas adult pigs seem to be the latent carriers (Wittmann and Hall, 1981). Different attenuated strains have been developed and are used with more or less success as vaccines (Bartha, 1961; Tatarov, 1968; Toma et al., 1979) to prevent the serious losses caused by the disease. Real protection of mammals against wildtype virus has not been proven.

Herpes simplex virus isolates of different origin could be separated according to the number and distribution of restriction endonuclease cleavage sites in their DNAs (Hayward et al., 1975). More recently this fingerprinting technique was used to follow the spread of HSV in the population (Buchman et al., 1979; Buchman et al., 1980). Meanwhile the restriction enzyme analysis of DNA was successfully applied to several other members of the herpesgroup, e.g., EBV (Dambough et al., 1980), CMV (Huang et al., 1980), BHV (Engels et al., 1981; Ludwig, 1982), EHV (Studdert et al., 1982), herpesvirus saimiri (Desrosiers and Falk, 1982) and VZV (Martin et al., 1982). As with other DNA viruses (Wadell et al., 1980; Faras et al., 1980) the goal of these DNA analyses was to correlate differing clinical entities with genome types or variations in the genome (Engels et al., 1981; Studdert et al., 1982; Pauli et al., 1982).

Restriction enzyme analysis of PsR virus isolates elucidated genome differences and resulted in a differentiation of wildtype isolates and vaccine strains (Herrmann, 1981; Ludwig et al., 1981; Gielkens and Berns, 1981; Lomnici pers. comm.). Similar differences between wildtype and vaccine strains have been observed using BHV-1 (Engels et al., 1981), EHV-1 (Studdert et al., 1982), and VZV (Martin et al., 1982).

The purpose of this report is to see whether the observed heterogeneity in PsR viruses could be split up into defined genome types. The study was extended to 150 strains, obtained from different parts of the world. The results show that four major genome types emerge in this serologically uniform virus and that these genome types seem to result from the evolution of viruses in distinct geographic regions.

RESULTS

The origin and designation of PsR virus isolates used in this study are listed in Table 1. All viruses were grown on mink lung cells and were used for these investigations at the third to fifth passage from isolation. Viral DNA was extracted

TABLE 1   Origin and description of PsR virus strains

Number of strains	Origin and description	Date of isolation	Animal	Genome group
1	Denmark Korsør (Borgen H.C.)	1962	cattle	III
2	Denmark (Bitsch V.)	1981	pig, cattle	III
1	USA DEK (Plummer G.)	1969 or earlier	not known	II
4	(Schleswig-Holstein (Zimmermann Th.)	1967	pig	Ii*
16	as above	1980	pig,dog, cat	Ii; II, IIi
3	as above	1981	pig	Ii, II
31	as above	1982	pig,dog, cat, cattle, mink	mainly II, IIi (5), Ii (2)
23	Berlin (Hentschke and own isolations)	1979-1982	dog,cat	mainly II or IIi, few Ii
4	Belgium (Pastoret P.-P.)	1980	pig,cat, cattle	I
6	Oldenburg (Hirchert R.)	1980	pig,dog	Ii, II, IIi
29	Detmold (Ulrich L.)	1980	pig,dog, cat, cattle, bear,fox, sheep	mainly II or IIi, few Ii
7	Frankfurt (Frost J.W.)	1980	not known	Ii, II, IIi
3	Hannover (Ließ B.)	1978,1979	pig, cattle	I, II
2	Japan (Shimiza)	1981	pig	II
6	Thailand (Löhr; G.T.Z.)	1981	pig	II (1), IV
5	Sweden (Morein)	1982	pig, mink,fox	III
4	Vaccine strains (Toma B.)	gift		similar I

i*   intermediate

either from virions or from infected cells according to
previously published procedures (Darai et al., 1975; Pignatti
et al., 1979). DNAs were digested with the following
restriction endonucleases: Bam H I, Bst E II, Kpn I, Hind III,
and Bgl II. Using a PsR strain originally characterized by
Kaplan (1969) physical maps of the cleavage sites have been
published (Ben-Porat et al., 1979; Rixon and Ben-Porat, 1979;
Ben-Porat et al., 1980).

The 150 PsR virus strains used in this study could
clearly be grouped into four major genome types when Bam H I
was used as the discriminating enzyme (Fig. 1a, b). Bst E II
did not separate the groups I and II of this classification
(Fig. 2a). With the other enzymes: Kpn I (Fig. 2b), Bgl II or

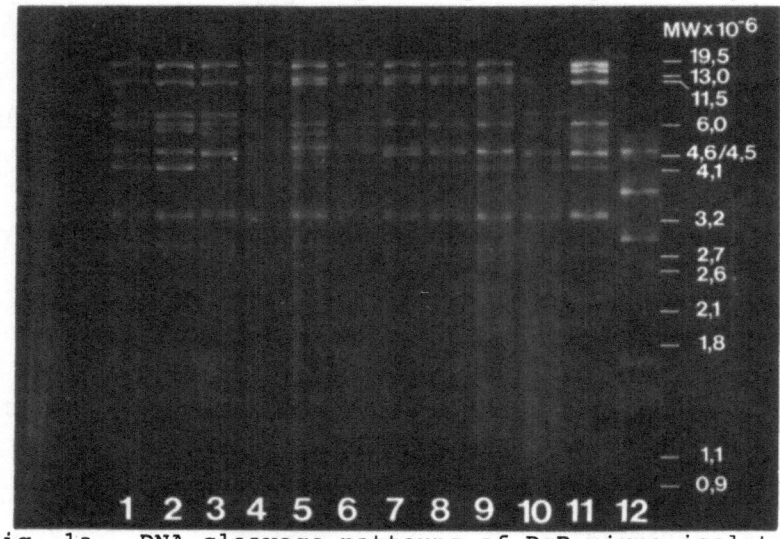

Fig. 1a   DNA cleavage patterns of PsR virus isolates
digested with restriction endonuclease Bam H I, indicating genome types (groups): Lane 1 genome type II intermediate; Lanes 2, 3 and 10 genome type II; Lanes 4, 5 and
6 genome type I intermediate; Lanes 7 - 10 genome type I;
Lanes 11 genome type III; Lane 12 molecular weight
marker. DNA fragments were separated by electrophoresis
on a 0.8% agarose gel at 40 V for 20 hours, stained with
ethidiumbromide (1µg/1) and photographed under UV
transillumination with a Polaroid Land camera.

Hind III (data not shown) only a limited distinction between
the viruses was possible. Isolates within the main groups vary

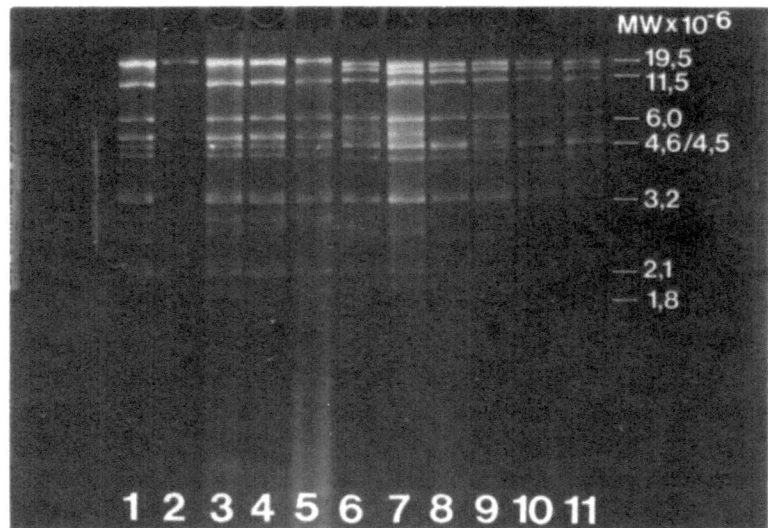

Fig. 1b   DNA cleavage patterns of PsR virus isolates digested
with restriction endonuclease Bam H I indicating genome types
(groups): Lanes 1 - 5 genome type IV; Lanes 6 - 11 genome type
III. Conditions of separation and visualization were as in
Fig. 1a.

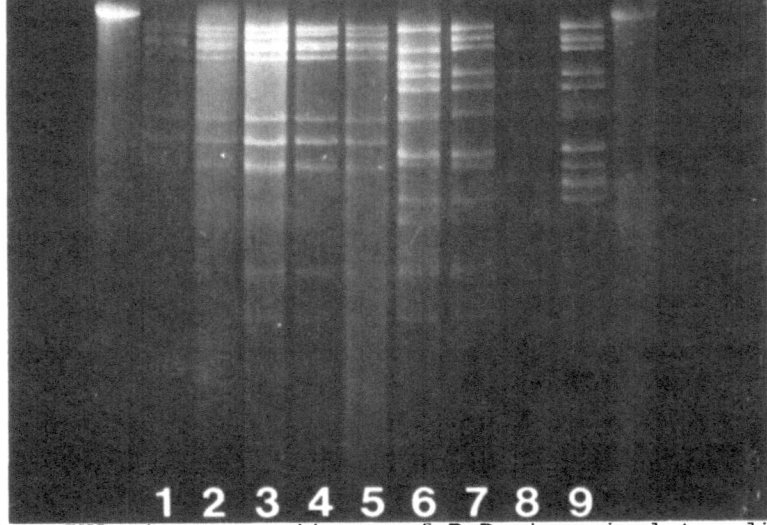

Fig. 2a   DNA cleavage patterns of PsR virus isolates digested
with restriction endonuclease Bst E II indicating the
different genome groups (designation according to Bam H I as
well as to Bst E II): Lanes 1 - 5 type IV (Bam H I) / type III
(Bst E II), Lane 6 type III (Bam H I) / type II (Bst E II)
                Lane 7 type II   (Bam H I) / type I v2 (Bst E II)
                Lane 8 type II   (Bam H I) / type I v2 (Bst E II)
                Lane 9 type I   (Bam H I) / type I v1 (Bst E II)
                Conditions were as in Fig. 1a.

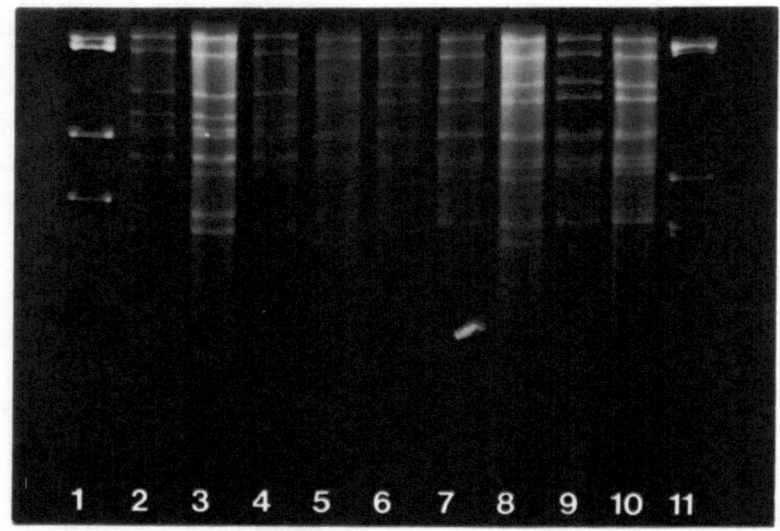

Fig. 2b   DNA cleavage patterns of PsR virus isolates
digested with restriction endonuclease Kpn I, conditions
as in Fig. 1a.

slightly according to their epizootiological relatedness. The
observed genome types correlate with certain geographic areas.
The group I viruses are similar to or identical with the
published Bam H I DNA pattern (Rixon and Ben-Porat, 1979); the
group II strains lack one fragment (No. 2) of group I but
possess two new fragments (above and below fragment 4). The
two groups represent viruses found in Middle Europe (Germany
and Belgium). Intermediates of the two genome types do exist
(Fig. 1a): variations of group I have an additional fragment
below fragment 4, and variations of group II have only one new
fragment above fragment 4. The frequency of genome type II
together with its variation was about 75% in all the isolates.
The distribution of the genome types and their intermediates
must be seen in connexion with the time of the virus
isolation. Virus strains isolated 10 years ago or prior
(except strain DEK, which belongs to group II) are very
similar or identical to the group I, whereas all the recent
isolates, collected after 1979, resemble the group I variation
(except 4 isolates derived from Belgium). In 1980 and 1982,
when two collections of strains from the same area of Germany

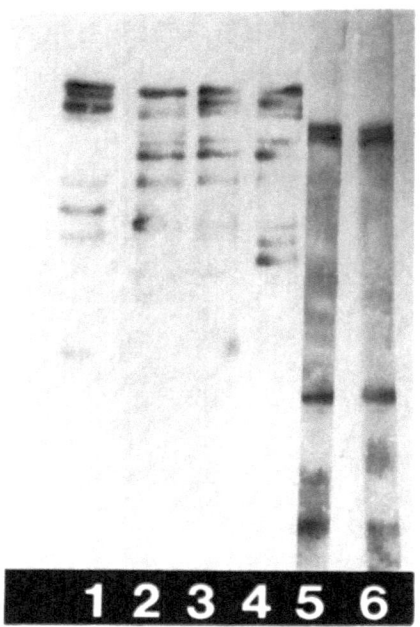

Fig. 3   Hybridization of PsR DNAs of different genome
groups using the Southern blot technique:
Lane 1 PsR DNA of group IV; Lane 2 PsR DNA of group III;
Lane 3 PsR DNA of group II; Lane 4 PsR DNA of group I;
fragments of Bst E II digests transferred to gene screen
membrane (NEN) were hybridized to nicktranslated ³H
labelled PsR DNA of group II and exposed to Kodak X-ray
film (- 70°C, for 10 days).
Lanes 5 and 6 Adeno 2 DNA Bst E II fragments hybridized
to nicktranslated Ad 2 DNA ³H labelled.
(We are grateful to B. Ehlers for performing the
hybridization experiments).

were compared (see Table 1, Zimmermann), an obvious shift in
the distribution of groups was observed. The frequency of
genome type II was highest in the collection of strains
received in 1982.

The groups III (genome type III) and IV (genome type IV)
are strictly limited to isolates originating from Northern
Europe (Denmark, Sweden) and Thailand, respectively. The group
III genome differed from group I only slightly in the Bam H I
DNA pattern but was quite distinct in the Bst E II pattern.
The group IV genome, however, differed widely in the

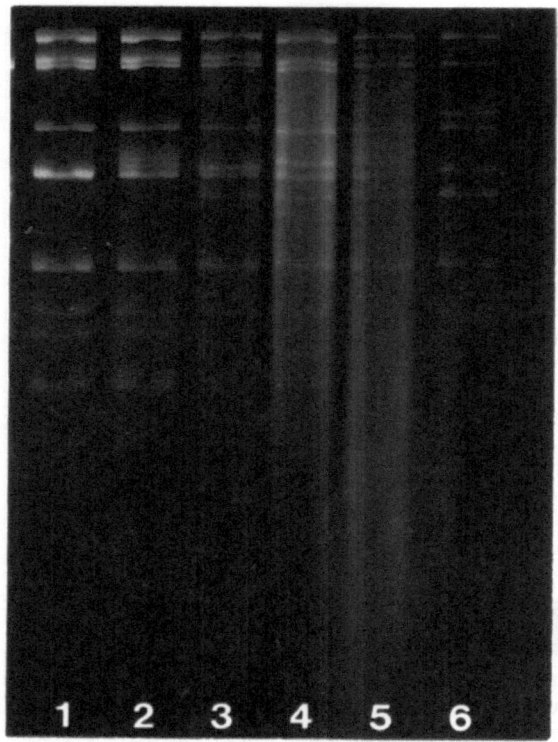

Fig. 4a   DNA
cleavage patterns of
PsR virus vaccine
strains and wildtype
isolates digested
with restriction
endonuclease Bam H I:
Lanes 1 - 4 vaccine
strains
(1 Bartha; 2 Dessau;
both lack fragment
No. 7 indicated as
triangle; 3 Tatarov;
4 Alfort). Lanes 5
and 6 represent
wild-type isolates.
Conditions as in Fig.
1a.

distribution of cleavage sites of both enzymes (Fig. 1b, 2b).
To ensure that the viruses were still PsR viruses,
hybridization experiments were done using the Southern blot
technique (1975). Nick-translated DNA of all four genome types
recognized the DNA fragments of each type. A representative
experiment where labelled DNA of the group II genome was used
is shown in Fig. 3. All the strains used for these studies
could be neutralized by PsR virus specific antisera.
Investigations to discriminate different genome groups by more
refined techniques are in progress.

The 150 strains represent viruses from Aujeszky's Disease
outbreaks or from latently infected animals, since part of our
isolates came from diseased dogs, cats or other carnivores
which had eaten meat of healthy pigs. To see whether the
widely used vaccine strains could be discriminated,
representative strains were included in this investigation.

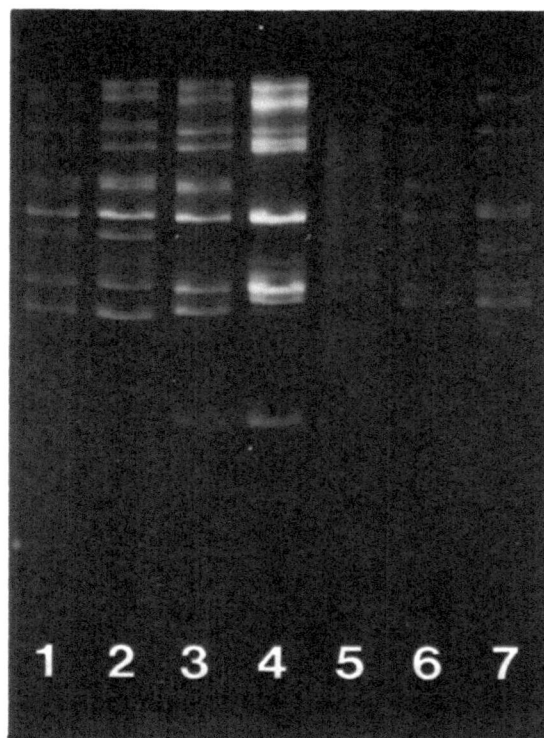

Fig. 4b DNA cleavage patterns of PsR virus vaccine strains and wildtype isolates digested with restriction endonuclease Kpn I: Lanes 1 and 2 represent wild-type isolates; Lanes 3 and 4, vaccine strains Bartha and Dessau, which both lack fragment I and have instead an additional fragment of lower molecular weight (all indicated by tri-angle); Lane 5 molecular weight marker; Lanes 6 and 7 vaccine strains Alfort and Tatarov. Conditions as in Fig. 1a.

Only the Bartha and Dessau strains were significantly different in their DNA pattern. Both viruses lack fragment 7 of the Bam H I DNA pattern, and the Kpn I fragment I, which is known to map in the same genomic region, is also lost. However, in the Kpn I digest a new fragment of lower molecular weight appears (Fig. 4a, b). Moreover, the corresponding high molecular weight fragments obtained after cleavage with Bgl II (D, E) show significant shifts compared to the standard type pattern (not shown). Based on the known PsR virus genome maps, our findings with Bartha and Dessau strains indicate that these DNAs have a deletion in the short unique region of the genome (Fig. 5a, b), the size of which is estimated to be 2.5 x 10^6 Daltons at maximum. The two other vaccine strains, named Alfort and Tatarov, are more or less similar to wildtype strains (Fig. 4a, b). Generally speaking, all the vaccine strains can be grouped as type I.

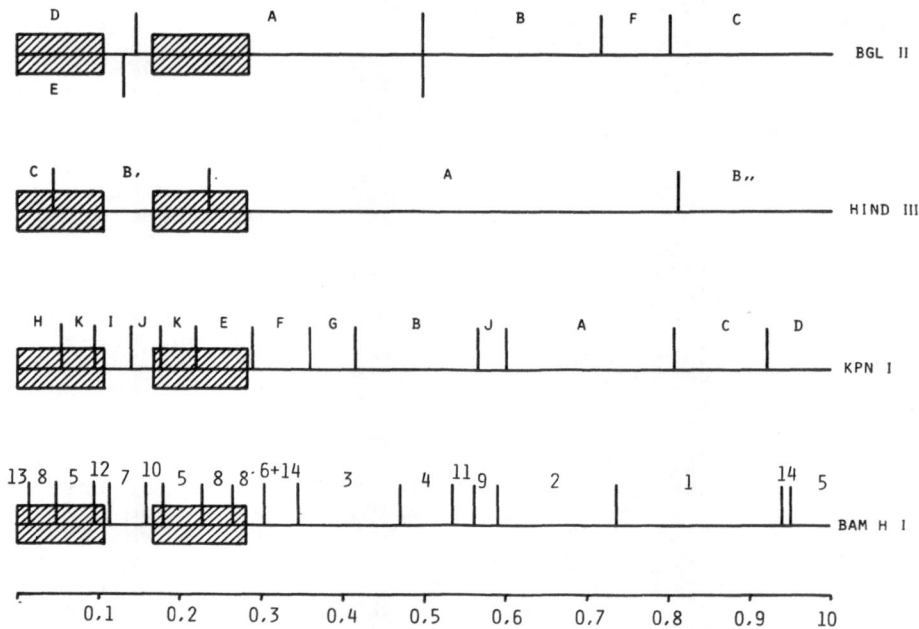

Fig. 5a   Physical maps of the restriction endonuclease
cleavage sites in the genome of PsR virus DNA according
to T. Ben-Porat (Rixon and Ben-Porat, 1979; Ben-Porat et
al., 1979; Ben-Porat et al., 1980).

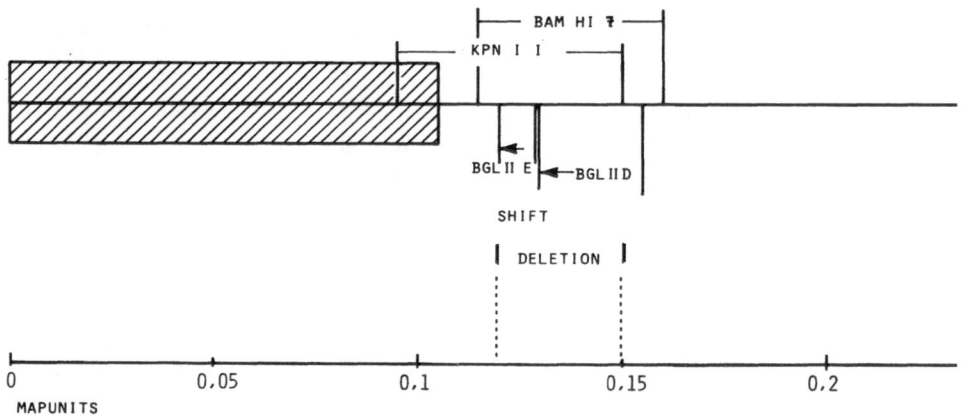

Fig. 5b   Part of the genome map of PsR virus: estimated
deletion region of the vaccine strains Bartha and Dessau.

DISCUSSION

A representative collection of PsR viruses of different countries, including vaccine strains, could be subdivided into four genome types. The findings indicate a clustering of distinct genomes peculiar to certain geographic regions. Nevertheless, within the genomic groups additional, slight variability can be observed, which is mainly due to molecular weight differences, and only in a few cases to the gain or loss of fragments. Although PsR viruses with different biological properties were isolated (Bartha, 1961; Lloyd and Baskerville, 1978), the virus is still considered to be serologically uniform. These studies have shown a considerable heterogeneity among PsR viruses. At the moment there is no definite correlation between genomic structure and virulence of these viruses. And so far the different genome types cannot be associated with distinct clinical entities. Much more work is necessary to map biologically important functions on the genome, before such genomic differences can be correlated to certain clinical manifestations of Aujeszky's Disease. This may prove to be difficult, since this virus is highly virulent in the vast majority of animal species, which die in a short time after infection. The rapid course of the disease certainly prevents the detection of more defined clinical symptoms.

Efforts to use the DNA fingerprinting technique to find out which genomes may be correlated with certain kinds of clinical symptoms were successful in equine herpesviruses (Studdert et al., 1982), and also to some extent in bovine herpesviruses, where the 'IBR-like' and the 'IPV-like' genomes could be separated (Engels et al., 1981) and the 'IBR-like' genome seems also to be responsible for abortion (Pauli et al., 1982). The most definitive studies, where genome types could be associated with defined diseases, were done with adenoviruses (Wadell et al., 1980). The successive appearance of different adenovirus genome types during an epidemic outbreak might serve as a model for similar investigations with herpesvirus genomes.

An investigation of 22 herpesvirus saimiri isolates using strains from different sources in South America has failed to establish distinct geographic subtypes (Desrosiers and Falk, 1982). The fact that four genome types of PsR viruses have been found in a representative number of isolates received from different geographic regions of the world may be explained in the following way: in contrast to the situation in HSV-1 and HSV-2 infections where worldwide exchange of genomes occurs, resulting in a huge heterogeneity in the virus genomes (Buchman et al., 1980), the epidemiology of Aujeszky's Disease is quite different. The rearing of pigs and the exchange of animals over great distances during the last decade contributes to the distribution of populations which were kept in regional areas before. Therefore an exchange of viruses of different genome types was a rare event until now and only a limited number of variants exists. In HSV-1 and 2 throughout their existence multiple recombinant events could readily occur, and additional mutations may have contributed to an accumulation of persisting variants in the human population (Buchman et al., 1980). Today the crowding of pigs favors the transmission of viruses from the always present latent carriers. During these severe outbreaks a higher recombination rate between genomes can be postulated. Otherwise, as suggested for herpesvirus saimiri (Desrosiers and Falk, 1982), successive reinfections may promote recombination. In such an epidemiological situation the occurrence of intermediates can be explained. Nevertheless it remains surprising that one genome group is by far more frequent than all the others. The stability of herpesvirus genomes as shown for HSV (Roizman pers. comm.) is also confirmed for PsR virus, since we were unable to detect any changes in the DNA cleavage pattern during 100 serial cellpassages. Therefore the natural mutation rate is only of minor importance to the variability of the PsR genome.

The most prominent finding of this investigation is that PsR viruses, although collected over 20 years, preserve a limited genome heterogeneity, which enables us to group PsR

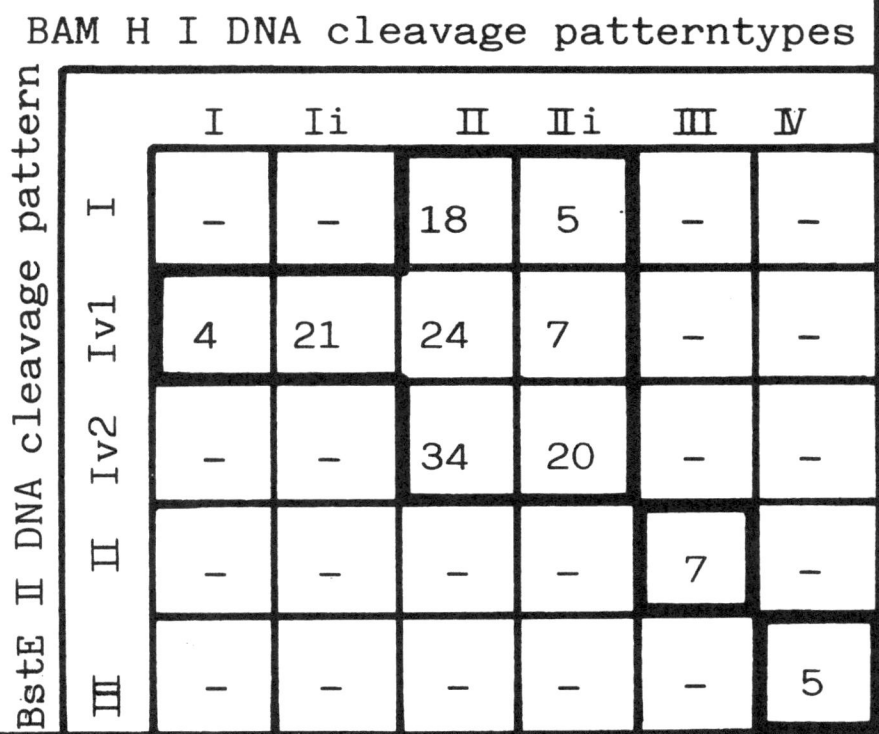

Fig. 6   Distribution of PsR virus isolates to the
different genome groups based on the cleavage patterns of
the restriction endonucleases Bam H I and Bst E II.

virus strains in four major genome groups (Fig. 6). This study
demonstrates the capability of modern DNA technology in
elucidating epidemiological backgrounds.

REFERENCES

Aujeszky, A. 1902. Über eine neue Infektionskrankheit bei
    Haustieren. Zbl. Bakt. Parasiten- und Infektionskrank-
    heiten, 32, 353-357.
Bartha, A. 1961. Versuche zur Reduzierung der Virulenz des
    Aujeszky-Virus. Magy. Allatorv. Lap., 16, 42-45.
Ben-Porat, T., Rixon, F.J. and Blankenship, M.L. 1979.
    Anaylsis of the structure of the genome of pseudorabies
    virus. Virology, 95, 285-294.
Ben-Porat, T., Veach, R.A., Ladin, B.F. 1980. Replication of
    herpes virus DNA: VI. Virions containing either isomer
    of pseudorabies virus DNA are infectious. Virology, 102,
    370-380.
Buchman, T.G., Roizman, B. and Nahmias, A.J. 1979. Demonstrat-
    ion of exogenous genital reinfection with herpes simplex

type 2 by restriction endonuclease fingerprinting of viral DNA. J. of Inf. Dis., 140, 295-304.

Buchman, T.G., Simpson, T., Nosal, C., Roizman, B. and Nahmias, A.J. 1980. The structure of herpes simplex virus DNA and its application to molecular epidemiology. Ann. of the New York Acad. of Sci., 354, 279-290.

Dambough, T., RaabTraub, N., Heller, M., Beisel, C., Hummel, M., Cheung, A., Fennewald, S., King, W. and Kieff, E. 1980. Variations among isolates of Epstein-Barr virus. Ann. of the New York Acad. of Sci., 354, 309-325.

Darai, G., Lorentz, A., Kammer, K. and Munk, K. 1975. The fate of herpes simplex virus type 2 DNA during abortive infection at 42°C of human embryonic lung cells. Virology, 68, 92-104.

Desrosiers, R.C. and Falk, L.A. 1982. Herpesvirus saimiri strain variability. J. Virol., 43, 352-356.

Engels, M., Steck, F. and Wyler, R. 1981. Comparison of the genomes of IBR- and IPV virus strains by means of restriction enzyme analysis. Arch. Virol., 67, 169-174.

Faras, A.J., Krzyzek, R.A., Ostrow, R.S., Watts, S.L., Smith, D.M., Anderson, D.L., Quick, C.A. and Pass, F. 1980. Genetic variation among papillomaviruses. Ann. of the New York Acad. of Sci., 354, 60-79.

Gielkens, A.L.J. and Berns, A.J.M. 1981. Differentiation of Aujeszky's Disease virus strains by restriction endo-nuclease analysis of viral DNAs. In "Current Topics in Vet. Med. and Animal Sci.", Vol. 17: Aujeszky's disease (Eds. G. Wittman and S.A. Hall). (Martinus Nijhoff Publishers, The Hague/Boston/London).

Hayward, G.S., Frenkel, N. and Roizman, B. 1975. Anatomy of herpes simplex DNA: Strain differences and heterogeneity in the locations of restriction endonuclease cleavage sites. Proc. Nat. Acad. Sci. USA, 72, 1768-1772.

Herrmann, S. 1981. Differentiation of pseudorabies virus strains. In "International Workshop on Herpesviruses" (Eds. A.S. Kaplan, M. La Placa, F. Rapp and B. Roizman). (Esculapio Publ. Co., Bologna, Italy). p. 21.

Huang, E.S., Huong, S.M., Tegtmeier, G.E. and Alford C. 1980. Cytomegalovirus: Genetic variation of viral genomes. Ann. of the New York Acad. of Sci., 354, 332-346.

Kaplan, A.S. 1969. Herpes simplex and Pseudorabies viruses. Virol. Monographs, 5. (Springer Verlag, Berlin).

Lloyd, G. and Baskerville, A. 1978. In vitro markers to differentiate an avirulent from a virulent strain of Aujeszky's disease virus. Vet. Microbiol., 3, 65-70.

Ludwig, H. 1972. Untersuchungen am genetischen Material von Herpesviren. Microbiol. Immunol., 157, 186-211.

Ludwig, H., Heppner, B. and Herrmann, S. 1981. The genomes of different field isolates of Aujeszky's Disease. In "Current Topics in Vet. Med. and Anim. Sci.". Vol. 17: Aujeszky's Disease (Eds. G. Wittmann and S.A. Hall). (Martinus Nijhoff Publishers, The Hague/Boston/London).

Ludwig, H. 1982. Bovine herpesviruses. In "The Herpesviruses IB", Compr. Virol. (Ed. B. Roizman). (Plenum Press, New York and London), in press.

Martin, J.H., Dohner, D.E., Wellinghoff, W.J. and Gelb, L.D.
    1982. Restriction endonuclease analysis of varicella
    zoster vaccine virus and wild-type DNAs. J. med. Virol.,
    9, 69-76.
Pauli, G., Gregersen, J.P., Storz, J. and Ludwig, H. 1982.
    Biology and molecular biology of latent bovine herpes-
    virus type 1 (BHV 1). CEC Symposium on "Latency of
    Herpesviruses", Tübingen, Sept. 2123 (this issue).
Pignatti, P., Cassai, E., Meneguzzi, G., Chenciner, N. and
    Milanesi, G. 1979. Herpes simplex virus DNA isolation
    from infected cells with a novel procedure. Virology, 93,
    260-264.
Rixon, F.J. and BenPorat, T. 1979. Structural evolution of
    the DNA of pseudorabies defective viral particles.
    Virology, 97, 151-163.
Roizman, B., Carmichael, L.E., Deinhardt, F., deThe, G.,
    Nahmias, A.J., Plowright, W., Rapp, F., Sheldrick, P.,
    Takahashi, M. and Wolf, K. 1981. Herpesviridae.
    Definition, provisional nomenclature, and taxonomy.
    Intervirol., 16, 201-217.
Southern, E.M. 1975. Detection of specific sequences among
    DNA fragments separated by gel electrophoresis.
    J. Mol. Biol., 98, 503-517.
Studdert, M.J., Simpson, T. and Roizman, B. 1982. Different-
    iation of respiratory and abortigenic isolates of equine
    herpesvirus 1 by restriction endonucleases. Science, 214,
    562-564.
Tatarov, G. 1968. Apathogener Mutant des AujeszkyVirus indu-
    ziert von 5Jodo2Deoxyuridin (JuDR). Zentralbl. Vet.
    med. B, 15, 847-853.
Toma, B., Brun, A., Chappuis, G. et Terre, J. 1979.
    Propriétés biologique d'une souche thermosensible (Alfort
    26) de virus de la maladie d'Aujeszky. Rec. Méd. vét.,
    155, 245-252.
Wadell, G., Hammarskjöld, M.L., Windberg, G., Vasanyi, T.M.
    and Sundell, G. 1980. Ann. of the New York Acad. Sci.,
    354, 16-42.
Wittmann, G. and Hall, S.A. (Ed.) 1981. Aujeszky's Disease.
    Current Topics in Vet. Med. and Anim. Sci. Vol. 17
    (Martinus Nijhoff Publishers, The Hague/Boston/London).

THE ROLE OF THE CARRIER PIG IN THE EPIDEMIOLOGY OF AUJESZKYS DISEASE

J.B. McFerran, R.M. McCracken, C. Dow
Department of Agriculture, Northern Ireland Veterinary
Research Laboratories Stormont, Belfast, BT4 3SD,
Northern Ireland

ABSTRACT

Investigations on a large breeding unit suggested waves of infection probably centred in the farrowing house. Eradication was achieved on the basis of the selection of serologically negatively pigs.

Using dexamethasone, carriers could be reactivated and in contact pigs became infected. However the efficiency of excretion is very low. It is suggested that infection under the cover of maternal anti-body may have a major place in the epidemiology of the disease.

INTRODUCTION

The importance of carriers in Aujeszky's disease has long been suspected. Thus Nikitin (1961) recognized that pigs, especially sows, although clinically healthy, could introduce disease into clean farms. Howarth (1969) suggested that changes in wether were important in reactivating latent virus.

However McFerran and Dow (1964) using anaphylactic shock or dietetic stress and Sabo (1969) using cortisone, hypo and hyperthermia or explant cultures of tonsillar tissue failed to detect reactivated virus.

Recently latency has been demonstrated in hydrocortisone treated pigs (Sabo and Rajcani, 1976). They injected between 500 mg and 1,000 mg cortisone over a 5 day period. They could not detect virus excretion. They did demonstrate virus in tissues taken from both the cortisone treated and control pigs by tissue explants. As they were unable to detect virus from animals infected with other strains they postulated genetic differences in virus isolates.

Virus was isolated from non immunologically suppressed pigs using explant cultures and co-cultivation from pigs up to 13 months following infection (Beran et al., 1980). Using

7,500 mg prednisolone distributed over 4 days, to
immunosuppress pigs Wittmann et al. (1982) obtained virus
excretion from days 4 to 11. They could not detect virus in
organs by direct means but were able to demonstrate virus in
the lungs and CNS by co-cultivation. Virus has also been
demonstrated in tissues of immunosuppressed (Rziha et al.,
1982) and non-immunosuppressed pigs (Gutekunst, 1979) using
hybridization techniques.

Vaccination does not prevent the establishment of
latency. Pigs vaccinated with an attenuated vaccine and then
challenged 3 weeks after vaccination were treated after 90
days with 400-600 mg dexamethasone. Virulent virus was
recovered from tonsil swabs on 4 occasions and also from the
tonsils and lungs by cocultivation. No vaccine virus was
found in the non-challenged vaccinated pigs (Mock et al.,
1981). Inactivated vaccine also did not prevent the
establishment of carriers (Gutekunst, 1979).

Davies and Beran (1980) described the case of a sow
which had been infected 19 months earlier. Spontaneous virus
shedding by the sow was detected on days 3 to 8
post-parturition, and a serological response from 4 to 64
occurred. However both the sow's litter and introduced
sentinal pigs were not infected.

Therefore although it is clear that carriers occur in
Aujeszky's disease their exact role has not been established.
In particular when they break down do they excrete enough
virus to infect in contacts? A second question of importance
is that carriers have only been demonstrated following a
primary clinical infection. However in a number of breeding
farms studied there was no evidence of clinical disease, in
spite of persistent infection. Of course this might be
because the virus strains were relatively mild and/or the pig
was infected when old enough not to show signs. Furthermore
carriers seem to excrete virus in or around the farrowing
unit. Two possible routes of infection seemed possible. One
was that in utero infection occurred with the production of
immune-tolerant persistent carriers. The second was that

infection occurred under the cover of maternal antibody. The first possibility was rejected because no evidence of persistent increased foetal mortality was evident and also from antibody surveys there was no evidence of consistent virus spread in growing pigs as might be expected from a persistently excreting carrier animal.

These investigations were undertaken in an attempt to elucidate some of these problems.

MATERIALS AND METHODS
Detection of antibody

The presence of antibody to Aujeszky's disease virus was detected by adding 200 $TCID_{50}$ of virus to doubling dilutions of serum in microtitre plates. There were 2 wells for each serum dilution. Following 1-hr incubation at $37^{O}C$, Vero cells were added to each well. The plates were sealed with transparent tape and the test read at 2, 4 and 6 days. Sera known free of antibody and with low and high titres of antibody were included as controls. The titres are expressed as the final serum dilution which neutralised 100 $TCID_{50}$ (30-300 $TCID_{50}$) virus in this test.

Detection of virus

Swabs were placed Earles lactalbumin medium with 0.1% bovine albumin. They were immediately centrifuged and the supernatent inoculated into 2 cultures of primary pig kidney cells. Isolates were identified as herpesviruses using the electron microscope and confirmed as Aujeszky's disease using the serum neutralisation test.

THE EPIDEMIOLOGY OF THE DISEASE ON A LARGE BREEDING FARM

A large breeding unit with approximately 450 sows was established in 1967 to produce hybrid pigs. It had a complicated breeding programme involving Large White, Landrace, Welsh, Hampshire and Peitran pigs. In 1969 it had an outbreak of disease which was not reported to us, but which may have been Aujeszky's disease (AD). In 1972 a confirmed outbreak occurred. Sows went off their food for 2 to 3 days and many were sneezing. About 10 days later most of the pregnant sows aborted. This was followed in about a week's time by high mortality in the pigs unter 3 weeks of age and lower mortality in the older ages. Pigs over 32 kg did not die and only about 30% showed any signs of disease.

A further small outbreak occurred in 1975 confined to a few gilts and their litters in the farrowing house and the overall losses from AD were considered minimal. A number of serious outbreaks of AD had occurred in herds buying apparently healthy breeding stock from this farm and as this was of considerable commercial importance the organisation sought our advice on possible eradication. They could not slaughter the entire herd and restock because of their valuable genetic stock and an eradication programme had to cause the minimum of disruption to their production.

Following farrowing the pigs were either weaned at 3 weeks into a cage rearing system or at 5 weeks. At 32 kg weight they were divided between the fattening house or the test house. In the test house further genetic selection was made and the rejects were transferred to the fattening house. At approximately 85 kg liveweight the pigs went for slaughter except those selected in the test house for sale or breeding, in which case the females were moved to the gilt house.

As a first step, in June 1975, animals were bled throughout the herd shortly after the recent clinical disease outbreak. It was evident that infection was widespread (Table 1). Previous experimental studies had indicated that titres of 32-256 could be expected after primary infection and titres of 500-4000 were achieved if the pigs were reinfected after 80 to 90 days (McFerran, unpublished). The range of titres in the farrowing house indicated reinfection in some sows and this was borne out by the fact that no female with one or two litters had titres in excess of 128. Titres indicating primary infection were found in some of the pregnant gilts. If infected during pregnancy abortion would be expected. It is now known if they were infected before becoming pregnant or if they were infected early in

TABLE 1   Results of testing a breeding herd for serum
           neutralising antibodies to Aujeszky's disease
           virus

House	Number of samples		Titre	
	Tested	%Positive	Range	Mean
June 1975				
Farrowing house	23	100	16-4000	128
Gilt house	15	47	4-128	58
Fattening house	21	48	4-16	5.2
Test house	34	44	2-8	4.2
Bacon factory	27	41	2-8	5.1
March 1976				
Farrowing house				
Sows	22	82	8-128	23.5
1st litter gilts	20	10	2 at 4	4
Gilt house	20	10	1 at 4, 1 at 8	6
Fattening house	27	70	4-64	21.4
Test house	19	0	-	-
Bacon factory	35	11	4-16	5

pregnancy, had early foetal deaths and had returned to
service. Studies on pigs at different ages on the farm showed
that maternal antibody fell down to undetectable levels in
some pigs. However other pigs still kept low levels of
antibody and even at around 26 weeks of age 41% of blood
tested at the bacon factory had low titre antibody.

A further sampling was undertaken in March 1976 just
before eradication was commenced. There were much lower
titres in the farrowing house and none of the gilts tested
had evidence of recent active infection (ie they had titres
of 4). It was concluded from this that active infection was
now absent in the farrowing house. A fall in titre from
500-4000 down to 32-128 and from 32-256 down to 4-16 can be
expected in 3-6 months time (McFerran, unpublished; Mock et
al., 1981). This view was reinforced by the titres in the
gilt house, and no titres were found in the test house. In
the fattening house however there was evidence of active
infection still continuing. As pigs were continually moving
from the rearing areas to both the test and fattening house,

it is assumed that the focus of infection was in the
fattening house and this was kept going by each week's new
susceptible intake. It was interesting that in spite of the
close proximity of other houses no viral spread from house to
house was occurring.

Therefore at 32 kg the potential breeding animals were
tested at a 1:2 serum dilution for antibody. If negative they
were moved to a separate house in batches of 50. After a
further 3 weeks they were retested. If still negative they
were moved to a different farm, kept in isolation and
retested after a further 3 weeks. If still negative they were
then mixed with the other pigs which had come through the
same programme.

In a few cases, reactors were found after the first
negative test. In all cases these titres were low and may
have represented non-specific reactions. However these
reactors were removed and the group retested twice at 3 week
intervals, before being moved to the clean farm.

When enough pigs were present on the clean farm a final
serological test was carried out, the old unit was destocked,
cleaned, disinfected and left empty for one month. It was
then restocked with pregnant gilts from the clean farm.

From this, and other studies, the following deductions
were made.

1. Infection may well have occurred under the cover of
    maternal antibody. This would explain the lack of
    clinical signs in many farms.

2. Carriers developed persistent low antibody titres.
    There was no evidence of carrier pigs failing to
    develop neutralising antibody.

3. Spread on the farm, at least with the traditional
    Northern Ireland strains of ADV was poor and
    required relatively close contact between pigs.
    This is reinforced from other field observations in
    Northern Ireland where there is no evidence yet of
    aerial spread form farm to farm. In a few cases
    there is indication of spread by fomites or by

human movement but in the majority of cases disease appears following the purchase of an apparetently healthy animal.

EXPERIMENTAL DEMONSTRATION OF CARRIERS

Experimental Design

A total of thirty six pigs were used. Thirty two were infected intranasally at six weeks of age with 0.5 ml of NIA.1 virus, titre $10^{6.5}$ TCID$_{50}$. The 19 survivors were kept in isolation for 70 days. Then 14 of these pigs were injected with 30 mgm dexamethasone intramuscularly. The remaining 5 infected pigs were kept as controls. In addition 4 uninfected pigs which had been kept in isolation were now added to the group.

Immediately following the dexamethasone treatment nasal swabs from all 23 pigs were taken, and thereafter at alternate days until 14 days post injection (pi). Ocular and vaginal or preputial swabs were taken at 4, 8 and 12 days pi and blood at 0, 8, 13 and 55 days pi.

RESULTS

Following infection, all 19 pigs developed antibody. When bled before the dexamethasone treatment, titres varied from 16 to 64 (Table 2). Following the treatment, titres of five pigs (13, 14, 28, 37 and 128) showed a four fold antibody rise. Of the 4 non-infected control pigs no response was seen in the first 14 days after injection, but at the 55 day bleeding 2 had developed very low level titres and one had a titre of 64.

Virus was isolated from the nasal swabs of 3 pigs (numbers 36, 37 and 41) at 2 days pi and at 4 days pi from the nasal swab of pig 36. No isolates were made from any other swabs.

DISCUSSION

The antibody rise in the five pigs was only four fold. Three of these pigs (14, 37 and 38) were treated with

TABLE 2 Serum neutralising antibody titres in infected and in-contact pigs, following treatment with dexamethasone, 70 days after infection with Aujeszky's disease virus

Pig number	Treatment	Days after injection of Dexamethasone			
		0	8	13	55
13	I	16	32	32	64
14	D	32	32	64	128
17	D	32	32	32	64
23	D	64	64	64	64
28	I	16	32	32	64
30	I	32	32	32	32
31	D	64	32	64	64
34	D	64	128	128	64
36	D	32	32	32	64
37	D	32	32	32	128
38	D	16	16	32	64
41	D	64	64	64	64
44	I	64	64	64	32
45	D	64	32	64	64
46	I	64	64	64	64
47	D	64	64	64	64
48	D	32	32	32	64
49	D	64	64	64	64
50	D	64	32	64	128
16	C	<2	<2	<2	<2
18	C	<2	<2	<2	2
25	C	<2	<2	<2	2
39	C	<2	<2	<2	64

D - dexamethasone injected pigs
I - infected pigs, not injected with dexamethasone
C - control non-inoculated pigs

dexamethasone. It cannot be determined if the titres of pigs
13 and 28 rose due to spontaneous unmasking of latent virus
or because they were infected by the dexamethasone treated
pen mates. It should be noted that virus was isolated from
two pigs which did not show a rise in antibody titre.

Taken together the rise in antibody titre, the
demonstration of virus excretion and the antibody produced by
pig 39 indicate that virus was reactivated in sufficient
titre to spread. The virus recovery pattern is similar to
that described by Mock et al. (1981), and the increase in
serum neutralisation titres is similar in timing to that
found by Wittmann et al. (1982). It is not surprising that
the process does not seem very efficient, because we find
that following introduction of AD virus into a breeding unit,
antibody usually disappears after a few years unless the herd
is relatively big - ie 50 sows or more.

Control pig 39 clearly became infected, but it is less
clear what happened to pigs 18 and 25. They developed titres
of 2, which is considerably less than would be expected
following a primary infection. One possibility was they were
only infected by a minimal amount of virus and did not
undergo a full scale infection. This possibility is now being
investigated.

INFECTION OF PIGS UNDER THE COVER OF MATERNAL ANTIBODY
Experimental Design

Fifteen 6 week old pigs, the progeny of 2 gilts were
used. These gilts were survivors of a previous experiment,
and had been vaccinated once at 6 weeks of age and then
challenged after 2 weeks with virulent virus (McFerran et
al., 1982). In the last month of pregnancy they had been
vaccinated once with an oil adjuvant vaccine. At 6 weeks of
age the progeny were bled and each infected intranasally with
1 ml of NIA.1, titre $10^{6.5}$ $TCID_{50}$.

At 15 weeks after infection, the pigs were divided into
3 groups. Group 1 (4 pigs) were twice injected with 30 mgm
dexamethasone, 2 days apart. Group 2 (4 pigs) were infected

with <u>Salmonella cholerae-suis</u> intranasally. Group 3 (7 pigs)
were left as controls and housed separately. In addition 2
serologically negative pigs were introduced into both groups
1 and 2 in order to detect any excreted virus.

RESULTS

At challenge the piglets had high levels of antibody
(Table 3) ranging from 48 to greater than 256. Following
infection there was no evidence of any disease, not even a
mild febrile response or transient inappetance. The only
evidence of infection was from reisolation of virus from the
nasal mucosa.

In spite of the infection, titres continued to fall for
the next 2-4 weeks. They then remained at these levels until
the 15th week following challenge. At this stage the titres
ranged from 3 to 48 except for pig 309 which had jumped from
a titre of 8 at 11 weeks to 256 at 15 weeks.

Following the treatments at 15 weeks post-infection it
was clear that some pigs in each group had developed rising
titres. Thus in the dexamethasone treated group 3 pigs had
greater than 4 fold rises in titre, whiles one pig did not
respond. In the Salmonella infected group all 4 pigs
responded with rising antibody titres. Two of the control
infected group (pigs 305 and 313) showed 4 fold or greater
rising titres in addition to pig 3o9.

A serologically negative control pig in each group
developed antibody, indicating virus spread to these animals.

DISCUSSION

Pigs infected under the cover of maternal antibody do
not necessarily respond with active antibody production even
though virus is excreted. This confirms earlier work
(McFerran and Dow, 1973).

The pigs were given dexamethasone in order to attempt to
reactivate latent virus. <u>Salmonella cholerae-suis</u> was used
for the same purpose especially since in fattening units,
mixed infections with AD virus were often found.

TABLE 3   Results of testing sera for neutralising antibody to Aujeszky's disease virus. Pigs with high levels of maternal antibody were challenged at 6 weeks with $10^{6.5} TCID_{50}$ NIA-1

Pig Number	Treatment at week 15	Weeks following infection												
		0	2	3	4	5	6	7	9	11	15	18	20	23
50	None. In contact controls introduced at week 15										NT	24	24	24
95											NT	<2	<2	<2
195											NT	<2	<2	<2
94											NT	4	8	16
303	Two intramuscular injections of 30 mg dexamethasone, at a 48 hour interval	128	64	32	24	16	16	24	12	24	32	48	256	768
307		128	16	48	24	24	24	16	24	12	16	32	64	192
315		192	48	48	24	24	24	12	16	24	8	6	6	6
316		96	16	12	12	12	16	12	24	32	12	192	192	96
302	Intranasal inoculation of Salmonella cholerae suis	>256	64	64	64	48	48	24	32	24	8	64	32	192
306		256	96	32	24	12	16	12	8	6	6	96	48	48
308		48	16	48	16	24	32	16	32	32	32	48	96	256
301		256	48	48	24	12	12	8	6	12	4	6	24	96
304	None	128	96	12	32	12	12	12	6	6	3	NT	3	3
305		>256	96	32	32	24	24	16	16	16	6	NT	512	768
309		64	16	16	8	16	8	8	8	8	256	NT	NT	128
310		256	48	48	48	32	48	16	16	32	48	NT	32	48
311		>256	96	64	32	32	12	12	4	6	6	NT	12	16
313		256	48	32	48	24	24	16	12	16	8	NT	128	192
314		128	16	16	16	32	48	24	16	32	32	NT	64	64

NT = Not tested

It is evident from these results that carriers do indeed occur. Furthermore one pig, not artificially stimulated showed a rising titre between 11 and 15 weeks. It is not, clear from these results if this pig then infected other pigs in the same group or if they also spontaneously broke down. Certainly by 20 weeks after challenge (ie when they were 26 weeks of age) 3 of the 7 pigs in the control group were showing evidence of active infection. At this age on the farm studied, these pigs would have been in the gilt house and it was not uncommon to find similar titres in this house.

Virus excretion was not studied, in case the act of taking samples would damage the mucosa and aid virus spread.

We concluded from the results presented and from other unpublished studies on herds suffering natural infection that infection under the cover of maternal antibody with subsequent reactivation of virus at farrowing may play a significant part in the epidemiology of Aujeszky's disease.

REFERENCES

Beran, G.W., Davies, E.B., Arambulo, P.V., Will, L.A., Hill, H.T. and Rock, D.L. 1980. Persistence of pseudorabies virus on infected swine. J. Am. Vet. Med. Ass., 176, 998-1000.

Davies, E.B. and Beran, G.W. 1980. Simultaneous shedding of pseudorabies virus from a clinically recovered post-parturient sow. J. Am. Vet. Med. Ass., 176, 1345-1347.

Gutekunst, D.E. 1979. Latent pseudorabies virus infection in swine detected by RNA-DNA hybridization. Am. J. Vet. Res., 40, 1568-1572.

Howarth, J.A. 1969. A serological study of pseudorabies in swine. J. Am. Vet. Med. Ass., 154, 1583-1589.

McFerran, J.B. and Dow, C. 1964. The excretion of Aujeszky's disease virus by experimentally infected pigs. Res. Vet. Sci., 5, 405-410.

McFerran, J.B. and Dow, C. 1973. The effect of colostrum derived antibody on mortality and virus excretion following experimental infection of piglets with Aujesky's disease virus. Res. Vet. Sci., 15, 208-214.

McFerran, J.B., McCracken, R.M. and Dow, C. 1982. Comparative studies with inactivated and attenuated vaccines for protection of fattening pigs. In "Aujeszky's disease" (Ed. G. Wittmann and S.A. Hall). (Nijhoff, The Hague). pp. 163-170.

Mock, R.E., Crandell, R.A. and Mesfin, G.M. 1981. Induced latency in pseudorabies vaccinated pigs. Can. J. Comp. Med., 45, 56-59.

Nikinit, M.G. 1961. Pigs as carriers of Aujeszky's disease virus (in Russian). Veterinarya, 38, 32-36.

Rziha, H.-J., Döller, P.C. and Wittmann, G. 1982. Detection of Aujeszky's disease virus and viral DNA in tissues of latently infected pigs. In "Aujeszky's disease" (Ed. G. Wittmann and S.A. Hall). (Martinus Nijhoff, The Hague). pp. 205-210.

Sabo, A. 1969. Persistence of perorally administered virulent pseudorabies virus in the organism of non-immune and immunized pigs. Acta. virol., 13, 269-277.

Sabo, A. and Rajcani, J. 1976. Latent pseudorabies virus infections in pigs. Acta. Virol. Prague, 20, 208-214.

Wittmann, G., Rziha, H.-J. and Döller, P.C. 1982. Occurrence of clinical Aujeszky's disease in immunosuppressed latently infected pigs. In "Aujeszky's disease" (Ed. G. Wittmann and S.A. Hall). (Martinus Nijhoff, The Hague). pp. 211-214.

LATENCY OF VIRULENT AUJESZKY'S DISEASE VIRUS IN PIGS IS
NOT PREVENTED BY PASSIVE OR ACTIVE IMMUNIZATION

J.T. van Oirschot
Central Veterinary Institute, Department of Virology,
39, Houtribweg, 8221 RA Lelystad, The Netherlands

ABSTRACT
    The NIA-3 strain of Aujeszky's disease virus (ADV)
established latent infections in seronegative pigs, in pigs
having high or low levels of maternal antibody and in
intranasally vaccinated pigs. One to 4 months after the
primary infection latency of ADV was demonstrated by in vitro
and in vivo reactivation procedures.
    Explants of trigeminal ganglion produced infectious ADV
after 4 days in culture. Administration of high doses of
corticosteroids to previously infected pigs resulted in
shedding of virus in oral secretions after a lag period of
4-11 days. The recrudescent shedding was not accompanied by
severe clinical signs. In a number of pigs the recurrent
infection resulted in a rise of neutralizing antibody. Most
pigs re-excreted ADV to such a level that in contact pigs
became infected.
    The findings reported here indicate that pigs, whether
immunized or not at the time of virulent ADV infection, must
be regarded as potential shedders of ADV.

INTRODUCTION

    Establishment of latency is a characteristic feature of
herpesvirus infections. The pig is considered to be the
natural host of Aujeszky's disease virus (ADV), although other
animal species can also be infected. Several strains of ADV
have been shown to induce latent infections in pigs (Sabo and
Rajcáni, 1976; Gutekunst, 1979; Beran et al., 1980; Mock et
al., 1981;, Wittmann et al., 1982). In most studies
seronegative pigs were used. Mock et al. (1981) demonstrated
that pigs vaccinated with modified-live vaccine failed to
prevent the production of latency of virulent virus. The
present study was conducted to investigate the establishment
of latency and subsequent reactivation of the virulent NIA-3
strain of ADV in seronegative, passively or actively immunized
pigs.

MATERIALS AND METHODS

Pigs

Pigs were from the Dutch Landrace minimal disease herd of
the Central Veterinary Institute. The herd is free of
antibodies to ADV, except for a number of sows that are
vaccinated twice a year with inactivated vaccine (Geskyvac,
Roger Bellon, France) to produce piglets with maternal
antibody. Pigs were housed in isolation pens and observed
daily for clinical signs.

Vaccination and infection

Pigs were intranasally vaccinated by instilling 0.5 ml of
a suspension, containing 10^6 plaque forming units (PFU) per ml
of the Bartha's K strain, drop by drop into each nostril. The
vaccine virus was grown on secondary pig kidney (PK2) cells.
Pigs were infected or challenge-exposed intranasally, as
described above, with 10^5 PFU of the virulent Northern Ireland
Aujeszky three (NIA-3) strain (McFerran and Dow, 1975; kindly
provided by Dr.J.B. McFerran, Belfast, Northern-Ireland),
passaged 6 times in PK2 cells.

Corticosteroid treatment

Pigs involved in the in vivo reactivation experiments
were given dexamethasone or prednisolone (1.5 mg and 15 mg per
kg of body weight, respectively) during 4 consecutive days. To
prevent secondary bacterial infections, pigs which developed
signs of illness were treated with antibiotics for 5 days.

Sampling procedures, virus titration and virus-neutralization
test

Oropharyngeal fluid (OPF) samples were collected,
processed and assayed for infectious ADV as described
elsewhere (De Leeuw et al., 1982). Isolates were identified by
neutralization with a specific ADV-antiserum.

Pigs were bled from the anterior vena cava before and at
weekly intervals after vaccination, infection or
corticosteroid treatment. The sera were tested for

neutralizing ADV-antibody in duplicate in a microtitre system, using PK2 cells and a virus serum incubation period of 24 hours at 37^OC. Titres are expressed as the $\log_{10}$ of the reciprocal of the final serum dilution inhibiting cytopathic effect in 50% of the cultures.

In vitro reactivation

Four 6-month-old pigs and 2 pigs of 2 months of age, which were all seronegative, were infected with NIA-3 virus and killed 4 weeks later. Trigeminal ganglia, tonsil and olfactory bulbs were removed for in vitro detection of latent ADV. Three pigs were given 20 mg dexamethasone for 4 days prior to slaughter. Three pigs (Nos. 892, 893, 896) with maternal antibody were infected at 3 weeks of age. Four months later they were given prednisolone. One month after treatment they were killed and their trigeminal ganglia examined for latent ADV.

Tissues to be assayed for latent ADV were removed under sterile conditions and minced into 1 to 2 mm pieces. In the explant method a few drops of chicken embryo extract were added to the pieces of tissue, which were then placed in culture-tubes precoated with chicken plasma. The pieces were allowed to adhere for 1 hour and thereafter the culture medium, consisting of Hanks' BSS, 10% of lamb serum and 100 IU of penicillin and 100 IU of streptomycin, was added to the tubes. In the co-culture method small tissue fragments were placed on a monolayer of PK2 cells, in Eagle's MEM supplemented with 2% lamb serum and antibiotics. Once a week the tissue fragments were transferred to fresh monolayers. The medium of explanted and co-cultured tissue was changed twice a week during at least 3 weeks, and tested for ADV, as described previously (De Leeuw et al., 1982). Tissue homogenates were prepared as 10% suspensions in Hanks' BSS with 0.5% lactalbumin hydrolysate, and 10 times the concentration of antibiotics used in the culture medium. After centrifugation for 10 minutes at 1200 x g, the supernatant was assayed for ADV.

In vivo reactivation

Experiment 1. Six pigs (Nos 634, 651, 652, 653, 656, 660) were infected at 6 months of age. Three months later they were housed individually and treated with corticosteroids. In each pen an additonal, sentinel pig was in contact. The pigs were swabbed every other day for 21 days after the initiation of corticosteroid treatment (days post treatment (DPT 21). The sentinel pigs were swabbed when showing clinical signs. Pigs 652 and 656 underwent a second corticosteroid treatment 1 month after the first one. Another 3 pigs (Nos 892, 893, 896) also used in the in vitro reactivation experiment, were infected at 3 weeks of age. Four months later they were also placed in separate pens, and then treated with corticosteroid. OPF-samples were collected daily for 3 weeks after treatment.

Experiment 2. Four pigs with maternal antibody were vaccinated intranasally at 10 weeks of age. Challenge-exposure was done 2 months later. Ten weeks after challenge, the pigs were given prednisolone. They were then housed separately and one sentinel pig was introduced into each pen. Pigs were mouth-swabbed daily for 3 weeks. Pig 8045 received two prednisolone treatments, 1 month apart.

RESULTS

In vitro reactivation

The explant culture technique, the co-cultivation technique and the tissue suspension technique were compared for detection of ADV in tonsils, olfactory bulbs and trigeminal ganglia from 6 pigs infected intransally 3 weeks previously. ADV was demonstrated in ganglionic tissue from 2 pigs by the explant culture and co-cultivation method, but not in tissue homogenates of ganglia (Table 1). No virus could be detected in tonsils and olfactory bulbs. The pigs from which virus was recovered had received dexamethasone. Oropharyngeal swabs were virus negative on the day of slaughter.

The individual supernatants of explant cultures were assayed for infectious ADV. Table 2 shows that virus was not detected until 4 days after the initiation of culture. The cultures of 391 RG and 616 RG produced ADV for at least 18 and 11 days, respectively.

In our hands the explant culture technique was less laborious than the co-cultivation technique. Therefore, in

TABLE 1   In vitro reactivation of latent ADV.

Tissue	Detection-method*		
	TS	EC	CC
Olfactory bulb	0/6**	0/6	0/6
Tonsil	0/6	0/6	0/6
Trigeminal ganglion	0/6	2/6	2/6

*   TS: tissue suspension; EC: explant culture;
     CC:co-culture
** Positive/total examined

further experiments we used the explant culture method for the detection of latent ADV in vitro.

In the above experiments we cultured 30-50% of the ganglionic tissue. In the next experiment the entire ganglionic tissue of 3 pigs, which proved to be latently infected, was cultured and the culture tubes were individually assayed for ADV. Seven out of 10 cultures from the right ganglion of pig 892 released virus into the supernatant, whereas its left

TABLE 2   Virus titres in supernatants of explanted
           trigeminal ganglia.

Pig no.	Tissue	Days of culture								
		0	2	4	7	9	11	14	17	21
391*	RG**	-	-	1.8	3.6	3.6	3.6	2.7	2.3	1.1
	LG	-	-	-	-	-	-	1.8	2.8	-
616	RG	-	-	5.3	5.2	4.2	nd	3.4	nd	nd

*   Pig 391 was 6 months and pog 616 2 months of age
     when infected.
** RG: right ganglion; LG: left ganglion
nd not done

ganglion was negative. ADV was recovered from 1 out of each of
5 cultures from both ganglia of pig 893 (Table 3). No virus
was recovered from cultured ganglia of pig 896.

TABLE 3   Reactivation of ADV in explant cultures of
           the entire ganglionic tissue

Pig no.	Trigeminal ganglion	Positive/ total	In vivo reactivation
892	L	0/10	+
	R	7/10	
893	L	1/5	+
	R	1/5	
896	L	0/5	+
	R	0/5	

In vivo reactivation

Experiment 1. The pigs which had high, low or no maternal
antibody showed mild to severe signs of AD after primary
infection, and virus was excreted for at least 10 days.
Corticosteroid treatment at 3-4 months post infection resulted
in clinical disease in 4 out of 9 pigs. Pig 656 had fever on
DPT 4-7. The most prominent sign in the other pigs (651, 893,
896) was respiratory distress, starting around DPT 14.

Reactivation of ADV was evidenced by virus shedding in 6
out of 9 pigs (Table 4), and in one pig (652) indirectly, by
the development of antibody to ADV in its sentinel pig. Virus
was recovered from OPF after a lag period of 4-11 days. The
recurrent ADV infection resulted in raised neutralizing
antibody levels in 4 pigs.

The sentinels of pigs 651, 652, 656 became infected, as
shown by the production of antibody to ADV. The sentinel of
pig 651 developed fever and a slightly reduced appetite on DPT
14-16 and excreted virus about the same time. The other
sentinel pigs remained healthy. Pig 634, which had virus in

its OPF for at least 3 days, did not transmit ADV since its contact control remained serologically negative.

Experiment 2. The pigs intranasally vaccinated with Bartha's K strain developed mild signs of AD after challenge

TABLE 4   In vivo reactivation of ADV in pigs with high, low or no maternal antibody.

Pig	Symptoms		Virus in OPF*		Maternal	Antibody response	
no.	Inf.	Sent.	Inf.	Sent.	antibody titre	Inf.	Sent.
634	−	−	+	nd	−	−	−
651	+	+	+	+	0.60	−	+
652	−	−	−	nd	0.30	−	+
653	−	−	−	nd	−	−	−
656	+	−	+**	nd	0.30	+	+
660	−	−	−	nd	0.30	−	−
892***	−		+		2.10	+	
893***	+		+		2.25	+	
896***	+		+		2.10	+	

*   Oropharyngeal fluid samples
**   Pig 656 had virus in OPF only after the second treatment
*** No pigs placed in contact
nd   not done

and virus was detected in OPF samples for 6 days. Results of this experiment are shown in Table 5. After corticosteroid treatment pig 8056 had pyrexia on DPT 8-12 and shed virus at the same time. Its entinel pig showed mild signs of disease on DPT 11-14, excreted virus on DPT 10-16 and elicited neutralizing antibody to ADV. The other pigs showed neither clinical signs nor viral excretion after the corticosteroid course. Pig 8045 was given a second treatment and a mild fever and diarrhoea was noticed on DPT 6-11. ADV was recovered from its OPF on DPT 6-7. Its sentinel pig showed highly elevated body temperatures on DPT 9-14 and was slightly depressed on DPT 12-13. Its OPF sample contained high concentrations of ADV from DPT 8-15. This pig developed neutralizing antibody to ADV.

More detailed results of the in vivo reactivation experiments will be published elsewhere.

DISCUSSION

The results of the present study demonstrate that the virulent NIA-3 strain of ADV can establish latent infections in seronegative pigs, in pigs with maternal antibody and in intranasally vaccinated pigs. That ADV persists in a latent state is strongly suggested by the failure to isolate virus from trigeminal ganglia homogenates, whereas explanted fragments of the same tissue produced infectious virus. In addition, ADV was not detected in mouth swabs on the day of slaughter. Latency of ADV is also indicated by the observation that there are lag periods after in vitro and in vivo reactivation.

In the present study reactivation of ADV has been accomplished by in vitro and in vivo methods. Explanted fragments of trigeminal ganglia from infected pigs released virus into the supernatant fluid. To obtain optimal results it seems necessary to culture the entire tissue of both ganglia, since in one pig only 2 out of 10 cultures produced ADV, while in another pig no virus was found in one ganglion. Thus, these findings suggest that generally in latent ADV infections a low proportion of ganglion cells are infected. In other herpesvirus infections, the percentages of latently infected neurons are estimated to be between 0.1 and 10% (Ackermann et al., 1981; Walz et al., 1976; Klein, 1982).

The administration of high doses of corticosteroids to infected pigs resulted in reactivation of ADV, as evidenced by viral shedding. In a number of pigs the artificially induced recurrent ADV infection was symptomless whereas other pigs developed clinical signs. However, in some pigs the symptoms were probably due to the corticosteroid course, since there was no apparent correlation between appearance of signs and periods of virus shedding.

The results of in vitro and in vivo reactivation are not in complete agreement. Pig 896 shed virus after immunosuppressive treatment, but virus was not recovered from its cultured ganglia. Plausible explanations for this discrepancy are either that ADV was latently present in the trigeminal ganglion but was simply not reactivated during the culture period, or that the virus resided in other tissues.

The recrudescent virus spread to susceptible pigs. The sentinel pigs that became infected, generally showed mild or no signs of AD. This is an unexpected finding, since the NIA-3 strain of ADV is highly virulent. However, pigs infected by contact may show less severe signs of AD, because the dose of virus transmitted is probably low (Baskerville, 1971). To determine whether ADV has changed during the reactivation process, the DNA's of the different isolates have been analyzed with Bam HI restriction-endonuclease. The results of these analyses are reported separately (Gielkens, proceedings of this seminar).

The recrudescent virus excreted by the pigs that were vaccinated and subsequently challenge-exposed, proved to be the virulent NIA-3 strain, as shown by restriction-endonuclease analysis of the DNA. No evidence was obtained for simultaneous shedding of vaccine virus. It is not surprising that virulent ADV induced latency in vaccinated pigs, since it is well-known that ADV can replicate in (intranasally) vaccinated pigs (McFerran et al., 1979; De Leeuw et al., 1982). In addition, Mock et al. (1981) have already reported ADV latency in parenterally vaccinated pigs.

The inability to detect recrudescence of Bartha's K strain of ADV is in keeping with our findings that Bartha virus could not be recovered from intranasally vaccinated pigs, using in vivo and in vitro methods successfully employed in reactivation of virulent ADV (to be published). These results suggest that Bartha virus is not readily reactivated or does not persist at all in intransally vaccinated pigs.

Maternal antibody also failed to prevent the induction of latency of ADV in pigs. Establishment of latency under cover of passive immunity has also been shown in herpes simplex virus infection in mice (Sekizawa et al., 1980). On the other hand, in herpes simplex virus infection of guinea pigs maternal antibody exerted a protective effect on the development of latency (Tenser and Hsiung, 1977).

In conclusion, virulent ADV can establish latency in pigs, irrespective of whether or not the pigs are seronegative, passively, or actively immunized. Reactivated virus can spread to susceptible pigs. Thus, infected pigs, whether immunized or not, must be regarded potential shedders of ADV.

ACKNOWLEDGEMENTS

The author thanks D. de Jong, A.D.N.H.J. Huffels and W.A.M. van Rossum for skillful technical assistance.

REFERENCES

Ackermann, M., Peterhans, E. and Wyler, R. 1981. DNA of bovine herpes virus type 1 (BHV-1) is present in trigeminal ganglia of latently infected calves. Proc. 5th. international congress of virology, Strassbourg, France.

Baskerville, A. 1971. A study of the pulmonary tissue of the pig and its reaction to the virus of Aujeszky's disease. PhD Thesis, Queens Univ., Belfast.

Beran, G.W., Davies, E.B., Arambulo, P.V., Will, L.A., Hill, H.T. and Rock, D.L. 1980. Persistence of pseudorabies virus in infected swine. JAVMA, 176, 998-1000.

De Leeuw, P.W., Wijsmuller, J.M., Zantinga, J.W. and Tielen, M.J.M. 1982. Intranasal vaccination of pigs against Aujeszky's disease. 1. Comparison of intransal and parenteral vaccination with an attenuated vaccine in 12-week-old pigs from immunized dams. Vet. Quarterly, 4, 49-55.

Klein, R.J. 1982. The pathogenesis of acute, latent and recurrent herpes simplex infections. Arch. Virol., 72, 143-168.

McFerran, J.B. and Dow, C. 1975. Studies on immunisation of pigs with the Bartha strain of Aujeszky's disease virus. Res. Vet. Sci., 19, 17-22.

McFerran, J.B., Dow, C. and McCracken, R.M. 1979. Experimental studies in weaned pigs with three vaccines against Aujeszky's disease. Comp. Immun. Microbiol. infect. Dis., 2, 327-334.

Mock, R.E., Crandell, R.A., Mesfin, G.M. 1981. Induced latency in pseudorabies vaccinated pigs. Can. J. Comp. Med., 45, 56-59.

Sabó, A. and Rajčani, J. 1976. Latent pseudorabies virus infection in pigs. Acta Virol., 20, 208-214.

Sekizawa, T., Openshaw, H., Wohlenberg, C. and Notkins, A.L. 1980. Latency of herpes simplex virus in absence of neutralizing antibody; model for reactivation. Science, 210, 1026-1028.

Tenser, R.B., Hsiung, G.D. 1977. Pathogenesis of latent herpes simplex virus infection of the trigeminal ganglion in guinea pigs: Effects of age, passive immunization, and hydrocortisone. Infect. Immun., 16, 69-74.

Walz, M.A., Yamamoto, H. and Notkins, A.L. 1976. Immunological response restricts number of cells in sensory ganglia infected with herpes simplex virus. Nature, 264, 554-556.

Wittmann, G., Rziha, H.J., Döller, P.C. 1982. Occurrence of clinical Aujezsky's disease in immunosuppressed latently infected pigs. In: Wittmann, G., Hall, S.A. (eds): Aujezsky's disease. Curr. Top. Vet. Med. Anim. Sci., 17, 211-214. Martinus Nijhoff Publishers.

OCCURENCE OF PSEUDORABIESVIRUS DNA IN
LATENTLY INFECTED PIGS

H.-J. Rziha, T. Mettenleiter, G. Wittmann
Federal Research Institute for Animal Diseases
P.O.Box 1149, 7400 Tübinben, Federal Republic of Germany

ABSTRACT
     After experimental infection of swine we determined the
time of establishment of PrV latency. Results of virus
recovery and virus reactivation from organs of latently
infected animals are presented. For the detection of latent
viral DNA different techniques of molecular hybridization
were preformed (in situ hybridization, reassociation kinetic,
Southern blot analysis). The occurrence of the viral genome
is demonstrated in several neural tissues. In addition the
presence of PrV DNA is suggested in white blood cells of
latently infected pigs.

INTRODUCTION
     One major charateristic of herpesviruses is their
ability to establish latency in the infected host. After
primary infection pseudorabiesvirus (PrV) persists in a
latent state in the recovered pigs (Sabo, 1969; Sabo and
Grunert, 1971; Sabo and Rajcani, 1976; Beran et al., 1980;
Davies and Beran), as e.g. herpes simplex virus (HSV) in man.
The latent virus can be reactivated by exogeneous or
endogeneous stimuli, and subsequently shed without clinical
signs (Sabo and Rajcani, 1976; Beran et al., 1980; Mock et
al., 1980; Davies and Beran, 1980; Rziha et al., 1982;
Wittmann et al., 1982). In animal models it could be shown
that the main source of latent HSV are the sensory ganglia of
the infected host (Stevens and Cook, 1971). During the latent
state viral DNA could be detected in the central nervous
system (Sequiera et al., 1979; Cabrera et al., 1980; Fraser
et al., 1981). Also prV and PrV DNA is still present in
neural tissues, especially in the trigeminal ganglia of the
latently infected pigs, though virus cannot be recovered
(Gutekunst, 1979; Gutekunst et al., 1980; Beran et al. 1980;
Rziha et al., 1981).
     The latent HSV genome seems to persist rather in a
non-infectious form than that a low-level chronic infection
does occur. Evidence for such a static state comes from

experiments which show that (1) temperature sensitive mutants of HSV are able to establish latency in tissues at the non-permissive temperature (Lofgren et al., 1977; McLennan and Darby, 1980); (2) treatment with antiviral drugs inhibiting the viral DNA replication did not affect the virus reactivation rate from latently infected ganglia (Field et al., 1979; Blyth et al., 1980); (3) during latency no viral transcription could be observed as compared to the acute phase of infection (Puga et al., 1978). However, a limited viral gene expression was demonstrated in the sensory neurons of humans and rabbits (Green et al., 1981; Galloway et al., 1982). Moreover, HSV thymidine kinase activity was found in the ganglia of latently infected mice (Yamamoto et al., 1977). Recently the expression of this viral enzyme is suggested to play a possible role by the invasion of HSV into the ganglia, and therefore by the establishment of latency (Tenser et al., 1981). However, which mechanisms may actually regulate the initiation, the maintenance, and the reactivation of latency, is still unclear.

There are 2 reasons giving rise to investigate PrV latency in more detail. It displays one important problem with respect to a successsful virus eradication programme, and on the other hand, it provides the opportunity to study virus-host relationships during herpesvirus latency in a natural host. The following experiments were initiated in order to determine (1) at which time after experimental infection of pigs the latent state of PrV will be established, (2) to define more precisely the range of tissues harbouring the latent virus, and (3) to investigate the presence and state of the latent viral genome.

RESULTS AND DISCUSSION
1. Establishment of latency

Pigs were intranasally infected with a virulent PrV strain (Phylaxia), and at different times after infection (p.i.) part of the animals was killed. Virus recovery was performed by co-cultivation of various tissue fragments with

TABLE 1: Virus recovery from latently infected pigs. For a viurs reactivation part of the animals were immunosuppressed (+IS) by the application of prednisolone (1250 – 1875 mg per animal) for 4 consecutive days. Virus isolation was performed by co-cultivation of tissues fragments with permissive MDBK or BHK cells, essentially according to BERAN et al. (1980).

| Organ tissues | Times p.i. (weeks) | | | | | | | | | | | | | |
| | 5 | | 7 | | 11 | | 12 | | 26 | | 36 | | 64 | |
	-IS[a]	+IS	-IS	+IS	-IS	+IS	-IS	+IS	-IS	+IS	-IS	+IS	-IS	+IS
Lungs	2/4[b]	2/2	0/1	1/1	0/4	3/4	0/2	0/2	0/3	2/2	0/2	1/3	0/2	1/2
Nasal mucosa	nt[c]		nt		0/4	2/4	0/2	1/2	0/3	0/2	0/2	2/3	0/2	2/2
Tonsils	2/4	2/2	0/1	1/1	0/4	3/4	0/2	1/2	1/3	2/2	0/2	0/3	0/2	1/2
Lymph nodes	2/4	2/2	0/1	1/1	0/4	2/4	0/2	1/2	0/3	2/2	0/2	2/3	nt	
Brain stem	2/4	2/2	0/1	1/1	0/4	3/4	1/2	2/2	3/3	2/2	0/2	0/3	0/2	1/2
Trigeminal ganglia	nt		nt		0/4	nt	0/2	1/2	0/3	2/2	0/2	1/3	0/2	0/2
Medulla	nt		0/1	1/1	0/4	1/1	0/2	2/2	1/3	2/2	0/2	2/3	0/2	0/2
Olfactory bulb	nt		0/1	1/1	0/4	1/1	0/2	1/1	2/3	2/2	0/2	1/3	0/2	1/2
Spinal cord	nt		0/1	1/1	0/4	nt	0/2	2/2	0/3	2/2	0/2	1/3	nt	

a IS: immunosuppression

b no. of positives / no. of animals tested

c nt: not tested

permissive indicator cells (Rziha et al., 1982; Wittmann et al., 1982). In order to prove the reactivity of latent virus the other part of the animals was treated with prednisolone for 2 - 4 consecutive days, and also tested for the occurrence of infectious PrV. The results of these experiments are given in Table 1. Beyond 7 weeks p.i. virus could be no more re-isolated from various organ tissues of the non-treated animals (-IS), except single cases. In contrast, after immunosuppression of the pigs virus recovery succeeded readily up to 64 weeks p.i. (+IS). The identity of the recovered virus was occasionally proven by restriction enzyme analysis of the viral DNA (data not shown). From these results we conclude that in our system a latent PrV infection will be established beyond 7 weeks p.i. At later times p.i. virus recovery was only achieved by immunosuppressive

TABLE 2   Detection of PrV DNA by in situ cytohybridization in organ tissues of latently
infected pigs.

Organ samples	Times p.i. (weeks)					
	5	6	7	11	13	26
Tonsils	0	0	–	–	–	–
Lymph nodes	0	0	0	–	–	–
Lungs	0	0	–	–	–	–
Brain stem	0	0	–	–	–	–
Trigeminal ganglia	nt[a]	0	nt	0	0	0
Spinal cord	–	–	0	0	nt	0
Vagus nerve	nt	nt	0	0	nt	nt
Maxillar nerve	nt	nt	0	0	nt	nt

[a]   nt :   not tested

treatment of the latently infected animals. Furthermore, the experiments could imply the presence of latent PrV in a non-infectious form. However, we cannot absolutely exclude a

very low persistent or abortive virus multiplication, which
might be not detectable by this assay.

2. Presence of viral DNA

Organ tissues of the latently infected,
non-immunosuppressed pigs were further analyzed for the
presence of viral DNA. For this purpose in situ
cytohybridizations were performed on frozen thin sections of
various organ tissues (Brahic and Haase, 1978; Rziha et al.,
1982). Purified viral DNA was in vitro radioactively labeled
(Rigby et al., 1977), and used as a radioactive probe. Its
fidelity was confirmed in reconstruction experiments by the
Southern blotting technique (Souther, 1975). In addition, for
each set of experiments control hybridizations were done on
sections of organs of uninfected pigs (Fig. 1a, b). Multiple,
heavily labeled cells were found after hybridization of
sections of tonsils (Fig. 1c, d) and lungs (Fig. 2) of
acutely infected animals. Some results of hybridizations with
organ tissues of latently infected pigs are shown in Figure 3
and 4. Very single cells can be detected displaying the
presence of viral DNA. The results of the in situ
cytohybridization studies are summarized in Table 2. This
table comprises only those results which were undoubtedly
positive. From these data it becomes apparent that the latent
viral DNA persist predominantly in the neural tissuses of the
infected animals. Obviously latent PrV was not segmented only
to certain ganglia. It could be also demonstrated in other
neural tissues of the latently infected animals, as e.g. in
the presence of latent HSV in the ganglia of mice (Walz et
al., 1976). From the number of specific grains after in situ
hybridization a rough calculation of the amount of PrV DNA
per positive cell nucleus could be made. According to the
specific activity of the radioactive probe, to the exposure
time, and to the estimated hybridization efficiency (Gall and
Pardue, 1971) between 1 to 5 viral genome copies were
present.

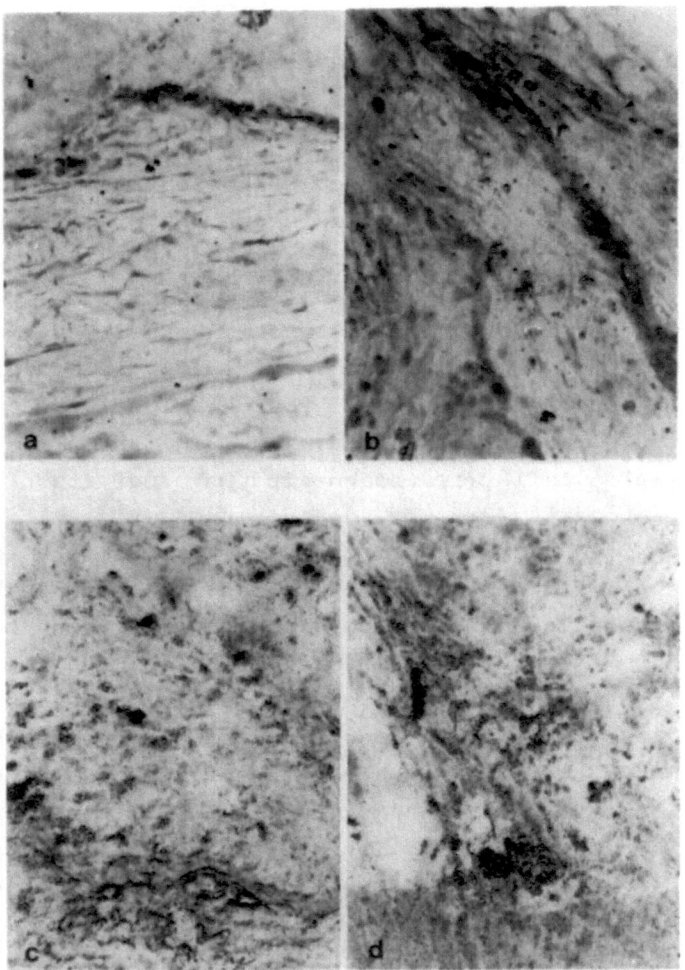

Fig. 1: In situ cytohybridization of frozen thin
sections of tonsils of an uninfected pig (a and b), and
of tonsils of an acutely infected pig (c and d).

3. Qantification of the amount of viral DNA

In order to determine more precisely the amount of viral
DNA during the latent state we investigated DNA samples of
different neural tissues by liquid hybridization
(reassociation kinetic). The organ DNA was extracted and in

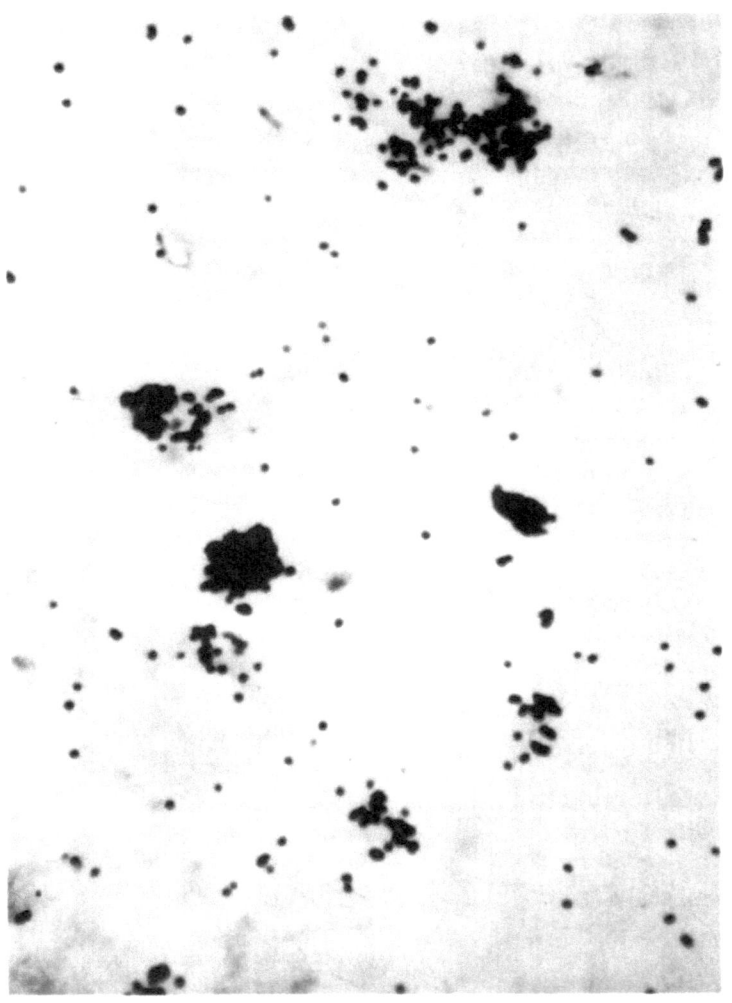

Fig. 2   Detection of PrV DNA in a lung tissue section
of an acutely infected animal (7 days p.i.).

solution hybridized with purified viral DNA, which was <u>in</u>
<u>vitro</u> radioactively labeled with ^{32}P-nucleotides to a
specific activity of 2 - 5 X 10^8 cpm/ug. In 2 cases a
relatively high concentration of the latent PrV DNA (5 - 6
genome copies/cell) was demonstrated in the brain and in the
cortex of animals 13 weeks p.i. (Rzhia <u>et al.</u>, 1981).
However, in further studies of 10 other DNA samples tested

436

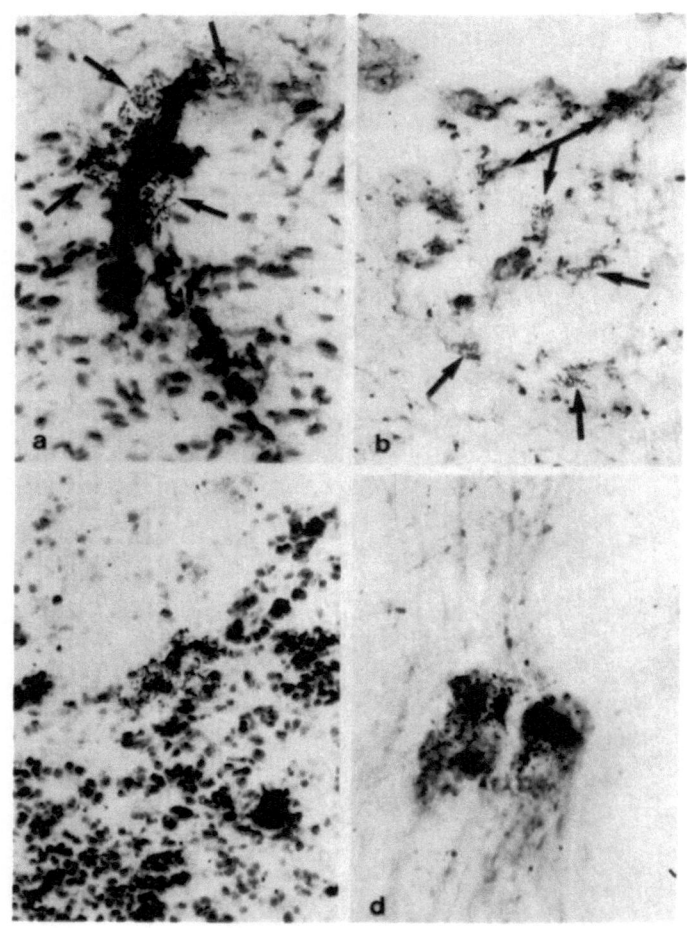

Fig. 3   Detection of PrV DNA in cells (arrows) of the
vagus nerve of 2 animals 7 weeks p.i. (a and b), and in
cells of lymph nodes (c) and tonsils (d) of a pig 5
weeks p.i.

only 0.2 - 0.5 genome copies/cell or less could be found.
These data show that generally the amount of the latent PrV
DNA in neural tissues is very low. Therefore these results,
as well as the _in situ_ hybridization data described might
favour the suggestion that the latent PrV occurs in a
non-replicable form. An explanation for the presence of the
relatively heavy load of viral DNA in the 2 cases mentioned

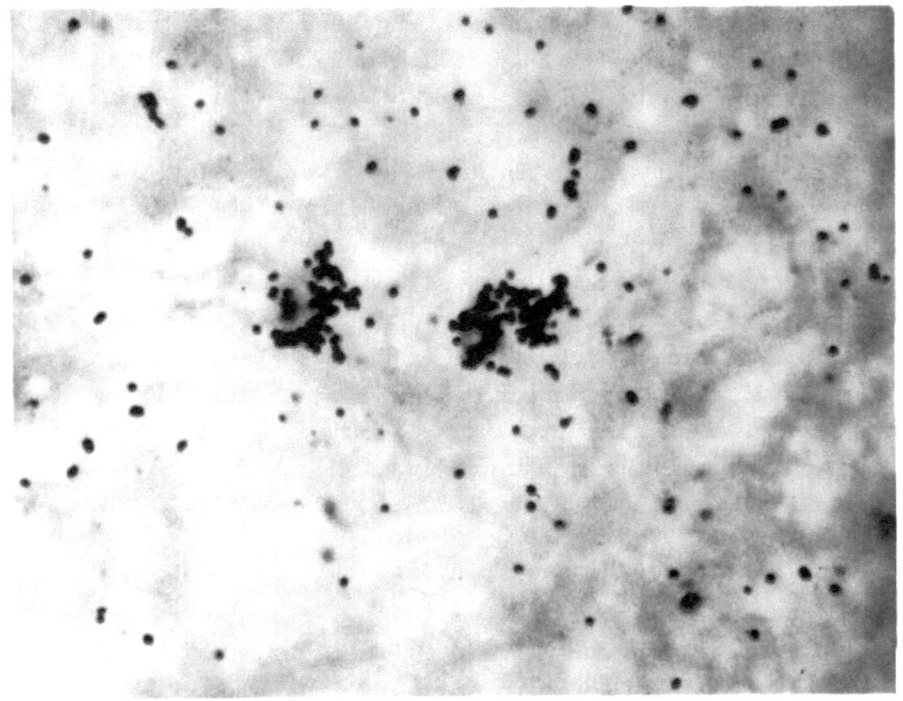

Fig. 4   Two cells displaying PrV DNA in a section of
the spinal cord of a pig 11 weeks p.i.

above remains speculative (defective viral DNA ?). Actually
no virus rescue could be achieved with both neural tissue
specimens.

4. Blot hybridizations

Investigations for the presence and the state of the
latent PrV DNA were initiated using the Southern blot
technique (Southern, 1975). The DNA samples were cleaved with
restriction enzymes generating only a small number of
virusspecific fragments (Hind III, Bgl II, Xba I), in order
to increase the sensitivity of the test. All hybridizations
were performed under stringent conditions. As an example, a
reconstruction experiment is shown in Figure 5. There we were
able to detect less than 0.5 genome copies (Fig. 5). A

preliminar result of a blot hybridization is shown in Figure 6. Hind III-cleavage of the viral DNA (lane 1 and 10) results in the generation of 3 virusspecific bands. The hybridization of the Hind III-digested DNA of different neural tissues is demonstrated in lanes 3 to 9 of the Figure (for details see Figure legend). Additionally the DNA of unseparated white blood cells of a latently infected pig was tested (lane 2). In all cases a relatively weak hybridization was found with DNA fragments comigrating with the largest Hind III fragment A of the PrV DNA (about 50 md). A more pronounced hybridization signal exhibits a DNA fragment corresponding in size to the second PrV Hind III fragment B/B'. In all cases the smallest viral fragment C was missed. Because this fragment represents a terminal fragment of the viral genome, it could be of particular interest. The other terminal fragment comigrates with the Hind III fragment B (Ben-Porat and Rixon, 1979). The lack of terminal fragments would be the first indication to the possible state of the latent herpesvirus genome (integration, circularization). However, in the moment it remains rather speculative, since our data are very preliminar. Further studies using cloned PrV DNA fragments have to confirm these results. Thus we cannot totally exclude possible homologies between regions of the viral genome and cellular DNA sequences (Maitland et al., 1981; Peden et al., 1982; Puga et al., 1982).

Finally, our blot hybridizations might indicate that the viral genome is also present in white blood cells of latently infected animals (Fig. 6, lane 2), which were negative in the co-cultivation assay. Weak positive hybridization signals were found after cleavage of those DNA samples with other endonucleases, too (data not shown). It might be possible that others than neural tissues are involved during latency (Fraser et al., 1981; Scriba, 1981). To elucidate these opened questions further studies are necessary, which are, however, complicated by the paucity of the PrV genome in the latent state.

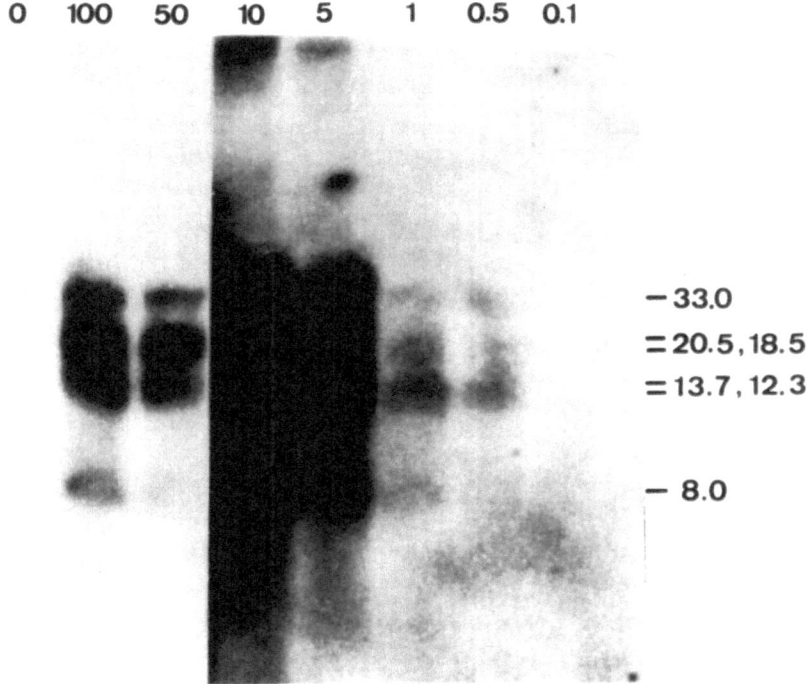

Fig. 5   Southern blot hybridization of a
reconstruction experiment after Bgl II digestion. In
each lane the indicated amounts of PrV genome
equivalents are cleaved in the presence of calf thymus
DNA (20 ug). After gel electrophoresis (0.6 % agarose)
and transfer to a nitrocellulose filter hybridization
was performed with in vitro ³²P-labeled PrV DNA. The
molecular weights (md) of the viral DNA fragments are
indicated on the right.

ACKNOWLEDGEMENTS

The technical assistance of Mrs. B. Bauer is gratefully
acknowledged. This work was supported by the Deutsche
Forschungsgemeinschaft.

HIND III

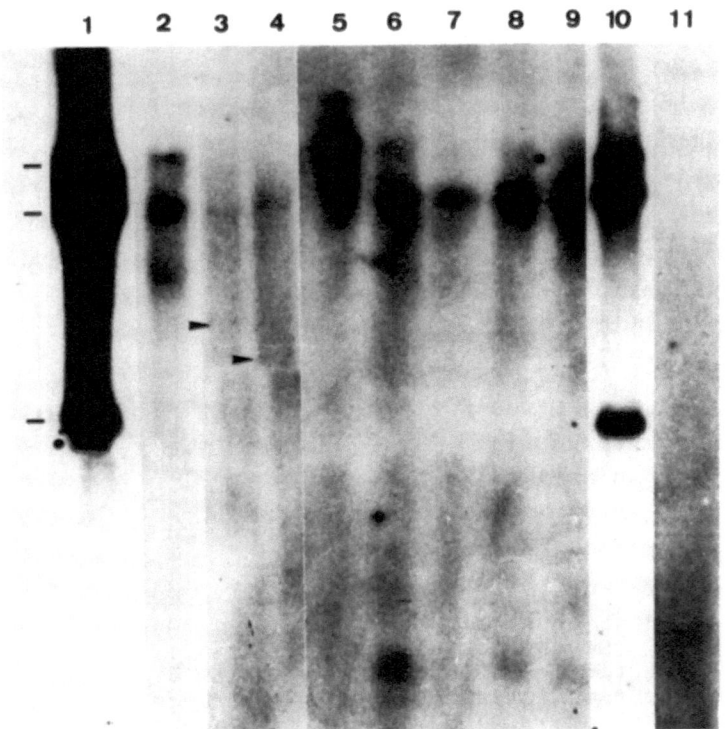

Fig. 6   Blot hybridization following Hind III
digestion of DNA (20 ug) obtained from organ tissues of
different latently infected pigs. Lane 1 and 10
represents a positive control of 10 and 1 viral genome
equivalent, respectively, in the presence of 20 ug calf
thymus DNA. Lanes: (2) white blood cells, 6.5 months
p.i., after immunosuppression; (3) and (4) brain stem,
6.5 months p.i.; (5) trigeminal ganglia, 5 months p.i.;
(6) medulla, 6 months p.i.; (7) spinal cord, 5 months
p.i.; (8) and (9) spinal cord, 6 months p.i.; (11) brain
stem of an uninfected pig as a negative control. The 3
virusspecific Hind III DNA fragments are indicated on
the left.

LITERATURE

Ben-Porat, T. and Rixon, F.J. 1979: Replication of herpesvirus DNA. III. Analysis of concatemers. Virology, 94, 61-70.

Beran, G.W., Davies, E.B. Arambulo, P.V., Will, C.A., Hill, H.T. and Rock, D.L. 1980. Persistence of pseudorabies virus in infected swine. J.Am.Vet.Assoc., 176, 998-1000.

Blyth, W.A., Harbour, D.A. and Hill, T.J. 1980: Effect of Acyclovir on reccurrence of herpes simplex skin lesions of mice. J.gen.Virol., 48, 417-419.

Brahic, M. and Haase, A.T. 1978: Detection of viral sequences of low reiteration frequency by in situ hybridization. Proc.Nat.Acad.Sci. USA, 75, 6125-6129.

Cabrera, C.V., Wohlenberg, C., Openshaw, H., Rey-Mendez, M., Puga, A. and Notkins, A.L. 1980: Herpes simplex virus DNA sequences in the CNS of latently infected mice. Nature, 288, 288-290.

Davies, E.B. and Beran, G.W. 1980: Spontaneous shedding of pseudorabies virus from a clinically recovered post-parturient sow. J.Am.Vet.Med.Assoc., 176, 1345-1347.

Field, H.J., Bell, S.E., Elion, G.B., Nash, A.A. and Wildy, P. 1979: Effect of acycloguanosine treatment on acute and latent herpes simplex infections in mice. Antimicrob. Agents Chemother., 15, 554-561.

Fraser, N.W., Lawrence, W.C., Wroblewska, Z., Gilden, D.H. and Koprowski, H. 1981: Herpes simplex type 1 DNA in human brain tissue. Proc.Nat.Acad.Sci. USA, 78, 6461-6465.

Gall J.G. and Pardue, M.L. 1971: Meth.Enzymol., 21, 470-480.

Galloway, D.A., Fenoglio, C.M. and McDongall, J.K. 1982: Limited transcription of the herpes simplex virus genome when latent in human sensory ganglia. J.Virol., 41, 686-691.

Green, M.T., Courtney, R.J. and Dunkel, E.C. 1981: Detection of an immediate early herpes simplex virus type 1 polypeptide in trigeminal ganglia from latently infected animals. Inf.Immun., 34, 987-992.

Gutekunst, D.E. 1979: Latent pseudorabies virus infection in swine detected by RNA-DNA hybridization. Am.J.Vet.Res., 40, 1568-1572.

Gutekunst, D.E., Pirtle, E.C., Miller, L.D. and Stewart, W.C. 1980: Isolation of pseudorabies virus from trigeminal ganglia of a latently infected sow. Am.J.Vet.Res., 41, 1315-1316.

Lofgren, K.W., Stevens, J.G., Marsden, H.S. and Subak-Sharpe, J.M. 1977: Temperature-sensitive mutants of herpes simplex virus differ in the capacity to establish latent infections in mice. Virology, 76, 440-443.

Maitland, N.J., Kinross, J.H., Busuttil, A., Ludgate, S.M., Smart, G.E. and Jones, K.W. 1981: The detection of DNA tumour virusspecific RNA sequences in abnormal human cervical biopsies by in situ hybridization. J.gen.Virol., 55, 123-137.

McLennan, J.L. and Darby, G. 1980: Herpes simplex virus latency: The cellular location of virus in dorsal root ganglia and the fate of the infected cell following virus activation. J.gen.Virol., 51, 233-243.

Mock, R.E., Crandell, R.A. and Mesfin, G.M. 1980: Induced latency in pseudorabies vaccinated pigs. Can.J.Comp.Med., 45, 56-59.

Peden, K., Mounts, P. and Hayward, G.S. 1982: Homology between mammalian cell DNA sequences and human herpesvirus genomes detected by a hybridization procedure with high-complexity probe. Cell, 31, 71-80.

Puga, A., Rosenthal, J.D., Openshaw, H. and Notkins, A.L. 1978: Herpes simplex virus DNA and mRNA sequences in acutely and chronically infected trigeminal ganglia of mice. Virology, 89, 102-111.

Puga, A., Cantin, E.M. and Notkins, A.L. 1982: Homology between murine and human cellular DNA sequences and the terminal repetition of the S component of herpes simplex virus type 1 DNA. Cell, 31, 81-87.

Rigby, P.W., Dieckmann, M., Rhodes, C. and Berg, P. 1977: Labelling deoxyribonucleic acid to high specific

activity _in_ _vitro_ by nick translation with DNA
polymerase I. J.Mol.Biol., _143_, 363-393.

Rziha, H.-J., Döller, P.C. and Wittmann, G. 1981: Detection
of pseudorabies virus and viral DNA in organ tissues of
latently infected pigs. Int. Workshop on Herpesviruses,
Bologna, Italy, p. 147.

Rziha, H.-J., Döller, P.C. and Wittmann, G. 1982: Detection
of Aujeszky's disease virus and viral DNA in tissues of
latently infected pigs. In "Aujeszky's disease" (Ed. G.
Wittmann and S.A. Hall). (Martinus Nijhoff, The Hague).
pp. 205-210.

Sabo, A. 1969: Persistence of perorally administered virulent
Pr virus in the organisms of nonimmune and immune pigs.
Acta Virol., _13_, 229-235.

Sabo, A. and Grunert, S. 1971: Persistence of virulent
pseudorabies virus in herds of vaccinated and
nonvaccinated pigs. Acta Virol., _15_, 87-94.

Sabo, A. and Rajcani, J. 1976: Latent pseudorabies virus
infection in pigs. Acta Virol., _20_, 208-214.

Scriba, M. 1981: Persistence of herpes simplex (HSV)
infection in ganglia and peripheral tissues of guinea
pigs. Med.Microbiol.Immunol., _169_, 91-96.

Sequiera, L.W., Carrasco, L.H., Curry, A., Jennings, L.C.,
Lord, M.A. and Sutton, R.N.P. 1979: Detection of herpes
simplex viral genome in brain tissue. Lancet, _2_,
609-612.

Southern, E.M. 1975: Detection of specific sequences among
DNA fragments separated by gel electrophoresis.
J.Mol.Biol., _98_, 503-517.

Stevens, J.G. and Cook, M.S. 1971: Latent herpes simplex
virus in spinal ganglia of mice. Science, _173_, 843-845.

Tenser, R.B., Ressel, S. and Dunstan, M.E. 1981: Herpes
simplex virus thymidine kinase expression in trigeminal
ganglion infection: Correlation of enzyme activity with
ganglion virus titer and evidence of _in_ _vivo_
complementation. Virology, _112_, 328-341.

Walz, M.A., Yamamoto, H. and Notkins, A.L. 1976:
   Immunological response restricts number of cells in
   sensory ganglia infected with herpes simplex virus.
   Nature, <u>264</u>, 554-556.

Wittmenn, G., Rziha, H.-J. and Döller, P.C. 1982: Occurrence
   of clinical Aujeszky's disease in immunosuppressed
   latently infected pigs. In "Aujeszky's disease" (Eds. G.
   Wittmann and S.A. Hall). (Martinus Nijhoff, The Hague).
   pp. 211-214.

Yamamoto, H., Walz, M.A. and Notkins, A.L. 1977: Virol.
   specific thymidine kinase in sensory ganglia of mice
   infected with HSV. Virology, <u>76</u>, 866-869.

This work was supported by grant WI 619/2-2 from the Deutsche
Forschungsgemeinschaft.

LATENCY OF AUJESZKY'S DISEASE VIRUS (ADV) FOLLOWING CHALLENGE IN PREVIOUSLY VACCINATED PIGS

G. Wittmann, V. Ohlinger, H.J. Rziha

Bundesforschungsanstalt für Viruskrankheiten der Tiere,
Postfach 1149, D-7400 Tübingen,
Federal Republic of Germany

ABSTRACT

Pigs which were vaccinated with an inactivated ADV vaccine developed a latent ADV infection up to 18 months after ADV challenge. Latent virus could be demonstrated up to 6.5 months post infection by co-cultivation of different tissues (lungs, tonsils, olfactory bulb, brain stem, medulla). After this time, reactivation of latent virus was only achieved by immunosuppresion of the animals. Immunosuppression led to limited virus replication in nasal mucosa, tonsils, lymph nodes and central nervous system. In addition, ADV was detected in the nasal secretions.

Humoral and cellular immunity was investigated before and after immunosuppression of the animals. Before immunosuppression most of the animals displayed spontaneous cell-mediated cytotoxicity (SCC), antibody-dependent cell-mediated cytotoxicity (ADV-ADCC) and ADV-specific lymphocyte stimulation (ADV-LYST), and all animals had medium to high titres of neutralizing serum antibodies. After immunosuppression the number of pigs reacting in SCC and ADV-LYST assays was distinctly reduced, but the number of animals reacting in ADV-ADCC assays remained unaltered. A significant reduction of serum antibody titres occurred only in 2 of 12 animals one day after the end of immunosuppression.

INTRODUCTION

The establishment of ADV latency after infection of non-vaccinated pigs which have recovered from Aujeszky's disease (AD) is well documented (Gutekunst, 1979; Beran et al., 1980; Davies and Beran, 1980; Gutekunst et al., 1980; Rziha et al., 1981; Wittmann et al., 1982b). Since vaccination of pigs with inactivated ADV vaccines is commonly practised, the question arises as to whether or not latency will be established after these animals undergo virus challenge. This is an important point to consider in relation to the epizootiology and control of AD. We therefore investigated the

occurrence and reactivation of latent ADV following challenge
in previously vaccinated pigs. In addition, the humoral and
cell-mediated immune response of these animals was examined
before and after immunosuppression (IS).

METHODS and RESULTS

The first part of the experiments was designed to
investigate the appearance of ADV latency. Twenty-five pigs
vaccinated with a commercial, inactivated vaccine were
challenged intranasally with $10^{9.0}$ $TCID_{50}$ of the virulent ADV
strain Phylaxia two or six weeks after the second vaccination,
when 8-12 weeks old. At 3, 6.5, 11.5, 15, 16 and 22.5 months
post infection (p.i.), respectively, 2 or 3 pigs were killed,
and in parallel, 2 pigs were immunosuppressed on 4 consecutive
days by the application of 1250 mg or 1875 mg prednisolone, and
killed one or 3 days after the last prednisolone injection.

Olfactory bulb, brain stem, medulla, cervical, thoracic
and lumbar parts of the spinal cord, tonsils, retropharyngeal
lymph nodes (RLN) and lung were removed from the animals. In
addition to these organs, spleen, kidneys, inguinal lymph nodes
(ILN), nasal mucosa, vaginal and preputial mucosa, were removed
from the immunosuppressed animals.

Four non-vaccinated pigs were included in the studies 16
months after ADV infection. Two animals were killed without IS
and two animals after IS, and the organs removed.

For virus isolation from the specimens of the
non-immunosuppressed pigs co-cultivation of the tissue
fragments in the bovine kidney cell line MDBK was applied
(Beran et al., 1980), modified by the use of versene trypsin
(Scriba, 1981). For demonstration of ADV multiplication in the
tissues from all the immunosuppressed pigs the virus titration
(suspension) method in BHK cell monolayer cultures was used,
using 10% tissue homogenates and tenfold dilutions of them. We
wanted to demonstrate by means of this, the change form the
latent virus state into the active, replicating virus state.
The infectivity titres were calculated according to Kärber
(1931).

TABLE 1   ADV isolation from latently infected pigs.

Number of pigs	Months p.i.	Imm. suppr.	ND_{50}	pos./total[1]	Virus isolation from
Vaccinated pigs (group I)					
2	3	no	294	1/2	C: brain stem
2		yes	223-294 (97)	2/2	T: nasal mucosa, retroph. LNN, tonsils, medulla, cerv.cord (1.5 - 3.1)[2]
3	6.5	no	97-169	3/3	C: tonsils, lung, olf. bulb, brain stem
2		yes	72-97 (42-56)	2/2	T: tonsils, retroph.LNN, inguin. LNN, olf.bulb, brain stem, medulla, cerv. and lumbal cord (1.1 - 3.3)
2	11.5	no	72-97	0/2	C: negative
2		yes	32-256 (56-256)	2/2	T: olf.bulb, brain stem, cerv.cord (0.7)
3	15	no	188-388	0/3	C: negative
3		yes	97-169 (47-256)	2/3	T: brain stem (0.7)
2	18	yes	284-512 (389-512)	1/2	T: tonsils, retroph.LNN, (2.7 - 3.1)
2	22.5	no	128-512	0/2	C: negative
2		yes	294-389 (128-512)	0/2	T: negative
Non-vaccinated pigs (group II)					
2	16	no	14-18	0/2	C: negative
2		yes	11 (8-14)	2/2	T: nasal mucosa, tonsils, lung (0.1 - 5.1)

ND_{50} Neutralization titre, in brackets results after immunosuppression.

[1]   Numerator: Number of animals with positive ADV isolation. Denominator: Number of examined animals.

[2]   Range of virus amounts detected in the organs ($\log_{10}$ $TCID_{50}$/0.1 gr).

C   Co-cultivation method.

T   Titration method.

The inactivated ($56°C$, 30 min) sera of the animals were tested for antibodies in the neutralization test in the presence of guinea pig complement (Jakubik and Wittmann, 1978).

After ADV infection of the vaccinated pigs (group I) some animals did not show any signs of the disease whereas other animals displayed slight fever and slightly reduced appetite for a few days. In contrast, the non-vaccinated animals (group II) showed typical symptoms of Aujeszky's disease: fever, nasal discharge, loss of appetite, loss of voice and somnolence.

ADV could be isolated from the non-immunosuppressed pigs only by co-cultivation and never by the titration method. Virus was found in the olfactory bulb and the brain, in the tonsils and in the lung up to 6.5 months p.i. From 11.5 months onward, all attempts failed to isolate ADV from non-immunosuppressed pigs by co-cultivation (Table 1).

In contrast, ADV could be regularly isolated from immunosuppressed pigs up to 18 months p.i., however, virus isolation was unsuccessful after 22.5 months. Until 6.5 months p.i., ADV was most frequently found in these animals in the central nervous system, with no preference for any particular region, and also in the tonsils and the RLN. In addition, in one case only, ADV was detected in the ILN and in the nasal mucosa. The fact that virus titres up to $10^{3.3}$ $TCID_{50}$ per 0.1 gr were detected indicates the occurrence of virus multiplication. The ADV specificity of all isolates was ascertained by neutralization with ADV hyperimmune serum.

Since latency was demonstrable in non-immunosuppressed pigs up to 6.5 months p.i. and after immunosuppression up to 18 months p.i., one might conclude that ADV latency is reduced and disappears during the course of time. This assumption is supported by the fact that the frequency of positive ADV isolation from latently infected pigs decreased the longer the time after infection. However, the number of animals tested was relatively small. More sensitive experiments of the corresponding organ samples are in progress to detect viral DNA by molecular hybridization methods (Rziha et al., 1981).

With the non-vaccinated pigs ADV isolation by

co-cultivation was negative when examined 16 months p.i.
However, after immunosuppression ADV could be detected in the
nasal mucosa, the lung and in the tonsils, where a virus titre
of $10^{5.1}$ $TCID_{50}$/0.1 gr was found.

All the vaccinated animals showed fairly high titres of
neutralizing serum antibodies. After immunosuppression, the
antibody levels were significantly reduced in only two of 13
animals, when tested one day after the end of IS. In contrast,
the non-vaccinated pigs of group II yielded rather low
neutralization titres before and after IS when tested 16 months
p.i. This shows that even high titres of neutralizing serum
antibodies were of no influence on latent virus infection. This
is not surprising since the central nervous system (CNS) is
known to display only poor antibody-mediated and cell-mediated
defense mechanisms (Wolinsky and Johnson, 1980).

Some parameters of cell-mediated immunity were also
tested, namely cell-mediated cytotoxicity and lymphocyte
stimulation. For the former we used ^{51}Cr labelled non-infected
and ADV infected Vero cells as target cells and unpurified
white blood cells (WBC) as effector cells. Details of the
various tests will be published else where.

SCC reflects spontaneous cell-mediated cytotoxicity of the
effector cells against non-infected target cells. This may
reflect natural killer cell activity, but we did not verify
this.

ADV-CC reflects cell-mediated cytotoxicity of the effector
cells against ADV infected target cells. Probably, it primarily
reflects SCC against ADV infected target cells and, perhaps,
additionally low degrees of ADV-ADCC, since the presence of
antibody producing cells in the effector cell preparations
cannot be excluded. It seems unlikely that T-cell cytotoxicity
is participating since we used neither purified T-cells nor an
isogenic system.

ADV-ADCC reflects antibody dependent cell-mediated
cytotoxicity of the effector cells in co-operation with the
serum of the same donor against ADV-infected target cells. We
did not use the usual method with non-sensitized effector cells

TABLE 2   Cell-mediated immunity in latently infected pigs.
Percentage of reacting animals.

SCC[1]	total	68.4%[2]
	before IS	66.7%[3]
	after IS	22.2%[3]
ADV-CC[1]	total	21.1%
	before IS	11.1%
	after IS	11.1%
ADV-ADCC[1]	total	94.7%
	before IS	100 %
	after IS	100 %
N-ADCC[1]	total	36.8%
	before IS	44.4%
	after IS	11.1%
ADV-LYST[1]	total	78.9%
	before IS	77.8%
	after IS	11.1%
N-LYST[1]	total	15.8%
	before IS	11.1%
	after IS	11.1%

[1] Explanation see text.

[2] Values from 19 pigs without or before
immunosuppression (IS).

[3] Values from 9 pigs before and after IS.

of a normal pig and the antisera of the latently infected pigs, since we think that the in vivo situation is more reflected by the modified method.

N-ADCC is a control for the participation of non-ADV specific reactions in ADV-ADCC, e.g. by antibodies against non-viral vaccine constituents. We know from former experiments that traces of calf serum and BHK antigen are contained in the vaccine. The test procedure is according to ADV-ADCC but non-infected target cells were used.

ADV-LYST reflects stimulation of ADV sensitized lymphocytes by ADV-antigen.

N-LYST reflects stimulation of lymphocytes by non-viral control antigen, especially with regard to BHK antigen.

Table 2 shows that SCC was displayed in 68.4% of the 19 animals tested. Nine of them were immunosuppressed. Before IS 66.7% of them displayed SCC, whereas after IS SCC only occurred in 22.2% of the animals.

ADV-CC, that is, enhanced cytotoxicicty of effector cells against ADV infected target cells in comparison to SCC, occurred in 26.3% of the animals. In the immunosuppressed part of them, 22.2% reacted before and 11.1% after IS.

ADV-ADCC was displayed in 94.7% of the pigs. The 100% value was not reached because in one pig ADV-ADCC was a high as N-ADCC. From the immunosuppressed animals 100% displayed ADV-ADCC before and after IS.

N-ADCC occurred in 36.8% of the animals. From the immunosuppressed pigs 44.4% displayed N-ADCC before and 11.1% after IS. However, with one exception, N-ADCC was significantly lower than ADV-ADCC.

ADV-LYST was displayed in 79.0% of the animals. From the immunosuppressed animals 77.8% reacted before but only 11.1% after IS.

N-LYST occurred in 15.8% of the animals. Of the immunosuppressed animals 11.1% reacted before IS and after IS.

Rather similar results were obtained with non-vaccinated latently infected pigs as with the vaccinated pigs, with the exception that ADV-LYST was only present in one of the animals.

452

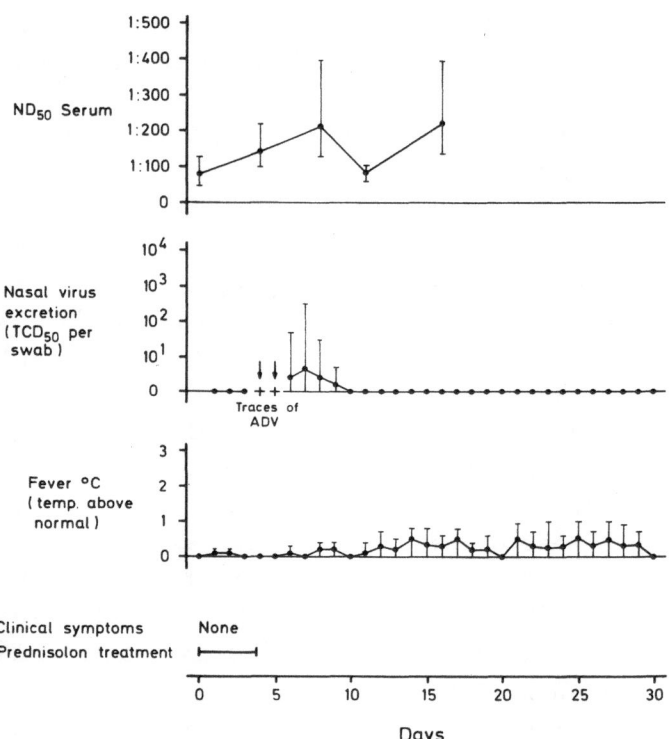

Fig. 1   Immunosuppression of latently ADV infected,
          vaccinated pigs, 13 months after infection.
          Clinical symptoms, virus excretion and neu-
          tralizing antibody titres (ND_{50}).
          Mean values of 4 animals with maximum and
          minimum range.

The results showed that the effect of immunosuppression on
the immune response of the animals was mainly pronounced in SCC
and ADV-LYST. In contrast, IS did not alter ADV-ADCC. This may
be connected with the fact that the neutralizing antibody
titres remained rather unaltered after IS. It remains to be
clarified whether or not the reduction of SCC and of the
stimulation response of sensitized lymphocytes to ADV is
correlated with the reactivation of latent virus. However,
according to the literature, relationships between SCC and the
severity of infection do seem to exist with different herpes
viruses (Ching and Lopez, 1979; Quinnan et al., 1982; Wittmann
et al., in press). On the other hand, neutralizing antibodies
were apparently not involved in the reactivation process,
because IS did not reduce serum antibody titres in the majority
of the animals and ADV-ADCC was not impaired at all by IS.

In the second part of the experiments we examined whether
or not clinical symptoms and virus excretion appear after
immunosuppression of latently infected, vaccinated pigs. Four
vaccinated pigs were i.n. infected with $10^{9.0}$ TCID$_{50}$ when 11-12
weeks old and immunosuppressed as described before 13 months
p.i. The results are summarized in Fig. 1.

The immunosuppressed animals displayed moderate fever,
which never exceeded one degree above normal. ADV was found in
the nasal secretions of 3 of the 4 animals. However, virus
excretion usually only lated a short time and only reached low
titres of between $10^{<0.1}$ and $10^{0.7}$ TCID$_{50}$ per swab. Only one
pig excreted higher amounts of virus with a maximum of $10^{2.5}$
TCID$_{50}$ from day 4 until day 8. From data available in the
literature, it might be expected that virus amounts of around
$10^{2.5}$ TCID$_{50}$ would be too small to infect immune pigs or
cattle, but high enough to infect non-immune pigs (Baskerville,
1972; Biront et al., 1982; Wittmann et al., 1982a).

Two prednisolone treated control animals, not shown in the
Figure, never showed any signs of illness. Their temperatures
were slightly elevated around day 17 and from days 21 to 28,
but the temperature never exceeded the normal level by more
than 0.5°C. No agent cytopathic for BHK cultures could be

detected in the nasal swabs of the control animals.

The reactivation of the latent virus state was also reflected serologically because the titres of neutralizing antibodies increased from values between 1:56 and 1:128 (mean titre 1:78) before IS, to values between 1:169 and 1:389 (mean titre 1:224) 16 days after IS.

CONCLUSION

Our experimental results demonstrate that there is always the risk of the presence of an unknown number of latently, ADV infected pigs even in vaccinated herds in the field. These animals can originate either from vaccinated pigs with pre-existing infection, or from vaccinated pigs which are subsequently infected. However, the number of latently infected pigs is certainly lower with vaccinated pigs than with non-vaccinated animals, because vaccinated pigs require much higher virus doses for infection (Wittmann et al., 1982a). Since the latent virus state of vaccinated pigs can be reactivated by stress, and limited virus excretion can occur, non-immune pigs may be infected. However, it is unlikely that sufficient virus is excreted to infect immune (vaccinated) pigs and cattle. Nevertheless, it is unlikely that AD can be eradicated by vaccination. Vaccination reduces the economical losses and reduces virus spread, but does not completely prevent it. (The paper has been published in detail in the Archives of Virology, 75, 29-41, 1983).

REFERENCES

Baskerville, A. 1972. The influence of dose of virus on the clinical signs of experimental Aujesky's disease in pigs. Brit. Vet. J., 128, 394-401.
Beran, G.W., Davies, E.B., Arambulo, P.V., Will, L.A., Hill, H.T. and Rock, D.L. 1980. Persistence of pseudorabies virus in infected swine. Am. J. Vet. Med. Ass., 176, 998-1000.
Biront, P., Vandeputte, J., Pensaert, M.B. and Leunen, J. 1982. Vaccination of cattle against pseudorabies (Aujeszky's disease) with homologous virus (herpes suis) and heterologous virus (herpes bovis 1). Am. J. Vet. Res., 43, 760-763.

Ching, C. and Lopez, C. 1979. Natural killing of herpes simplex virus type 1 infected target cells. Normal human response and influence of antiviral antibody. Infect. Immun., 26, 49-56.

Davies, E.B. and Beran, G.W. 1980. Spontaneous shedding of pseudorabies virus from clinically recovered post parturient sow. Am. J. Vet. Med. Ass., 176, 1345-1347.

Gutekunst, D.E. 1979. Latent pseudorabies virus infection in swine detected by RNA-DNA hybridization. Am. J. Vet. Res., 40, 1568-1572.

Gutekunst, D.E., Pirtle, E.C., Miller, L.D. and Stewart, W.C. 1980. Isolation of pseudorabies virus from trigeminal ganglia of a latently infected sow. Am. J. Vet. Res., 41, 1315-1326.

Jakubik, J. and Wittmann, G. 1978. Neutralizing antibody titres in pig serum after revaccination with an inactivated Aujeszky's disease virus (ADV) vaccine. Zbl. Vet. Med., B, 25, 741-751.

Kärber, G. 1931. Beitrag zur kollektiven Behandlung pharmakologischer Reihenversuche. Naunyn-Schmiedebergs Arch. exp. Path. Pharmak., 162, 480-483.

Quinnan, G.V., Manischewitz, J.E. and Kirmani, N. 1982. Involvement of natural killer cells in the pathogenesis of murine cytomegalovirus interstitial pneumonitis and the immune response to infection. J. gen. Virol., 58, 173-180.

Rziha, H.J., Döller, P.C. and Wittmann, G. 1981. Detection of pseudorabies and viral DNA in organ tissues of latently infected pigs. Abstr. Int. Workshop Herpesviruses, Bologna, p. 147.

Scriba, M. 1981. Persistence of herpes simplex virus (HSV) infection in ganglia and peripheral tissues of guinea pigs. Med. Microbiol. Immunol., 169, 91-96.

Wittmann, G., Ohlinger, V. and Höhn, U. 1982a. Die Vermehrung von Aujeszkyvirus (AV) in vakzinierten Schweinen nach experimenteller Infektion mit hohen und niederen Virusmengen. Zbl. Vet. Med., B, 29, 24-30.

Wittmann, G., Rziha, H.J. and Döller, P.C. 1982b. Occurrence of clinical Aujeszky's disease in immunosuppressed latently infected pigs. Current Topic Vet. Med. Animal Sci., 17, 205-210.

Wolinsky, J.S. and Johnson, R.T. 1980. Role of viruses in chronic neurological diseases. Comprehensive Virol., 16, 257-296.

SESSION IV

AVIAN HERPESVIRUSES

Chairman: L.N. Payne
Co-chairman: H.-J. Rziha

UBIQUITY AND PERSISTENCE OF MAREK'S DISEASE VIRUS
IN TUMOURAL AND NON-TUMOROUS EXPLANTS

F. Coudert, L. Cauchy

Institut National de la Recherche Agronomique
Station de Pathologie Aviaire et de Parasitologie
Centre de Recherches de Tours
Nouzilly, 37380 Monnaie, France

ABSTRACT

Marek's disease (MD) is a contagious disease of chickens characterized by the development of various lymphoid tumours. It is induced by a specific herpesvirus that multiplies in a variety of cells. The persistence of viral production is well documented in the skin cells around the feather follicules. In blood leucocytes and tumour cells the viral multiplication is rather of the abortive form. In this paper the presence of Marek's Disease Herpes Virus (MDHV) was investigated in various chicken tissues from tumorous and non tumorous organs. The explant culture technique was used from MD affected chicken organs. Virus particles were found by electron microscopy in numerous explants. After a latent period of three weeks the virus particles appeared and increased in number in both tumorous and non tumorous tissues (ovary, testis, nerve, kidney, lung, spleen, thymus, heart). They replicated in undifferenciated mononuclear cells which were not organ specific. They were seen up to 180 days of culture. In vivo assays of infectivity were negative for the explants but positive for migrating cells originating from the explants. No permanent cell lines were established at 37°C. The ubiquity and persistence of the MDHV is discussed. It could be related to the presence of an undifferentiated cell type which appeared and could be maintained in long term culture.

INTRODUCTION

Marek's Disease (MD) is a contagious disease of chickens characterized by the development of various lymphoid tumours. It is induced by a specific herpesvirus (Churchill and Biggs, 1967) that multiplies in vitro in some cells. Viral multiplication occurs during the life of the infected chickens whatever their tumorous condition. The persistence of viral production is well documented in feather follicle skin cells (Nazerian and Witter, 1970), in blood lymphocytes (Cauchy, 1970) and in tumour cells. In skin cells the Marek's Disease Herpesvirus (MDHV) multiplies actively and may be seen both as the naked (nuclear) form and the enveloped (cytoplasmic) form.

In the other cells the multiplication is rather abortive or repressed as was demonstrated by in vitro cultures olf lymphocytes (Cauchy and Coudert, 1972; Coudert and Cauchy, 1974), or by integration into the cellular genome of tumour cells (Nazerian et al., 1973).

Using long term cultures of explants of chicken tumours, it was previously shown that viral particles appeared after few days of culture in somme cells of tumour tissues (Coudert and Cauchy, 1975). Since in infected chickens the persistence of the virus is not dependent on the tumour growth, it was of interest to investigate explants of non tumorous tissues for the presence of MDHV and also to study possible enhancement of virus growth in tissues with tumour characteristics. In additon an attempt was made to determine which kind of tissue or cell supported viral multiplication and/or cell transformation.

MATERIAL AND METHODS

MD affected chickens

MD susceptible White Leghorn chickens were obtained from a parental flock free of MDHV, infected at one day old with the HPRS 16 strain that was maintained by in vivo passages. At 6 or 7 weeks of age about half of the chickens developed clinical signs of MD. Both clinically affected and asymptomatic chickens were killed and examined for gross MD lesions. Tumorous ovaries, testes and nerves, and non tumorous thymuses, spleens, kidneys, lungs, heart and feather follicle, were quickly processed by the explant culture technique for MDHV detection.

Explant culture technique

The organ culture technique of Trowell's grid procedure modified by Jensen (Jensen et al., 1964) and adapted by De Thé et al., 1970) for nasopharyngeal carcinoma tissue, was described previously (Coudert and Cauchy, 1975). Briefly small pieces of each organ were placed on gelatin foam (Spongostan, Ferrosan, Malmö, Sweden) mounted on a squarish filter paper and stainless steel grid in a Petri dish. The medium was RPMI 1640 with 20 per cent foetal calf serum. The cultures were

maintained at 37°C in a 5 per cent CO_2 atmosphere. Three weeks
later, the grids with explants were placed in other Petri
dishes in order to observe the development of cells which
migrated from the explants to the bottom of Petri dishes.
Migrating cells were harvested by scarping and centrifugation.
They were then fixed with osmium tetroxide and embedded in
EPON. Explants were removed, fixed and embedded as the
migrating cells.

Tests for MDHV detection - Herpesvirus Particles (HVP) and
Infectivity assay -

At the beginning of culture and at different intervals
thereafter (as indicated in Results), a total of 113 cultured
explants were examined by electron microscopy for the presence
of viral particles having the characteristics of herpesviruses.
A number of samples of migrating cells were also checked for
HVP.

For 3 explants and 6 samples of migrating cells a test of
infectivity was performed as following: explants were ground in
mortars with chilled medium and the suspension was injected
into chickens. Migrating cells were trypsinised, counted, and
injected immediately at a dose of 50,000 cells per chicken.

Injected chickens were reared in isolators for germ free
animals and observed for 10 weeks. Their organs were examined
for gross and microscopic MD lesions.

RESULTS

1. Viral Particles detection by electron microscopy

Out of the 20 different tissues examined, 13 of them
showed HVP in at least one explant studied during the long term
cultures.

HVP were never seen in cultures before day 18 except for
the feather follicle. Later HVP were seen at day 50, 100 and as
late as day 240 of culture.

From the tumorous tissues, 3/3 ovaries and 2/2 testis were
positive for a least one explant. In contrast, not one of the
17 explants from 3 tumorous nerves were positive. From the non

TABLE 1   Number of cultured tissues with Herpesvirus Particles
(HVP) by e. microscopy

	With HVP	Number tested
TUMOROUS TISSUES		
Ovaries	3	3
Testis	2	2
Nerves	O	3
NONTUMOROUS TISSUES		
Thymuses	2	3
Spleens	2	2
Kidneys	1	3
Lungs	1	2
Heart	1	1
Feather follicles	1	1
Total	13	20

tumorous tissue 2/3 thymuses, 2/2 spleens, 1/3 kidneys, 1/2
lungs, 1/1 heart, and 1/1 feather follicle were found positive.

In migrating cells one sample from a tumorous testis
cultured explant was positive and 2 samples of the same lung
explant which was cultured for 3 and 8 months respectively,
were HVP positive.

Viral particles appeared in all cases as unenveloped
virions in nuclei of living cells or within debris of lysed
cells in some long term cultures (Fig. 1 and 2).

2. Assays of infectivity

No explants were found to be infectious although they
contained HVP before treatment and injection. On the contrary
all migrating cells were infectious to chickens except for

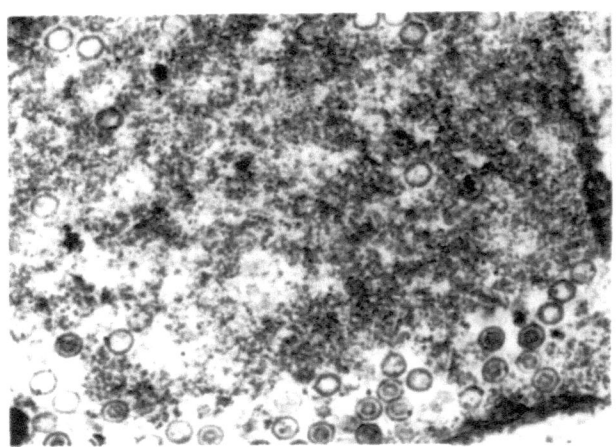

Fig. 1: HVP in migrating cells of lung explant cultured for
         110 days x 40,000.

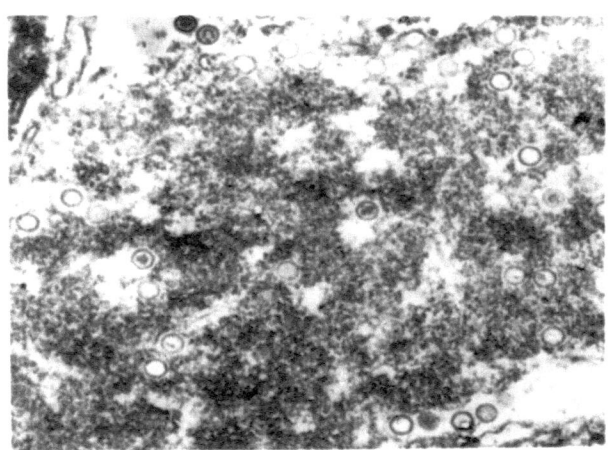

Fig. 2: HVP in lysed cells of kidney explant cultured for
         69 days x 32,500.

TABLE 2   Marek's disease infectivity of explants and
           migrating cells from long term cultures organs.

		Age of culture (Days)	HVP before Assay	MD positive Infected chickens
EXPLANTS				
Testis TT	11.I	180	+	0/11
Testis TT	17.IV	240	+	0/11
Thymus Thy	25.VI	180	+	0/11
MIGRATING CELLS				
Ovary OT	8.IV	70	0	0/5[a]
Testis TT	17.VI	120	+	5/6[a]
Thymus Thy	25.VI	180	0	3/5[a]
Thymus Thy	11.IV	70	0	4/4[a]
Lung 1) L.	17.IV	90	+	1/2[b]
2) L.	17.IV	240	+	8/8[a]

a : 50,000 cells were injected/chicken
b : only 100,000 cells were harvested and injected
    into 2 chickens (50,000 cells/chicken)

cells originating from a tumorous ovary. From a non tumorous
lung, infectious migrating cells were found at day 90 and 240
respectively. In the other cases, migrating cells were
infectious although electron microscopy was negative for HVP in
previous assays.

3. Nature of cells in cultured explants and migrating cells
     Organ specific cells disappeared from the explants at
various times but shortly after culture, as evidenced by
ovarian follicles, Sertoli cells and spermatides, nephrotic and
glomerular kidney cells, thymocytes, muscular cells, etc. Later
other cells which constituted the main cell population were
observed. These cells often appeared mononuclear, with numerous
inclusions in the cytoplasm, a round or lightly indented pale

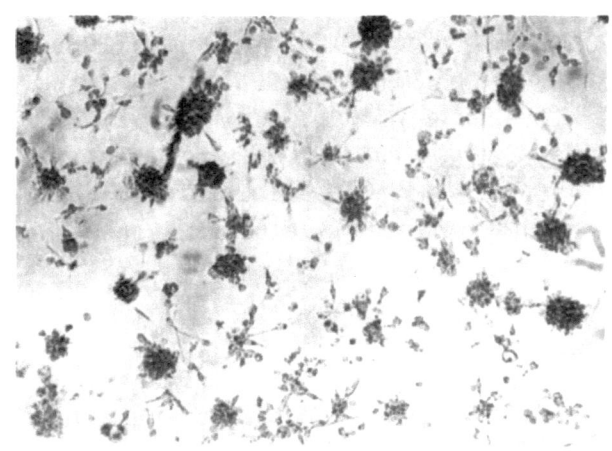

Fig. 3: Clusters of migrating cells of tumoral ovary explant cultured for 114 days x 120.

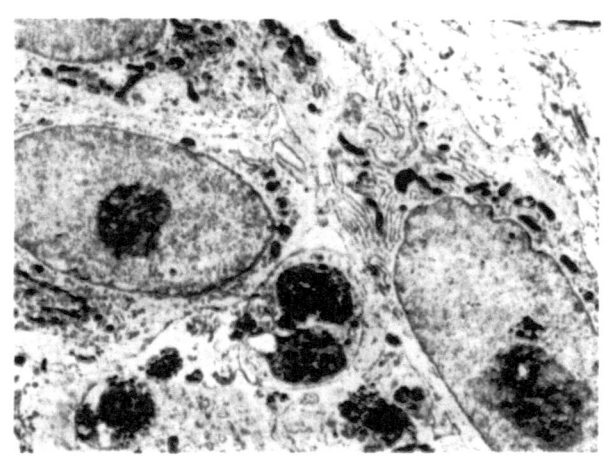

Fig. 4: Mononuclear cells of tumoral ovary explant cultured for 61 days x 4,600.

nucleus, a normal Golgi apparatus and a developed endoplasmic reticulum (Fig. 4). Their number decreased with time but some were still present at day 240.

After 1 or 2 weeks of culture fibroblastic cells began to migrate and to constitute monolayers on the Petri dish bottom. Subsequent waves of other larger cells migrated and formed clusters of round refringent cells which were loosely attached to the bottom (Fig. 3). Some of the migrating cells have been passaged several times at 37°C but their multiplication stopped within 5-6 months.

DISCUSSION

The explant technique was able to demonstrate HVP in a number of assays but not in all the samples despite careful electron microscopic examinations. Such results demonstrate the ability of MDHV to multiply in various tissues, thus supporting the ubiquitons character of MDHV. It was expected to find HVP in nonneuronal cells of nerves as shown by Pepose and al., 1981. The failure of our results with nerves could be due to the in vitro swelling of collagenic fibers which restricted the number of viable cells. Such alteration was also found in feather follicles in which explants were negative after a first positive culture.

The in vitro persistence of MDHV multiplication could indicate that life long target cells exist in both tumorous and non tumorous tissues. However MDHV is known to actively multiply in epithelial skin cells during the life of infected chickens. However the mechanism of that persistent infection is not still clear. Persistent cell-associated viremia was supported by the blood lymphocytes but previous reports (Coudert and Cauchy, 1974) failed to demonstrate viable lymphocytic cells in cultures older than a month. These results were not consistent with the long persistence of blood lymphocytes in the explants. However the mononuclear cells which were found to be infected in long term cultures were undifferentiated rather than lymphocytic cells. Our opinion is that one type of cell, perhaps reticular, undifferentiated, and of mesodermal origin, which could exist in all the tissues of chickens, maybe able to support the albeit poor multiplication of MDHV. This kind of cell had some similarities in morphology with the migrating cells, which were described previously. Unfortunately there was a discrepancy in the infectivity between the explants cells and the migrating cells, probably because the former cells were rare and/or destroyed by the treatment before injecting into the chickens.

A question remains about the mechanism by which the productive MDHV infection could be maintained for such a long time in cultures in vitro. Is the MDHV production normally repressed and transiently derepressed according to the stage of specific differentiation of the target cells? It might be of interest to know whether a relationship could exist between repressed MDHV multiplication in undifferentiated cells and oncogenic transformation.

CONCLUSIONS

Such results corroborate the presence of MDHV in many organs and could offer a new explanation of the persistence of viremia in infected chickens. The multiplication of MDHV is not dependent of a tumorous environment. The target cell for viral production seems to be a type of undifferentiated mononuclear cell which was able to grow in very long term culture.

ACKNOWLEDGEMENTS

Jacques Richard et Jean Courtens were thanked for their excellent technical assistance.

REFERENCES
Cauchy, L. 1970. Recherches virologiques, expérimentales et infrastructurales sur une néoplasie: la maladie de Marek (Thèse Sci. Nat. Paris) (Tours, Ed. du CIUM). 79p.
Cauchy, L. and Coudert, F. 1972. Particules de type Herpès de la maladie de Marek dans les lymphocytes infectés et maintenus in vitro. C.R. Acad. Sci. Paris, 274, 1864-1866, série D.
Churchill, A.F. and Biggs, P.M. 1967. Agent of Marek's Disease intissue culture. Nature, 215, 528-530.
Coudert, F. and Cauchy, L. 1974. La maladie de Marek. Production virale et transformation dans les lymphocytes en cultures. Rec. Méd. Vét., 150, 413-418.

Coudert, F. and Cauchy, L. 1975. Virus replication and cell modifications in organ cultures of tumor tissue from chickens with Marek's Disease. J. natl. Cancer Inst., 55, 47-51.

De Thé, G., Ho, H.C., Kwan, H.C., Desgranges, C. and Farre, M.C. 1970. Nasopharyngeal carcinoma (NPC). I. Types of cultures derived from tumor biopsies and non tumorous tissues of chinese patients with special reference to lymphoblastoid transformation. Int. J. Cancer, 6, 189-206.

Jensen, F.C., Gwatkin, R.B.L. and Biggers, J.D. 1964. A simple organ culture method which allows simultaneous isolation of specific types of cells. Exp. Cell. Res., 34, 440-447.

Nazerian, K. and Witter, R.L. 1970. Cell-free transmission and in vivo replication of Marek's Disease Virus. J. Virol., 5, 388-397.

Nazerian, K., Lindahl, T., Klein, G. and Lee, L.F. 1973. Deoxyribonucleic acid of Marek's disease virus in virus-induced tumors. J. Virol., 12, 841-846.

Pepose, J.S., Stevens, J.G., Cook, M.L. and Lampert, P.W. 1981. Marek's disease as a model for the Landry-Guillain-Barré Syndrom. Latent viral infection in nonneuronal cells accompagnied by specific immune response to peripheral nerves and myelin. Am. J. Path., 103, 309-320.

EXPERIMENTAL MAREK'S DISEASE IN TURKEYS AND THE
ESTABLISHMENT OF TURKEY LYMPHOID CELL LINES

P.C. Powell, L.N. Payne, K. Howes, B.M. Mustill,
M. Rennie and M.A. Thompson
Houghton Poultry Research Station, Houghton,
Huntingdon, Cambs., PE17 2DA, UK.

ABSTRACT
    Marek's disease (MD) has been induced in turkeys by the inoculation of large doses (5×10^4 plaque forming units) of a virulent strain of MD virus (GA) but not of two other virulent strains (HPRS 16 and JM). The disease differed from both the acute and classical forms of MD seen in chickens and the most prominent findings were lymhocytic leukaemia and lymphoid and reticular hyperplasia in the spleen and liver. None of the early histological changes (lymphoid cell destruction and reticuloendothelial cell hyperplasia) reported in chickens were observed, and haematological changes were less pronounced.
    Eight lymphoid cell lines have been cultured from the leukaemic blood and spleens of affected turkeys. The lines share a common morphology and express MD-associated tumour surface antigen, MATSA. On the basis of lack of immunofluorescent staining with specific anti-T cell, anti-B cell or anti-turkey immunoglobulin antisera the lines have been characterised as T-cells.

INTRODUCTION

    Marek's disease (MD) is a lymphoproliferative disease of chickens characterised by lymphoid infiltration of the peripheral nerves and visceral organs (see Payne et al., 1976). The disease is caused by a herpesvirus (MDV) and infection is associated with the expression of virus-specific antigens, particularly in the lymphoid organs of susceptible chickens. In addition, a MD-associated tumour surface antigen (MATSA) is induced on lymphoid cells, as a result, it is assumed, of malignant transformation of the cells. It has been shown previously that experimental inoculation of pathogenic MDV can cause a lymphomatous disease in turkeys (Paul et al., 1977; Elmubarak et al., 1981). We have confirmed and extended these earlier observations and we have, in addition, established several lymphoid cell lines which have been characterised as T-cells.

MATERIALS AND METHODS

Experiments 1 and 2 were concerned with the experimental induction of disease in 2 commercial strains (designated A and B) of turkeys by inoculation of 3 strains of MDV (GA, HPRS 16, JM).

Experiment 3 was designed to study the pathogenesis of the disease, following the basic schemes of Payne and Rennie (1973 and 1976). Groups of poults were inoculated at 10 days old with 5×10^4 plaque forming units (pfu) of cell-associated MDV (GA strain) and control poults housed separately were sham injected. At intervals after infection 5 infected and 2 control turkeys were killed. The body weights and weights of the bursa, thymus and spleen were determined. The following tissues were examined histologically for evidence of reticulum cell hyperplasia, lymphoid proliferation and intranuclear inclusion bodies: feather follicle, breast muscle, heart muscle, liver, kidney, lung, proventriculus, gonad, adrenal, thyroid, spleen, bursa, thymus and sciatic and brachial plexuses. Frozen sections of the bursa, thymus, spleen, liver, proventriculus and feather follicle were examined with chicken anti-MDV fluorescein-conjugated antiserum for the presence of viral antigens. Suspensions of blood mononuclear cells and of spleen, bursa and thymus cells were assayed on chicken kidney cell monolayers for the presence of infectious virus (Powell and Rowell, 1977). Smears of these suspensions (fixed and unfixed) were also examined with specific antiserum for viral antigens. At each sampling time heparinised and citrated blood was collected from 5 infected and 5 control turkeys. Total and differential white cell counts were made and mononuclear cells were examined in the indirect immunofluorescence test for staining with specific anti-MATSA, anti-turkey T-cell, anti-turkey B-cell and anti-turkey immunoglobulin antisera. The anti-MATSA antiserum was prepared by injecting rabbits with a chicken lymphoblastoid cell line (MDCC-HP1) as described by Powell and Rennie (1978); the other antisera were prepared according to the method of Hudson and Roitt (1973).

At 7, 21 and 35 days after infection 9 infected and 9

control poults were inoculated with 1 ml of a 10% suspension of sheep erythrocytes and with 0.25 ml of a suspension of killed Brucella abortus containing 5×10^9 organisms. Seven days after each injection the birds were bled and the serum assayed for agglutinins.

Establishment of cell lines

Single cell suspensions from splenic tumours or from the buffy coats of leukaemic birds were cultured by a liquid culture technique described by Payne et al. (1981).

RESULTS

Preliminary results are given below; a definitive account will appear in a later paper.

MD mortality

It was found in earlier experiments that the dose of virus normally administered when infecting chickens (10^3 pfu) failed to induce any lesions in turkeys and, on the basis of the lack of any serological response and the failure to reisolate virus, apparently did not infect the birds. Two commercial strains of turkeys were inoculated with large doses of 3 different strains of MDV and mortality was observed over a 5 month period. The results (Table 1) showed that the GA strain of MDV, but not HPRS 16 or JM, when administered as a large dose, caused lymphoma formation and death. Dead birds had grossly enlarged livers and spleens; gross lesions in other visceral organs were not common.

MD pathogenesis

Following inoculation with GA virus, randomly selected groups of turkeys were killed at twice weekly or weekly intervals. The results of the observations made on these birds are summarised in Table 2. No birds showed clinical signs of disease until after 31 days post-infection, and the first deaths occurred at 38 days post-infection. The most striking

TABLE 1   Marek's disease mortality in turkeys

Experiment	Turkey strain	Virus strain	Dose per poult	Mortality
1	A	GA	4.5×10^4	2/2
	A	HPRS 16	6.2×10^4	0/9
	A	JM	6.3×10^4	0/18
	B	GA	14.3×10^4	17/20
2	B	GA	10.0×10^4	9/11

finding was the lack of significant histological and virological changes in the early stages of the disease. Virus was isolated sporadically at very low titre from suspensions of lymphoid cells during the course of the experiment, and viral antigens were observed in frozen sections rarely and then only towards the end of the experiment. Histologically, no changes were observed in the sampled birds until 38 days after infection when regression of the bursa and thymus was prominent and lymphoid proliferation was observed in some visceral organs. These changes in the lymphoid organs were reflected in the changes in the weights of the organs which were consistent with regression of the bursa and thymus and lymphoid proliferation in the spleen.

Histological examination of birds that died revealed proliferative lesions in many visceral organs. The infiltrating cells were a heterogeneous population in which small and medium lymphocytes, and reticulum cells were prominent (Fig. 1). These proliferative lesions were accompanied by degenerative changes in the bursa and the thymus. During the course of this study, lymphoproliferative changes were not observed in the peripheral nerves or feather follicle regions, but in subsequent experiments a few turkeys did develop lymphoproliferation typical of MD in the peripheral nerves.

TABLE 2 Pathogenesis of Marek's disease in turkeys

Number of poults (n/5) with

Days post infec- tion	lymphoid proliferation in												regres- sion of		virus iso- lated from				viral antigen in				
	F	M	H	L	K	Li	P	G	A	Tr	S	N	B	T	B	T	S	Pb	F	P	Li	B	T
3	Not done														0	0	0	0	0	0	0	0	0
6	0	0	0	0	0	0	0	0	0	0	0	0	0	0	0	0	0	0	0	0	0	0	0
10	0	0	0	0	0	0	0	0	0	0	0	0	0	0	0	0	1	1	0	0	0	0	0
13	0	0	0	0	0	0	0	0	0	0	0	0	1	0	0	1	0	0	0	0	1	0	0
20	Not done														0	0	0	0	0	0	0	0	0
24	0	0	0	0	0	0	0	0	0	0	0	0	0	0	0	0	0	0	0	0	0	0	0
31	Not done														0	0	1	1	0	0	0	0	0
38	0	0	0	0	0	0	1	0	0	1	1	0	3	1	0	0	0	0	0	0	0	0	1
45	0	0	0	0	0	0	0	0	0	0	0	0	5	3	0	0	0	0	0	0	0	0	1
52	0	0	0	2	1	0	1	1	1	1	2	0	3	2	0	0	0	0	0	0	0	2	2

F = Feather follicle
M = Muscle (pectoral)
H = Heart
L = Lung
K = Kidney

Li = Liver
P = Proventriculus
A = Adrenal
Tr = Thyroid
S = Spleen

N = Nerves
B = Bursa
T = Thymus
Pb = Periphera
G = Gonad

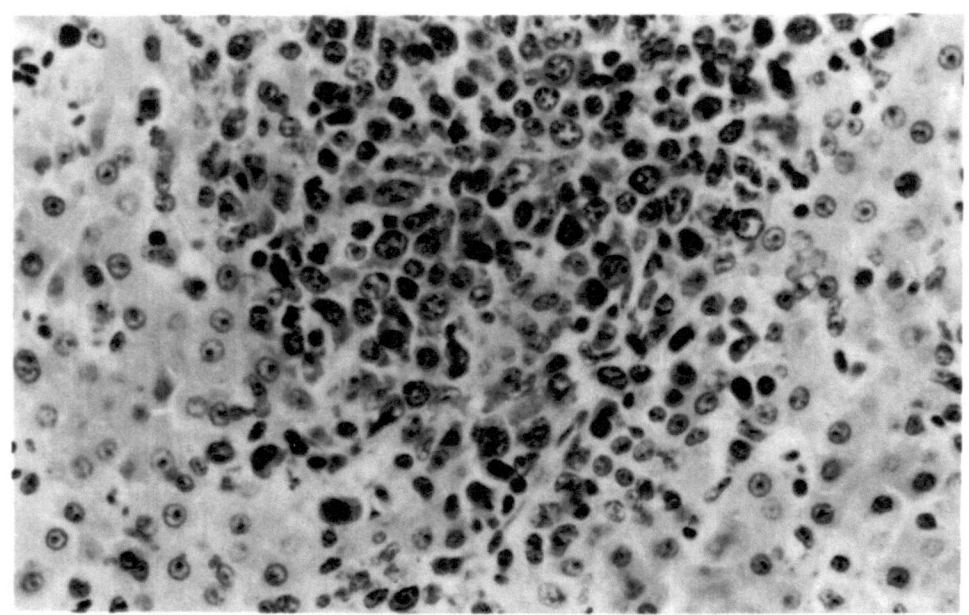

Fig. 1   Infiltrating lymphocytes and reticulum cells in
the liver of a turkey 64 days after infection with
Marek's disease virus (GA strain). H. & E., x 930.

Haematological changes

Infection had little effect on the total numbers of
mononuclear cells in blood suspensions from randomly sampled
birds (Fig. 2). However, some individual turkeys selected for
clinical signs of disease had greatly elevated mononuclear
cell counts. Blood from these birds contained large numbers of
medium and large lymphocytes and lymphoblasts. The percentages
of B-cells and T-cells in the blood were unaffected by
infection. The proportions of B-cells in uninfected and
infected turkeys remained constant throughout the period
studied, with average values of 14.4% $\pm$ 0.64 s.e.m. and 13.3%
$\pm$ 0.86 respectively. The equivalent values for T-cells were
77.5% $\pm$ 0.80 and 78.7% $\pm$ 0.82. The proportions of cells
expressing membrane immunoglobulins in control and infected
turkeys were 11.1% $\pm$ 0.80 and 10.2% $\pm$ 0.65 respectively.

Cells expressing MATSA were detected only in infected

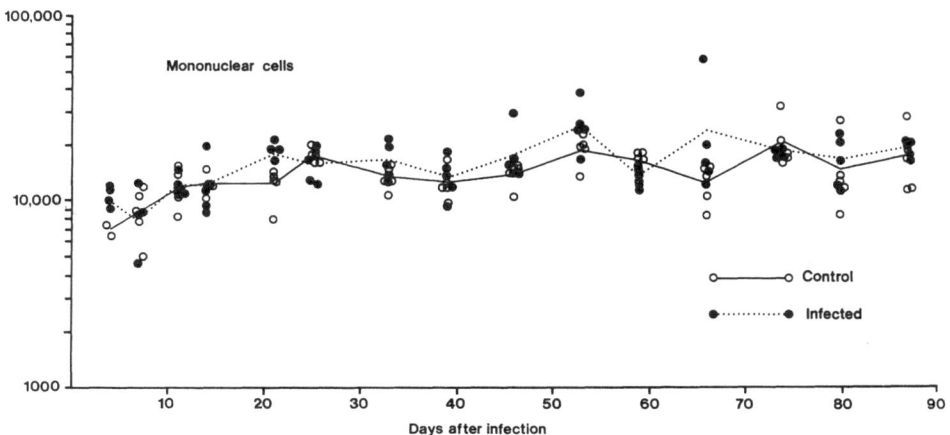

Fig. 2   Individual and mean numbers of mononuclear
cells (lymphocytes and monocytes) in the blood of
infected and control turkeys.

turkeys, but other than in leukaemic birds, the proportion of
peripheral blood lymphocytes positive did not exceed 4% and
more usually was less than 2%. Mononuclear cells from
leukaemic chickens, however, contained between 8% and 27%
MATSA-bearing cells.

Immunosuppressive effects of infection

Infection caused a significant ($p < 0.001$) depression in
the primary response to B. abortus antigen but the response to
sheep erythrocytes was unaffected (Table 3). Secondary and
tertiary antibody responses of infected turkeys to sheep
erythrocytes, but not to B. abortus, were also significantly
depressed ($p < 0.05$).

Establishment and characterisation of cell lines

A total of 8 cell lines have been established from
cultures of spleen cells or buffy coat cells from infected and
leukaemic turkeys. This represents a success rate of 73%. The
cell lines consist of a mixed population of medium and large

TABLE 3   Agglutinin responses to sheep erythrocytes and
           B.abortus in infected and control turkeys

	Sheep erythrocytes			B.abortus		
	1°	2°	3°	1°	2°	3°
In-fected	3.7±0.29*5.2±0.40		6.6±0.32	1.1±0.35	11.0±0.33	10.3±0.49
Con-trol	3.3±0.84	7.1±0.52	7.8±0.37	5.2±0.84	10.8±0.15	9.6±0.75

* mean $\log_2$ titre ± s.e.m.

lymphocytes with a few lymphoblasts (Fig. 3). The four cell
lines that have so far been tested appear to be producer cell
lines although the levels of virus expression indicated by
immunofluorescence or by isolation in tissue culture were very
low; chick inoculation experiments confirmed the presence of

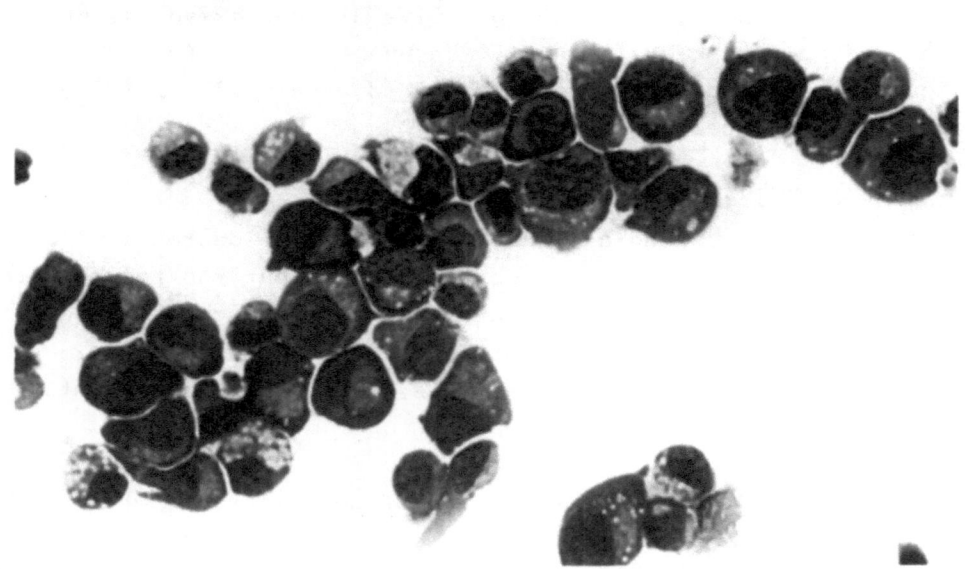

Fig. 3   Cells of the lymphoid cell line MDTC-HP114-1
derived from the leukaemic blood of an infected turkey.
May-Grünwald & Giemsa, x 930.

infectious MDV. All of the cell lines were examined for the presence of B-cell and T-cell antigens using specific antisera prepared in rabbits against turkey thymus cells, turkey bursa cells and turkey immunoglobulins. The mean percentage of cells expressing T-cell antigens was 85.2% (Table 4). Using a specific rabbit anti-MATSA serum raised against a chicken MD lymphoblastoid cell line (MDCC-HP1), the mean percentage of cells expressing MATSA was 60.9% (Table 4).

TABLE 4   Percentage of cells showing membrane fluorescence

Turkey cell lines	Antisera			
	anti-turkey T-cells	anti-turkey B-cells	anti-turkey immunoglobulin	anti-MATSA
MDTC-HP41-1	89.7	2.8	0.0	69.0
MDTC-HP41-2	90.2	0.0	0.0	70.4
MDTC-HP48-3	92.0	0.8	0.0	61.7
MDTC-HP114-1	73.1	2.1	0.4	53.7
MDTC-HP114-2	77.9	0.4	0.4	56.5
MDTC-HP115	88.3	0.4	1.8	59.2
MDTC-HP116	82.9	1.7	1.6	58.6
MDTC-HP117	92.2	0.0	0.8	55.0
MDTC-HP118	82.8	0.0	0.4	61.8
MDTC-HP119	83.3	6.0	2.6	63.1
Chicken cell line				
MDCC-HP3	11.3	6.2	0.0	53.5

Preliminary experiments have indicated that the cell lines release substances into the culture medium (i.e. lymphokines) which suppress the response of normal chicken spleen cells to concanavalin A. Surprisingly, the same samples of culture medium were found to enhance the response of normal chicken spleen cells to phytohaemagglutinin and to poke weed mitogen.

DISCUSSION

These observations confirm previous reports that inoculation of the GA strain of MDV into turkeys can cause a disease characterised by lymphoproliferation in the visceral organs and gross tumour formation. There were, however, many differences between the disease induced in turkeys and MD in chickens. There was no evidence of early histological changes in the lymphoid organs of the type described in susceptible strains of chickens (Payne and Rennie, 1973). This probably reflects a lack of significant virus replication in these sites, and is consistent with our failure, with very occasional exceptions, to detect virus or viral antigens. A lack of early virus replication would similarly account for our failure to observe any early haematological changes. Despite these negative features, there was a high incidence of lymphomatous disease, and it appears that clinical disease developed rapidly with few premonitory signs. The lack of significant early pathology may have been due to the fact that MDV is a naturally occurring virus of chickens, which does not normally infect turkeys. Although infection may be experimentally established, as indicated by the ultimate development of disease, it appears that non-productive infection and malignant transformation of lymphocytes occurs in the virtual absence of semi-productive infection and virus replication. There was also no evidence of productive infection in the feather follicles, of the type responsible for virus shedding in chickens. It is perhaps significant that it was not possible to rescue virus from lymphomatous material, and that the four cell lines tested contained very low titres of infectious MDV. This supports the notion that the preferred relationship between turkey lymphocytes and MDV is of the non-producer type.

The cell lines were characterised as belonging to the T-cell lineage on the basis of cell surface staining. This was not unexpected as all the established MD cell lines of chicken origin express T-cell antigens, and it is believed that T-cells are the targets for neoplastic transformation by MDV. This conclusion is, however, at variance with the findings of Nazerian et al. (1982) who characterised turkey lymphoblastoid cell lines as B-cells, on the basis of the reactions of the cells with anti-chicken T-cell, anti-chicken B-cell and anti-chicken immunoglobulin antisera; in our hands, such antisera did not give specific reactions with turkey cells.

There were differences between our observations on the
pathogenesis of the disease in turkeys and those of Elmubarak
et al. (1981) who, also using GA virus strain, described an
early lytic stage associated with viral antigen in the thymus
and spleen, consistent virus rescue from blood leukocytes, and
virus-induced immunosuppression. The virus titres were,
however, much lower (10 to 100-fold) than those found in
chickens, and the occurrence of viral antigen and of lytic
lesions (which were described as mild) was lower than in
chickens. These differences may be attributable to different
strains of turkey.

REFERENCES
Elmubarak, A.K., Sharma, J.M., Witter, R.L., Nazerian, K. and
    Sanger, V.L. 1981. Induction of lymphomas and tumor
    antigen by Marek's disease virus in turkeys. Avian Dis.,
    25, 911-926.
Hudson, L. and Roitt, I.M. 1973. Immunofluorescent detection
    of surface antigens specific to T and B lymphocytes in
    the chicken. Eur. J. Immunol., 3, 63-67.
Nazerian, K., Elmubarak, A. and Sharma, J.M. 1982.
    Establishment of B-lymphoblastoid cell lines from Marek's
    disease virus-induced tumors in turkeys. Int. J. Cancer,
    29, 63-68.
Paul, P.S., Sautter, J.H. and Pomeroy, B.S. 1977.
    Susceptibility of turkeys to Georgia strain of Marek's
    disease virus of chicken origin. Am. J. Vet. Res., 38,
    1653-1656.
Payne, L.N. and Rennie, M. 1973. Pathogenesis of Marek's
    disease in chicks with and without maternal antibody. J.
    Natn. Cancer Inst., 51, 1559-1573.
Payne, L.N. and Rennie, M. 1976. Sequential changes in the
    numbers of B and T lymphocytes and other leukocytes in
    the blood in Marek's disease. Int. J. Cancer, 18,
    510-520.
Payne, L.N., Frazier, J.A. and Powell, P.C. 1976. Pathogenesis
    of Marek's disease. Int. Rev. exp. Path., 16, 59-154.
Payne, L.N., Howes, K., Rennie, M., Bumstead, J.M. and Kidd,
    A.W. 1981. Use of an agar culture technique for
    establishing lymphoid cell lines from Marek's disease
    lymphomas. Int. J. Cancer, 28, 757-766.
Powell, P.C. and Rowell, J.G. 1977. Dissociation of antiviral
    and antitumor immunity in resistance to Marek's disease.
    J. Natn. Cancer Inst., 59, 919-924.
Powell, P.C. and Rennie, M. 1978. Marek's disease
    tumour-specific antigen induced by the herpesvirus of
    turkeys in vaccinated chickens. Vet. Rec., 103, 232-233.

PERSISTENCE OF VIRAL DNA IN MAREK'S DISEASE VIRUS-
TRANSFORMED LYMPHOBLASTOID CELL LINES

H.-J. Rziha and B. Bauer

Federal Research Institute for Animal Virus Diseases,
Paul-Ehrlich-Str. 28, D-7400 Tübingen, F.R.G.

ABSTRACT

The state of latent viral DNA in Marek's disease virus
(MDV) - transformed chicken cell lines was investigated. In
addition to integrated viral DNA sequences, free MDV DNA with
properties of plasmid molecules could be demonstrated in the
virus producer line MDCC-MSB1, as well as in the non-producer
line MDCC-HP2. In contrast, in the non-producer line MDCC-RP1
viral DNA appeared to be mainly associated with the cellular
DNA. Treatment of the cell lines with tetradecanoylphorbol
acetate (TPA) did not influence significantly the intracellular
state of the viral genome.

INTRODUCTION

Marek's disease (MD) is a highly contagious neoplastic
disease in domestic fowls. In vivo, virus infection leads to
the development of malignant lymphomas, apparently as a
consequence of an abortive infection of the T cells. The
lymphoid tumours of the infected animals are free of viral
antigens and virus particles, but viral DNA can be demonstrated
in single tumour cells (Nazerian et al., 1973; Ross et al.,
1981; Rziha, unpubl.). Chickens vaccinated with the apathogenic
herpesvirus of turkeys (HVT) can be protected against MD tumour
development by a still unknown mechanism. In view of the
protective role of HVT, and of the antigenic and immunologic
similiarities between HVT and MDV, it was very surprising that
both viruses lack major genome homologies. The DNA analysis of
MDV and HVT displays homologous equences only in the range of
1 - 5% (Hirai et al., 1979; Kaschka-Dierich et al., 1979a;
Tamaka et al., 1980; Nonoyama and Hirai, 1981; Rziha, unpubl.).
Several lymphoblastoid cell lines have been established
from MD tumours, but in vitro transformation of chicken

lymphoid cells by MDV has not yet been accomplished. All these cell lines share common properties, such as carrying T cell markers and expressing MD associated tumour surface antigens (MATSA). All established cell lines contain multiple copies of MDV DNA (Nazerian et al., 1973; Nazerian, 1979), but production of viral antigens and virus particles varies in the different cell lines. In contrast to the virus non-producer lines, some cell lines produce virus particles in a small percentage of the cell population. The existence of MD lymphoblastoid cell lines enables investigations of mechanisms leading to herpesvirus-induced transformation and viral persistence.

We report here our studies on the state of the persistent MDV DNA in a producer line, and in two non-producer lines. Additionally, induction experiments with the phorbol ester tetradecanoylphorbol acetate (TPA) are briefly reported.

METHODS

The two non-producer lines MDCC-HP2 (HP2, Powell et al., 1974) and MDCC-RP1 (RP1, Nazerian et al., 1977), as well as the producer line MDCC-MSB1 (MSB1, Akiyama and Kato, 1973) were investigated. The cells were maintained in culture as described previously (Rziha and Bauer, 1982). Virus-specific intracellular antigens were demonstrated by indirect immunofluorescence tests (v. Bülow and Schmid, 1979). Virus production was tested by co-cultivation of the cells on chick embryo fibroblasts (CEF) following plaque assays in 0.9% agarose-medium. Treatment with the phorbol ester TPA (20 ng/ml culture medium) was performed essentially as described (zur Hausen et al., 1978). MDV DNA was demonstrated by in situ cytohybridization using in vitro synthesized ^{3}H-labeled cRNA (Brahic and Haase, 1978, Moar and Klein, 1978). The following control experiments attested to the specificity of the hybridizations: (i) the MDV probe did not hybridize to uninfected CEF, and (ii) the reaction was greatly reduced after DNase treatment. The experiments for the investigation of the intracellular state of the viral DNA in the cell lines were recently published (Rziha and Bauer, 1982).

RESULTS AND DISCUSSION

All MDV-transformed cell lines investigated contain multiple copies of the viral genome (Nazerian et al., 1973; Nazerian, 1979). The number of genome equivalents per cell ranges from about 100 genomes in the producer line MSB1 to 10 - 20 genomes or less in the different non-producer lines. The occurrence of the viral DNA in these cells can be demonstrated by _in situ_ hybridization, as shown in Figures 1 and 2. The results indicated that nearly every cell of the MSB1

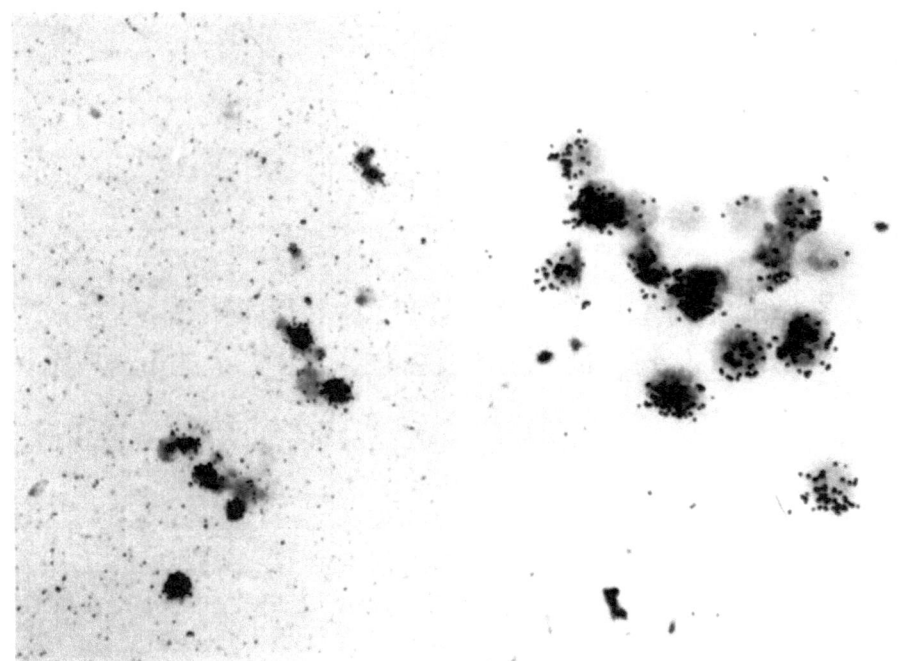

Fig. 1   In situ hybridization demonstrating MDV DNA in MSB1 cells. Autoradiographic exposure was for 2 weeks.

line (Fig. 1) and of the RP1 line (Fig. 2) contained viral DNA. Similar results have been published recently (Ross et al., 1981). In further experiments the three cell lines described were tested for inducibility of virus production, viral antigen, and viral DNA synthesis after treatment with the phorbol ester TPA (zur Hausen et al., 1978). Untreated control and TPA-treated cultures were assayed 2-7 days later. In the

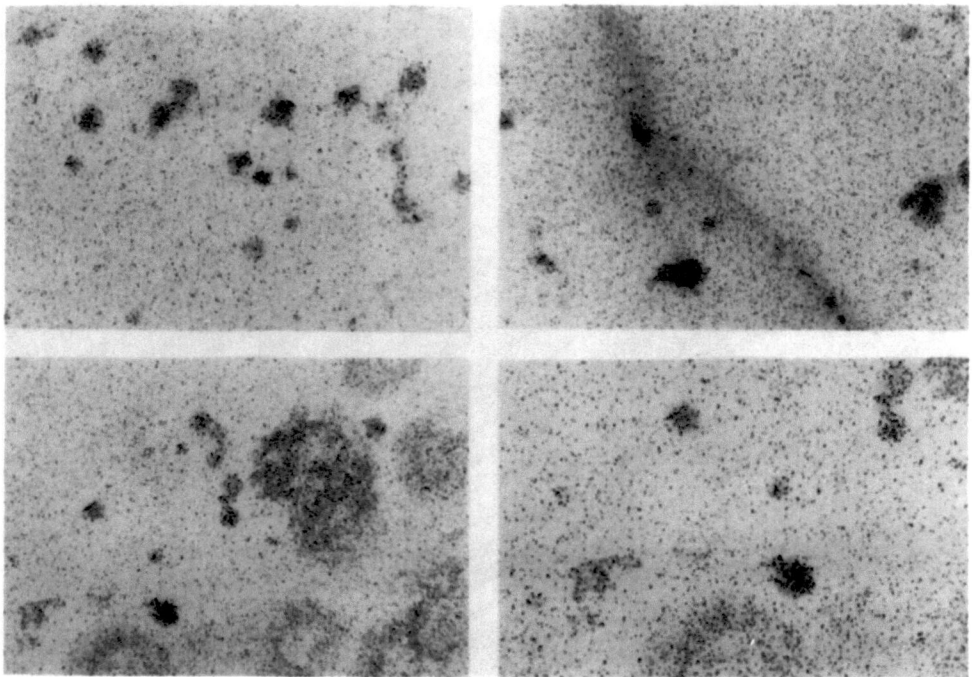

Fig. 2   In situ hybridization showing MDV DNA in RP1
cells. In order to enhance the sensitivity of the
hybridization, dextran sulphate (10% w/v) was added to the
annealing mixture. Autoradiographic exposure was for 5
weeks.

producer line MSB1, TPA caused a slight increase of
intracellular viral antigens as determined by indirect
immunofluorescence. A similar enhancement of virus replication
could be found after co-cultivation with CEF cultures, as well
as after in situ hybridization for MDV DNA (data not shown).
TPA treatment of the non-producer lines, however, did not
result in virus production, and no significant increase of
viral DNA synthesis and antigen expression could be observed.

How the viral genome is transmitted and maintained in the
MDV-transformed cells is an unsettled question. So far, the
state of MDV DNA in these cells has not been clearly defined.
In the low producer line MDCC-HP1, Kaschka-Dierich et al.
(1979b) suggested a stable association between the viral and
the cellular genome. On the other hand, they found both

integrated and free viral DNA in the MSB1 cells, but were
unable to show the existence of covalently closed circular DNA.
In contrast, viral plasmid DNA could be demonstrated in the
majority of the cells of the non-producer line MKT-1 (Tanaka et
al., 1978).

Therefore, we decided to investigate the state of MDV DNA
in two further non-producer lines, HP2 and RP1, respectively.
Additionally we included the producer line MSB1 in our studies,
which were recently published in detail (Rziha and Bauer,
1982). After gentle lysis of the cells, total DNA was
extracted, and fractionated on neutral CsCl-density gradients.
These experiments demonstrated viral DNA sequences in the MSB1
and HP2 cells banding at the density position of purified
virion DNA (1.705 g/ml), indicative of the existence of free
MDV DNA. After size reduction of the cell DNAs from the two
lines following re-centrifugation on neutral CsCl gradients a
large proportion of the DNA material was released, which banded
again at the density of free viral DNA. In the RP1 cells,
however, the vast majority of viral DNA was detected in the
cellular DNA range after shearing of the DNA or after
centrifugation under denaturing conditions (data not shown).
Therefore, we suggest that MDV DNA is mostly associated with
the cell genome of the RP1 cells, although definite evidence
for integration remains to be demonstrated. But both integrated
and free viral DNA was found in the MSB1 and HP2 cells. In
order to investigate the sedimentation properties of the free
MDV DNA, the corresponding CsCl fractions were pooled, and
further analysed by glycerol gradient centrifugation. The
results shown in Figure 3 are representative of both MSB1 and
HP2 DNA, since their hybridization profiles were nearly
identical. A prominent viral DNA peak was reproducibly detected
in the 100 S region of the gradient (Fig. 3, fraction 10),
representing about 30% of the free MDV DNA. This is expected
for the sedimentation of covalently closed circular molecules.
The presence of MDV plasmid DNA could be confirmed after
centrifugation of the 100 S DNA material in ethidium
bromide-CsCl-density gradients (Fig. 4). As shown in the

Figure, about 35% of the 100 S MDV DNA banded near the density
of the covalently closed supercoiled marker DNA (human
papovavirus DNA, BKV I, 1.60 g/ml). The remainder of the MDV
DNA was found at the density of open circular DNA (BKV II),
which could be due to mechanical breakdown.

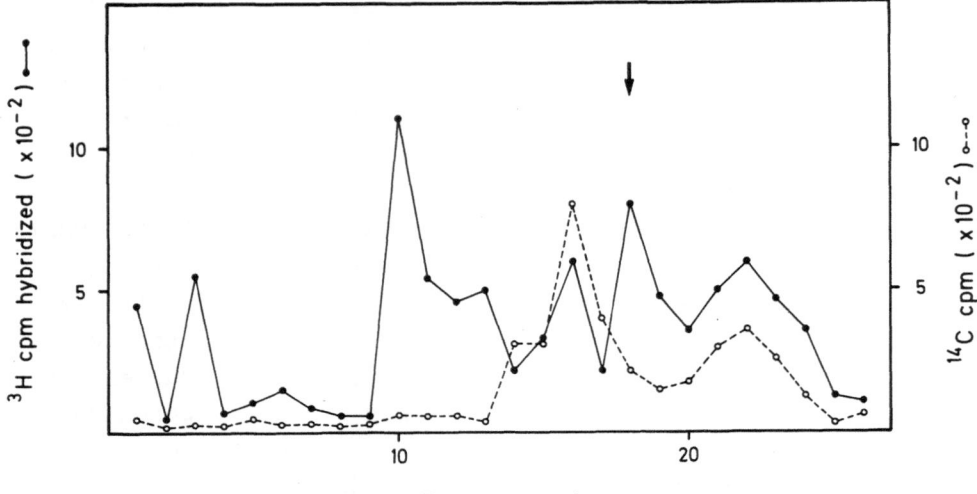

— Fraction number

Fig. 3   Glycerol gradient centrifugation of MDV DNA from
MSB1 and HP2 cells pre-fractionated in CsCl-density
gradients. Sedimentation was from right to left. The arrow
indicates the position of the 54 S marker DNA.

TPA treatment of the cells, as described above, did not
significantly influence the intracellular state of the viral
genome in the cell lines tested.

It has been well documented that the majority of the DNA
of other oncogenic herpesviruses, such as EBV (Adams, 1978),
and herpesvirus saimiri (Werner et al., 1977), exist as
circular plasmids. These studies demonstrate the presence of
circular viral DNA in two further MDV-transformed cell lines,
whereas in the third cell line tested (RP1) the viral DNA
seemed to be mainly associated with the cellular genome. The
failure to detect circular DNA in these cells might be due to
the low yield of viral DNA. Furthermore, the existence of
defective MDV DNA banding close to the cellular DNA density

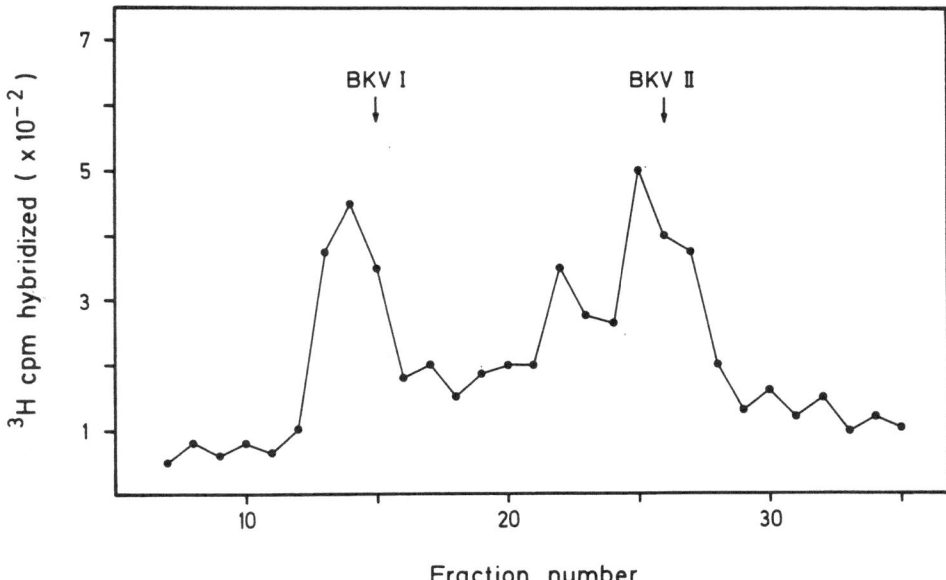

Fig. 4   Ethidium bromideCsCl-density gradient centrifugation of 100 S MDV DNA. The bottom of the gradient is
to the left.

region cannot be excluded (Tanaka et al., 1980). Finally, it is

possible that viral DNA occurs in a different intracellular

state in the different MDV-transformed cell lines. On the other

hand, since circular viral DNA can be found in cells

transformed by herpesviruses, one might speculate that the

plasmid form could be mandatory for a herpesvirus-induced

transformation.

(This work was supported by the Bundesministerium für Forschung

und Technologie, F.R.G., PTB 8066).

REFERENCES
Adams, A.   1978. The state of the virus genome in transformed
      cells and its relationship to host cell DNA. In "The Ep-
      stein Barr Virus" (Ed. Epstein, M.A., Achong, B.G.)
      (Springer-Verlag). pp. 155-178.
Akiyama, Y. and Kato, S.   1973. Continuous cell culture from
      lymphoma of Marek's disease. Biken's J., 16, 177-179.
Brahic, M. and Haase, A.T.   1978. Detection of viral sequences
      of low reiteration frequency by in situ hybridization.
      Proc. Natl. Acad. Sci. (USA), 75, 6125-6129.
Bülow, V. v. and Schmid, D.O.   1979. Antigenic characteristic

of Marek's disease tumour cells. Avian Pathol., 8, 265-277.

Hirai, K., Ikuta, K., Kato, S. 1979. Comparative studies on Marek's disease virus and herpesvirus of turkey DNAs. J. gen. Virol., 45, 119-131.

Kaschka-Dierich, C., Bornkamm, G.W., Thomssen, R. 1979a. No homology detectable between Marek's disease virus (MDV) DNA and herpesvirus of the turkey (HVT) DNA. Med. Microbiol. Immunol., 165, 223-239.

KaschkaDierich, C., Nazerian, K., Thomssen, R. 1979b. Intracellular state of Marek's disease virus DNA in two derived chicken cell lines. J. gen. Virol., 44, 271-280.

Lee, Y.S., Tanaka, A., Silver, S., Smith, M. and Nonoyama, M. 1979. Minor DNA homology between herpesvirus of turkey and Marek's disease virus? Virology, 93, 227-280.

Moar, M.H. and Klein, G. 1978. Detection of Epstein-Barr Virus (EBV) DNA sequences using in situ hybridzation. Biochim. Biophys. Acta, 519, 49-64.

Nazerian, K., Lindahl, T., Klein, G. and Lee, L.F. 1973. Deoxyribonucleic acid of Marek's disease virus in virus-induced tumours. J. Virol., 12, 841-846.

Nazerian, K., Stephens, E.A., Sharma, J.M., Lee, L.F., Lailitis, M. and Witter, R.L. 1977. A nonproducer T lymphoblastoid cell line from Marek's disease transplantable tumor (IMV). Avian Dis., 21, 69-76.

Nazerian, K. 1979. Marek's disease lymphoma of chicken and its causative herpesvirus. Biochim. Biophys. Acta, 560, 375-395.

Nonoyama, M. and Hirai, K. 1981. Organization and expression of the DNA of Marek's disease virus and of herpesvirus of turkeys. In "Herpesvirus DNA" (Ed. Y. Becker, M. Nijhoff Publishers). pp. 437-461.

Powell, P.C., Payne, L.N., Frazier, J.A. and Rennie, M. 1974. T lymphoblastoid cell lines from Marek's disease lymphomas. Nature, 251, 79-80.

Ross, N.L.J., DeLorbe, W., Varmus, H.E., Bishop, J.M., Brahic, M. and Haase, A. 1981. Persistence and expression of Marek's disease virus DNA in tumour cells and peripheral nerves studied by in situ hybridization. J. gen. Virol., 57, 285-296.

Rziha, H.J. and Bauer, B. 1982. Circular forms of viral DNA in Marek's disease virustransformed lymphoblastoid cells. Arch. Virol., 72, 211-216.

Tanaka, A., Silver, S. and Nonoyama, M. 1978. Biochemical evidence of the nonintegrated status of Marek's disease virus DNA in virustransformed lymphoblastoid cells of chicken. Virology, 88, 19-24.

Tanaka, A., Lee, Y.S. and Nonoyama, M. 1980. Heterogeneous population of virus DNA in serially passaged Marek's disease virus preparation. Virology, 103, 510-513.

Werner, F.J., Bornkamm, G.W. and Fleckenstein, B. 1977. Episomal viral DNA in a herpesvirus saimiri-transformed lymphoid cell line. J. Virol., 22, 794-803.

Zur Hausen, H., O'Neill, F.J., Freese, U.K. and Hecker, E. 1978. Persisting oncogenic herpesvirus induced by the tumour promotor TPA. Nature, 272, 373-375.

LATENCY OF PIGEON HERPESVIRUS 1 (PHV1)

H. Vindevogel*, P.P. Pastoret**, E. Thiry**
Faculté de Médecine Vétérinaire de l'Université
de Liège
*Clinique aviaire
**Service de Virologie
45, rue des Vétérinaires
B-1070 Bruxelles, Belgique

ABSTRACT

Pigeon herpesvirus 1 (PHV1) infection induces lesions in the upper digestive and respiratory tracts. It is the most common infection of pigeons in the E.E.C.

After experimental inoculation of squabs free of the infection, animals excrete high titres of infectious particles of PHV1 very soon and this excretion lasts a minimum of 7 to 10 days. The typical lesions appear 1 to 3 days after inoculation when viral excretion reaches its maximum. Mild episodes of recurrence (re-excretion of the virus) may occur spontaneously without clinical signs. High titres of antibodies do not prevent these recurrences and, conversely, recurrent episodes are not more frequent when the animals are nearly devoid of specific antibodies.

If experimentally infected pigeons are treated with cyclophosphamide a few months later, a viral excretion episode, nearly equivalent to that following primary infection, is provoked.

In a flock of pigeons naturally infected with PHV1, mature birds are asymptomatic carriers of the virus and they shed it from time to time. They may therefore transmit it to their offspring. Squabs become infected when they are protected from the disease by passive immunity of parental origin. Indeed, parental passive immunity, as in the other avian species, is conferred to the squabs through the egg yolk and protects it from the worst effects of infection. Therefore most of the squabs become latent carriers themselves after this initial infection although they are very soon devoid of detectable antibodies; nevertheless infection can be unmasked by cyclophosphamide treatment.

Clinical disease is therefore mainly observed during primary infection of young pigeons born to parents free of the infection or in carriers of the virus with the help of debilitating factors.

A strain of PHV1 has been attenuated by 100 passages on chicken embryo fibroblasts. The resulting attenuated strain multiplies in the animal to the same extent as the original wild strain and persists also after vaccination.

Previous infection of the pigeon with a wild strain of PHV1 prevents the occurrence of symptoms when they are re-infected.

Vaccination of pigeons either with the attenuated strain or with inactivated wild virus in oil adjuvant reduces viral excretion and symptoms after challenge with a virulent strain but is unable to prevent the establishment of latency as demonstrated by cyclophosphamide treatment of the animals. However, vaccination diminishes spontaneous viral re-excretion and therefore viral dissemination.

In conclusion, immunity, either passive or active, does not prevent the establishment of latent infection but helps to control the dissemination of the virus and protects from the disease resulting from infection. Under natural conditions, there is a sophisticated equilibrium between the virus and its host that prevents the occurrence of the disease.

INTRODUCTION

Since 1967, a herpesvirus (Pigeon herpesvirus 1, PHV1) has been isolated from pigeons affected with respiratory illness in numerous countries including Great-Britain, Belgium, France, Germany and Italy (Vindevogel, 1981).

Pigeon herpesvirus 1 infection is widespread in Belgium. Indeed, specific antibodies were detected by indirect immunofluorescence in the sera of 84% of clinically normal pigeons and by counter-immuno-electro-osmophoresis (C.I.E.O.P.) in 63% of the sera of pigeons affected with acute respiratory illness. PHV1 has been isolated in 60% of dove-cots permanently affected with respiratory troubles (Vindevogel et al., 1981; Vindevogel, 1981). A similar situation has been described in France and Germany (Heffels et al., 1981; Landré et al., 1982). PHV1 seems therefore to be frequently associated with respiratory distress in pigeons and we were able to reproduce the natural disease by experimental exposure of pigeons to the virus (Vindevogel et al., 1975; Vindevogel and Pastoret, 1981).

Classical signs of PHV1 infection are conjunctivitis, rhinitis and focal necrosis in mouth, pharynx and larynx. In addition, during natural outbreaks, lesions may be observed in the trachea, liver, spleen, kidney and pancreas (Vindevogel and Pastoret, 1981).

PHV1 has also been isolated from budgerigars where it provokes, naturally or experimentally, fatal hepatitis (Vindevogel and Duchatel, 1977; Vindevogel et al., 1980b).

PHV1 cannot be antigenically distinguished from Falcon herpesvirus and Owl herpesvirus but is antigenically dissimilar to Turkey herpesvirus (Turkey herpesvirus 1), Marek's disease virus (Phasianid herpesvirus 2), infectious laryngotracheitis virus (Phasianid herpesvirus 1) and duck plague herpesvirus (Anatid herpesvirus 1). PHV1 can also be clearly distinguished from Psittacine herpesvirus (Pacheco's disease virus) both from the point of view of its antigenic composition and biological properties (Purchase et al., 1972; Mare et Graham, 1973; Vindevogel et al., 1980b; Vindevogel, 1981).

EXPERIMENTAL INFECTION OF NORMAL PIGEONS (Vindevogel et al., 1980a)

For all experimental infections, squabs from parents free of the infection were used. After inoculation by pharyngeal painting of 10^5 pfu, the level of excretion of infectious particles in pharyngeal swabs was recorded as well the evolution of neutralizing antibodies and clinical signs.

a. Primary infection:

All the squabs excreted infectious particles 24 hours after infection with a maximum of excretion between the second and the fourth day. Excretion persisted generally seven to ten days. One squab died from the disease. Neutralizing antibodies appeared from the end of the first week following infection. The highest titre was observed on day 20 and then decreased slowly until day 90.

b. Spontaneous re-excretion:

After the first period of continuous excretion following the primary infection, spontaneous re-excretion without clinical signs was observed in several pigeons. High titres of specific antibodies did not prevent the occurrence of re-exretion and despite the episodes of re-excretion, specific antibodies decreased gradually.

c. Experimental re-excretion:

Ninety days after infection, the same birds were injected intraabdominally during four days with cyclophosphamide (10 mg/pigeon/day). All the pigeons re-excreted virus from 1 to 10 days after the beginning of the treatment. Two pigeons died

with signs and lesions of the natural disease. The two
surviving birds developed pharyngeal lesions associated with
lower levels of viral excretion. The cyclophosphamide treatment
led to a decrease in the titres of specific antibodies three
days after the last injection; this was followed by an increase
seven days later.

EXPERIMENTAL INFECTION OF DEBILITATED PIGEONS (Coignoul and
Vindevogel, 1980; Vindevogel et al., 1980a)

Cyclophosphamide treatment of pigeons produces a rapid
atrophy and an intense depletion of lymphoid cells in the bursa
of Fabricius. The thymus also shows reduced weight and
morphological degeneration but the T-cells system regenerates
more rapidly. Therefore, cyclophosphamide can be used to
debilitate pigeons before infection. To compare the evolution
of infection in debilitated pigeons", squabs free from the
infection were treated during four days with cyclophosphamide
seven days before primary infection with PHV1.

a. Primary infection:

Daily titration of virus in the pharyngeal swabs from
pigeons previously treated with cyclophosphamide showed a viral
excretion similar to that of control infected pigeons. However,
the cyclophosphamide treated pigeons showed a more severe
clinical disease with lesions of a more acute nature and a
similar but weaker serological response. Antibody titres became
non specific after two months.

b. Spontaneous re-excretion:

Several pigeons showed also spontaneous episodes of
re-excretion without clinical signs and these episodes were not
more frequent when the animals were nearly devoid of specific
antibodies.

c. Experimental re-excretion:

Ninety days after infection, pigeons were treated with
cyclophosphamide as in the control infected group. All pigeons

re-excreted infectious particles two to five days after the
first injection of cyclophosphamide. Three pigeons died within
the period of re-excretion with lesions of the disease; the two
remaining ones were asymptomatic despite the excretion of a
high level of infectious viral particles. Cyclophosphamide
treatment was first followed by a decrease of the titres of
specific antibodies and by an increase a week later, as in the
control infected group.

SUCCESSIVE EXPERIMENTAL EPISODES OF RE-EXCRETION (Vindevogel
and Pastoret, 1981)

Two groups of pigeons free from the infection were
inoculated with PHV1, one group being previously debilitated
with cyclophosphamide. Forty and eighty days after inoculation,
pigeons of both groups were treated with cyclophosphamide.
Attempts were made to isolate and titrate infectious particles
from pharyngeal swabs and blood samples during the primary
infection and the two episodes of experimentally provoked
re-excretion.

a. Primary infection:

Typical viral excretion patterns followed primary infection
in both groups. Signs and lesions were once again more intense
in the group previously treated with cyclophosphamide and virus
was isolated from blood of two pigeons belonging to this group.

b. Experimental re-excretion periods:

The cyclophosphamide treatment carried out 40 and 80 days
after infection were followed in all surviving birds, except
one, by a period of virus re-excretion nearly equivalent to
that following the initial infection and was sometimes
associated with clinical signs. During the first period of
re-excretion, virus was isolated from the blood of one pigeon
which died a few days later showing symptoms of encephalitis,
and virus was isolated from the brain.

494

SUCCESSIVE INFECTIONS WITH VIRULENT STRAINS (Vindevogel et al.,
1982a)

A group of squabs was infected with a virulent strain of
PHV1. Fifty six and hundred days after the initial infection,
the same pigeons were re-infected with an other virulent
strain. At each time of re-infection, other pigeons free of the
infection were infected with the same strain to serve as
control groups.

All the pigeons of the experimental group after initial
infection at day 0, as well as the animals of the first control
group at day 56 or of the second control group at day 100,
showed a classical pattern of viral excretion and clinical
signs of the disease.

After the first re-infection at day 56, three pigeons of
the experimental group demonstrated viral excretion equivalent
to that of the control group infected for the first time, but
except for one, this was without symptoms. The two remaining
animals did not excrete virus or show symptoms. A similar
situation was observed after the second re-infection on day
100.

Therefore, a previous exposure to a virulent strain
protects the animals against the clinical effects of a new
infection and this protection is sometimes sufficient to
inhibit further viral multiplication.

BEHAVIOUR OF AN ATTENUATED STRAIN (Vindevogel et al.,
1982b)

A wild strain of PHV1 has been serially passaged 100 times
in chicken embryo fibroblast cultures. Attenuation of the
strain was monitored by inoculation of budgerigars. Two groups
of pigeons were inoculated either with the wild initial strain
or with the attenuated one. Fifty six days after inoculation,
the animals inoculated with the attenuated strain were treated
with cyclophosphamide.

A similar pattern of viral excretion has been observed in
the two groups after primary infection, and animals of both
groups spontaneously re-excreted virus at the same level after

the initial period of excretion. After cyclophosphamide treatment, on day 56, of pigeons infected with the attenuated strain, all of them re-excreted virus. The attenuated strain remains therefore latent in infected pigeons as well as the virulent ones.

MODULATION OF RE-EXCRETION BY VACCINATION (Vindevogel et al., 1982b)

Several groups of pigeons were used to determine how vaccination of pigeons with an inactivated vaccine in oil adjuvant or with the attenuated strain influences infection and viral dissemination. Experiments were carried out to determine:

1) if a previous vaccination with an inactivated vaccine could prevent the establishment of a virulent strain in a latent state in the infected animals;

2) if a previous vaccination with an inactivated or attenuated vaccine could protect the animals from clinical symptoms and reduce viral excretion and dissemination after a first exposure to a virulent strain;

3) if vaccination could reduce the importance of spontaneous or experimental re-excretion if administered either after or before initial infection.

a. Vaccination with inactivated vaccine before infection:

As compared with a control group, the vaccinated pigeons excreted less viral particles during the infection, did not re-excrete virus spontaneously and re-excreted less virus after a cyclophosphamide treatment administered eight weeks after inoculation.

b. Vaccination with the attenuated strain before infection:

A similar situation, as the previous one, was observed.

c. Vaccination with inactivated virus after infection:

If vaccination was performed after infection, animals did re-excrete less virus than the control ones after a cyclophosphamide treatment performed eight weeks after infection.

d. General conclusions:

Both kinds of vaccination, performed before infection, either with an attenuated or an inactivated vaccine gave similar results and were efficient. Indeed, both of them were able to control primary excretion after infection and reduced symptoms but inactivated vaccine was unable to prevent the appearance of latent carriers. Both types of vaccination help to prevent spontaneous viral re-excretion and therefore help to control viral dissemination. Experimental re-excretion was also reduced if animals were vaccinated with inactivated vaccine after infection.

NATURAL TRANSMISSION OF THE INFECTION (Vindevogel and Pastoret, 1980)

Persistence and transmission of PHV1 under natural conditions were investigated in a dove-cot where the disease was diagnosed 13 months previously. At the beginning of our observations, pigeons had been clinically asymptomatic for 10 months and were rearing normal broods.

Mature pigeons possessed neutralizing antibodies and PHV1 was isolated from the pharynx of some of them. Yolk of eggs from the same pigeons contained neutralizing antibodies. PHV1 was also isolated from the pharynx of some squabs before weaning if they were reared by their parents. When squabs were reared in incubator, virus could not be isolated from pharyngeal swabs. All squabs examined after weaning were devoid of neutralizing antibodies but some of them were spontaneously excreting virus. After cyclophosphamide treatment, several squabs developed typical lesions and most of them shed virus.

In natural conditions, pigeons may therefore become latent carriers of the virus for a long time after recovery from natural infection. They transmit PHV1 to their offspring. The squabs become infected but are protected from the more severe effects of the infection by passive immunity of parental origin. Most of them become asymptomatic carriers themselves after this initial infection even if they were devoid of detectable neutralizing antibodies.

DISCUSSION

In natural or experimental conditions, pigeons infected with Pigeon herpesvirus 1 become latent carriers after recovery from the initial infection. Latent carriers may re-excrete the virus spontaneously without symptoms. High titres of specific neutralizing antibodies do not prevent the occurrence of re-excretion and conversely, recurrent episodes are not more frequent when the animals are nearly devoid of specific antibodies. Moreover, despite the episodes of re-excretion, specific antibodies decrease gradually.

A cyclophosphamide treatment performed after infection is followed by a period of viral excretion nearly equivalent to that following the initial infection. This period of re-excretion may be accompanied by lesions. Specific neutralizing antibodies first decrease and then reach a higher titre. This booster effect is probably due to the intense multiplication of the virus.

After experimental infection, virus usually remains confined near the site of inoculation. A transient viraemia may be observed during the primary infection and during episodes of re-excretion especially in squabs treated with cyclophospha-mide. Viraemia may thus occur but mainly in squabs weakened as in natural outbreaks by debilitating factors. Clinical disease is therefore principally observed in the primary infection of young pigeons free of the infection or in latent carriers with the help of debilitating factors.

In a flock of pigeons naturally infected with PHV1, some mature birds are latent carriers and transmit the infection to their offspring. The squabs reared by their parents, become infected but are protected from clinical disease by passive immunity of parental origin. They become themselves latent carriers although they are devoid of detectable neutralizing antibodies since the antibodies from parental origin quickly disappear.

Previous infection of the pigeon with a wild strain of PHV1 prevents the occurrence of symptoms when they are re-infected.

Vaccination of pigeons with an attenuated strain or with

inactivated virus in oil adjuvant reduces viral excretion and symptoms after challenge with a virulent strain but is unable to prevent the establishment of latency as demonstrated by cyclophosphamide treatment of the animals. However, vaccination diminishes spontaneous viral re-excretion and therefore viral dissemination. In conclusion, immunity, either passive or active, does not prevent the establishment of a latent infection but helps to control the dissemination of the virus and protects from the disease resulting from infection, or prevents generalization of the infection by viraemia.

In natural conditions, there is a sophisticated equilibrium between the virus and its host that prevents the occurrence of the disease.

REFERENCES
Coignoul, F. and Vindevogel, H. 1980. Cellular changes in the bursa of Fabricius and thymus of cyclophosphamide-treated pigeons. J. Comp. Path., 90, 395-400.
Heffels, U., Fritzsche, K., Kaleta, E.F. and Neumann, U. 1981. Serologische Untersuchungen zum Nachweis virusbedingter Infektionen bei der Taube in der Bundesrepublik Deutschland. Dtsch. Tierärztl. Wschr., 88, 97-102.
Landré, F., Vindevogel, H., Pastoret, P.P., Schwers, A., Thiry, E. and Espinasse, J. 1982. Fréquence de l'infection du pigeon par le Pigeon herpesvirus 1 et le virus de la maladie de Newcastle dans le nord de la France. Rec. Méd. Vét., sous presse.
Mare, C.J. and Graham, D.L. 1973. Falcon herpesvirus, the etiologic agent of inclusion body disease of falcons. Inf. Immun., 8, 118-126.
Vindevogel, H. 1981. Le coryza infectieux du pigeon. Thèse d'Agrégation de l'Enseignement Supérieur.
Vindevogel, H., Dagenais, L., Lansival, B. and Pastoret, P.P. 1981. Incidence of rotavirus, adenovirus and herpesvirus infection in pigeons. Vet. Rec., 109, 285-286.
Vindevogel, H. and Duchatel, J.P. 1977. Réceptivité de la perruche au virus herpès du pigeon. Ann. Méd. Vét., 121, 193-195.
Vindevogel, H. and Pastoret, P.P. 1980. Pigeon herpes infection: Natural transmission of the disease. J. Comp. Path., 90, 409-413.
Vindevogel, H. and Pastoret, P.P. 1981. Pathogenesis of pigeon herpesvirus infection. J. Comp. Path., 91, 415-426.
Vindevogel, H., Pastoret, P.P. and Burtonboy, G. 1980a. Pigeon herpes infection: Excretion and re-excretion of virus after experimental infection. J. Comp. Path., 90, 401-408.
Vindevogel, H., Pastoret, P.P., Burtonboy, G., Gouffaux, M. and Duchatel, J.P. 1975. Isolement d'un virus herpès dans un élevage de pigeons de chair. Ann. Rech. Vétér., 6, 431-436.

Vindevogel, H., Pastoret, P.P. and Leroy, P. 1982a.
    Comportement d'une souche atténuée du Pigeon herpesvirus 1
    et de souches pathogènes lors d'infections successives chez
    le pigeon. Ann. Rech. Vétér., sous presse.
Vindevogel, H., Pastoret, P.P. and Leroy, P. 1982b. Vaccination
    trials against pigeon herpesvirus infection (Pigeon
    herpesvirus 1). J. Comp. Path., sous presse.
Vindevogel, H., Pastoret, P.P., Leroy, P. and Coignoul, F.
    1980b. Comparaison de trois souches de virus herpétique
    isolées de psittacidés avec le virus herpès du pigeon.
    Avian Path., 9, 385-394.

SUMMARY

SESSION I :   HUMAN, SIMIAN, AND MURINE HERPESVIRUSES

Part 1:   Summarized by H. Openshaw and Marianne Scriba
Part 2:   Summarized by J.H. Subak-Sharpe and J.B. Hudson

Discussion at <u>part 1</u> of session I touched on many
aspects of herpes simplex virus (HSV) infection including the
effect of prior immunization on HSV challenge, the role of
immunity in the establishment and maintenance of latency, the
stimuli that induce reactivation, and the restriction enzyme
analysis of isolates from human ganglia. Instead of reviewing
all of these topics, this summary will focus on two aspects
that were discussed to some extent by all the speakers:
extra-ganglionic sites of HSV latency and the use of HSV
mutants in biological research.

At the latent stage of the infection, there is evidence
of HSV in human uterine ligament (<u>Subak-Sharpe</u>) and in eye
tissue of experimentally inoculated mice (<u>Openshaw</u>). Both of
these observations may be due to latency in neurons:
autonomic neurons in uterine tissue and retinal neurons in
the eye. However, reports at the conference also concerned
latency in non-neuronal tissue: footpad of the guinea pig and
mouse and spleen cells of tree shrews.

Experimental studies were summarized in the guinea pig
model after footpad inoculation of HSV (<u>Scriba</u>). At the
latent stage, explants of footpad tissue yielded virus with
or without recovery of HSV in the corresponding dorsal root
ganglia. These findings were attributed to a persistent
(i.e., low grade productive) infection of the footpad rather
than true peripheral latency. Compatible with this
interpretation is the short duration of explantation needed
for virus isolation (1-2 days) and the observation that short
term treatment of explants with phosphonoacetic acid prevents
isolation from footpad but not from ganglia.

More consistent with true peripheral latency are the experiments in the mouse model after footpad inoculation of HSV-2 but not HSV-1 (Subak-Sharpe). Depending on the temperature sensitive mutant used, isolation by explantation was achieved only from the footpad, only from lumbosacral dorsal root ganglia, or not at all.

Homogenates of footpad tissue were negative, and unlike the guinea pig model, a long time was required for the explants to yield virus (10-42 days).

Another example of probable extra neural latency comes from studies in tree shrews (Darai). In this model, animals received an intraperitoneal inoculation of a temperature sensitive mutant of HSV-1 or HSV-2 followed by an intraperitoneal challenge of the heterologous wild type virus. After challenge, virus could not be isolated from nervous system tissue but could be recovered by explantation of spleen cells. The isolates were shown to be intertypic recombinants that were not longer virulent for tree shrews.

In the general discussion, it was noted that work with lymphocytes provides some precedent for HSV latency in non-neuronal cells. Footpad tissue may also contain highly differentiated cells which are capable of harboring latent HSV, and reactivation may occur as the cells dedifferentiate in explant culture. It was speculated that the longer time required for a positive explant culture in the mouse compared to the guinea pig may reflect a species difference in growth rate of cells in the footpad explant rather than a difference in the state of the virus. Discussion also centered on whether peripheral latency occurs only in footpad and not other epithelial tissue, whether the difference in footpad latency of HSV-1 and HSV-2 is a general finding or a peculiarity only to the virus strains so far used in the mouse, and whether peripheral HSV latency has anything to do with the pathogenesis of recurrent disease.

The second aspect that we wish to emphasize in this summary concerns the use of HSV mutants to study the biology of latency. As noted previously, temperature sensitive mutants of HSV-2 differed not only in their ability to establish a latent infection but also in the site of latency (footpad and/or lumbosacral ganglia) (Subak-Sharpe). With some of these same mutants, latency could not be documented in tree shrews by nervous system explants (Darai). However, as previously noted, challenge with heterologous wild type virus resulted in the in vivo formation of intertypic recombinants (Darai).

Work with thymidine kinase deficient (TK⁻) mutants was presented (Becker, Schneweis, Scriba). After local inoculation, TK⁻mutants replicate well in cornea (Becker) but not in vaginal tissue (Schneweis). These mutants are virulent only in very young mice probably because cellular thymidine kinase is present in nervous tissue only during development (Becker). However, even in adult mice, prior immunization with TK⁻mutants does protect against a challenge of wild type virus in terms of mortality.

Consistent with published accounts, a latent nervous system infection could not be documented with TK⁻mutants. Two possibilities were discussed: either latency is not established or the explant technique fails to reactivate TK⁻mutants. Studies to detect HSV DNA in these models ultimately will make this distinction.

In conclusion, the present summary was intended to highlight certain surprising or discrepant findings in the biology of latent HSV infection. These findings underscore the importance of several experimental variables including the species, immune status, and strain of the experimental animal; the virus strain and mutant; and the route of inoculation.

Part 2 of session I was a heterogeneous one, involving descriptions of several different herpes viruses. Consequently this discussion deals separately with each presentation.

Bayliss reviewed the association between EBV (Epstein-Barr virus) antigen expression and various diseases.

In particular he drew attention to the association of NPC (nasopharyngeal carcinoma) with the lymphocytic-epithelial cell unction of the oropharynx viz: Waldeyer's ring. This helps to explain the apparent paradox that, while only B lymphocytes have receptors for EBV, the carcinoma arises in epithelial cells. However it is now known that EBV carrying lymphocytes can fuse with other cell types and thus could allow the viral genome to gain access to the epithelial cells. Furthermore this also reconciles Tseng Yi's observation of the correlation between NPC and the distribution of croton oil containing plants in southern China, since extracts of these plants, which are used for medicinal purposes, contain phorbol esters capable of activating EBNA in lymphocytes.

It is also of interest that in high risk patients VCA titers remain high, whereas in low risk patients the VCA titer decreases. Thus death usually follows treatment if the IgA anti-VCA rises.

Bayliss suggested further pursuit of possible associations between EBV and carcinomas in other organs where lymphocytic-epithelial junctions occur eg. tonsillar carcinoma and tongue cancer, by analogy with the NPC.

Another molecular approach which is being actively pursued is the identification of in vitro translation products from EBV specific mRNAs, obtained by hybridisation selection techniques with cloned viral DNAs. By this means it was shown that the portion of the viral genome which is complementary to cellular DNA contains the information for the 85k protein.

Fleckenstein reviewed the previous work and summarized recent results on the genome organization of herpesvirus saimiri (HVS) and herpesvirus ateles (HVA). Both viruses produce tumors from T-cells, although HVA immortalizes lymphocytes in vitro more readily.

The H-DNA tandem repeat, comprising 1.4kb, contains some short open reading frames, the longest having potential coding capacity for 85 amino acids, but does not appear to contain transcription signals. Thus it seems unlikely that these regions code for polypeptides. Fleckenstein suggests that they represent sites for cutting the DNA concatemers for encapsidation.

Tumors induced by both viruses contain various types of circular viral DNAs. Non-producer tumor cell lines contain circles with deletions in the L-region, whereas producer lines contain complete circular genomes.

In all non-producer lines the viral DNA was found to be heavily undermethylated. Although there were four specific undermethylated sites on the left portion of L DNA, these did not seem to correlate with transcription.

It is of interest that in two non-oncogenic strains of virus there were deletions at the left hand of the DNA and L insertions in the H region. These transpositions evidently interfered with tumor production but not transforming capacity.

No evidence was available so far for the presence of integrated viral DNA in addition to circles.

Fleckenstein also discussed the 2.8kb fragment of human CMV DNA which can oncogenically transform mouse cells in vitro. This DNA fragment has been sequenced and contains many TATA boxes and stop codons in all reading frames.

He suggested that herpes virus transformation may be a hit and run phenomenon, with the DNA circles related merely to persistence.

Modrow discussed immunity to HVS in natural and experimental hosts, and then proceeded to describe her recent studies on viral proteins. Accumulation of early (nonfunctional) proteins was examined with the use of the amino acid analogues azetidine and canavanine. HVS induced glycoproteins, phosphoproteins and structural proteins were identified. There were no apparent differences in the structural proteins of virulent and attenuated HVS strains. However there were some differences between the viral antigens found in the natural host and tumor bearing animals.

Darai compared the properties, pathogenesis and latency

of the tree shrew (tupaia) herpesviruses, THV 1-4. The Hind
III restriction endonuclease profiles of the four DNAs were
different, although they all had molecular weights of
approximately 130×10^6. Surprisingly he could find no
evidence for repeat sequences, or stem loops in renatured
DNAs. There was significant intertypic homology.

Some types could give malignant lymphomas in the natural
host and all produced lymphoid hyperplasia in newborn
rabbits. With THV-2 8% go on to produce malignant thymona.
Some THV types could subsequently be reactivated from B
lymphocytes of rabbit spleens. The restriction endonuclease
profile of the reactivated virus was the same as the parent
virus.

A novel finding not previously reported for
herpesviruses was the presence of a thymidine kinase activity
in purified THV virions. To date Darai has mapped the genome
of THV-2 and has produced a DNA library for this purpose.

Hudson reviewed the role of various factors involved in
persistent MCMV (Murine cytomegalovirus) infectens, by
considering studies on infected mice and cell lines infected
in vitro.

In mice of various strains, MCMV establishes a
productive infection in numerous tissues, although specific
cell types within a tissue may be spared. Dissemination of
the virus may be facilitated by a temporary and generalized
immunosuppression. Eventually a variety of anti-viral
responses help to terminate the acute phase of infection,
which is then replaced by a chronic type of infection in
certain tissues, and a true latent infection in others. Some
of the factors which are important in determining the
severity of the acute infection and the establishment and
duration of the chronic phase are: the strain and precise
history of the virus itself; age and strain of mice; the
presence of physical barriers to virus or immune cells;
macrophages, which may control virus dissemination or promote
persistence; and the immune status of the mouse.

The virus has frequently been reactivated from several

tissues of persistently infected mice. The two methods which have proven successful in reactivation are: immunosuppressive therapy of the animals; and explantation of tissues, usually in the presence of embryonic fibroblast cultures. These studies implicate the presence of virus-controlling factors in persistently infected animals.

Infections in vitro have been done on numerous cell lines of murine and non-murine origin. These studies have indicated the relevance of cell cycle parameters, and other host cell factors, in determining the extent of viral gene expression and persistence.

Koszinowski discussed the quantitation, state of activity, specificity and presence at various stages of infection of MCMV-induced cytolytic T-cells. During acute infection there were two populations of cytolytic cells. One population was active without in vitro antigen stimulation, and constituted one cell per 14,000 lymphoid cells, while the other population, which were stimulated by antigen in vitro, constituted one in 2,480 lymphoid cells. A massive 10^4 fold increase in virus dose only resulted in a ten-fold increase in the number of cytolytic T-cells.

An increase in the interleukin concentration resulted in increased cytolytic activity, which was due to the expansion of a different class of cells which non-specifically lysed rabies virus-infected targets as well as MCMV infected targets. Thus interleukin treatment expanded several sorts of memory cells. As expected the specifically lysed target cells showed H-2 restriction.

Persistently infected mice were reactivated by cyclophosphamide treatment. Forty days after the treatment infectious virus was detected in salivary glands, and one cell in 30,000 lymphoid cells were specifically cytolytic, in contrast to the non-reactivated mice, which remained free of infectious virus and cytolytic cells.

SESSION II :   BOVIDE, EQUIDE AND FELIDE HERPESVIRUSES

Part 1:   Summarized by P.-P. Pastoret and H. Ludwig
Part 2:   Summarized by Rosalind M. Gaskell and R.B. Burrows

   Part 1 of session II was mainly devoted to latency of
one of the major pathogens of cattle, bovid herpesvirus type
1 (BHV-1), with emphasis on molecular and epidemiological
aspects of its latency (Pastoret).
   As far as is known, all the other members of bovid
herpesviruses are also able to hide in the stage of latency.
On the basis of historical information, clinical and
serological knowledge, as well as recent molecular biological
investigations, such as restriction enzyme analysis of viral
DNA's the known herpesviruses of Bovidae have been tentatively classified as bovid herpesviruses types 1 to 6 (BHV-1 to
-6).
   This classification includes BHV-1, the virus responsible for infectious bovine rhinotracheitis/infectious
pustular vulvovaginitis; BHV-2, the virus causing bovine
herpes mammillitis; BHV-3, the virus involved in the African
form of malignant catarrhal fever; BHV-4 a group of isolates
of unknown etiological importance; BHV-5, the virus found to
be associated with ovine pulmonary adenomatosis ("jaagsiekte"); and BHV-6, the caprine (goat) herpesvirus (Ludwig).
   There was some discussion about the different clinical
forms of BHV-1 infections in cattle and about differences
between the isolates causing either infectious bovine
rhinotracheitis (IBR) or infectious pustular vulvovaginitis
(IPV). Evidence was presented showing that the isolates
causing the IBR form differ from those causing IPV on the
basis of restriction endonuclease cleavage patterns of the
viral DNA (Pauli).
   As already mentioned, most of those viral species have
been shown to remain latent in the recovered host, but
latency of BHV-1 is by far the most and the best investigated
model in this host species. This can be easily understood

since latency plays a prominent role in the epidemiology of infectious bovine rhinotracheitis (IBR), and since the etiological agent can easily be reactivated following glucocorticoid administration in latently infected cattle. Results from investigations performed in Denmark clearly demonstrated that latency is the rule rather than the exception in experimentally, as well as in naturally infected cattle (Bitsch). In some herds, periods as long as two years, elapse between infection and further spreading of the disease after reactivation. With regards to infection control, several problems are associated with vaccination (Nettleton). In fact, it seems likely that all the attenuated strains studied so far, reamin latent after vaccination and that vaccination does not prevent the installment of a virulent strain in a latent stage. Calves vaccinated with a live attenuated vaccine against IBR were later challenged with a field isolate of IBR virus. The calves were protected against clinical illness and the excretion of challenge virus was reduced. The same calves were later treated to provoke reactivation of latent virus.

Using different biological properties of the vaccine and the field virus, the reexcreted isolates were shown to be principally field virus, although vaccine virus could also be recovered. Restriction endonuclease analysis of some of those isolates confirmed that both the field and vaccine viruses had been reexcreted. The combined data show that cattle can be latently infected with two different strains of BHV-1, but it is still not clear whether recombination between attenuated virus strains and field virus occurs.

In order to pursue this problem further, the stability of the reactivated strains was studied. Genomes of the strains used for primary infection and reactivated viruses were compared after digestion with the restriction endonuclease, EcoRI, and no difference could be demonstrated between viruses isolated after successive reactivations in the same animal infected with only one strain. It was therefore concluded that the latent strains remain stable

(Thiry).

The problem of the possible emergence of recombinants was discussed in greater detail (Subak-Sharp). If recombination could occur between two field strains, and even if the recombinant virus is infectious and leads to a clinical disease, the significance of recombination would be less important than if recombination occurs between a field strain and a vaccine strain or between two vaccine strains. In order to obtain recombinants, the latently infected cells should harbor both parental viruses and the two parental strains should therefore invade the same cells in the same tissue. The problem was discussed according to data obtained with herpes simplex virus (human herpesvirus type 1) latency and Aujeszky's Disease/pseudorabies virus (suid herpesvirus 1) infection in pigs, where evidence exists that trigeminal ganglia cannot be invaded by two different strains of the same virus (Openshaw). For instance, the explanation as to why cattle can be infected with both a thermosensitive (ts) vaccine strain and a field virus strain may be that each virus invades a different tissue and consequently has a different site of latency.

Accordingly, the phenomenon of latent coinfections should be investigated using attenuated strains other than the ts mutant, e.g., a thymidine-kinase negative strain (Becker).

The site of BHV-1 latency in the body remains an important unsolved question. The finding that a thermosensitive vaccine strain, unable to invade the nervous system, can be reactivated, seems to indicate that this virus remains latent in epithelial cells. First attempts to give an answer have obviously shown that trigeminal ganglia as well as sacral ganglia of infected cattle may harbor the virus. These results were obtained by DNA in-situ-hybridization experiments (Ackerman). Whether the presence of viral DNA in neuron nuclei is indicative of a static or a dynamic stage of replication remained a matter of controversy. However, the question of whether or not this represents the only site of

latency remains still open (Subak-Sharpe, Becker, Ben Porat).
Suggestions were given for the use of cloned restriction
fragments amplified in bacteria for the detection of viral
DNA in tissues (Subak-Sharpe).

The work done in Denmark leads one to think that control
and eradication of BHV-1 is feasible and successful (Bitsch).
Nevertheless, vaccination is still useful since it prevents
clinical illness and immunized animals may be able to control
reexcretion. With this procedure the dissemination of virus,
even if reactivation occurs, is low.

Studies on the antigenic components of BHV-1 (Pauli) led
to a better understanding of the immune response of the
animal and a further improvement of vaccination procedures.
Here again, the discrepancy of being unable to differentiate
BHV-1 isolates by serological means was intensively discussed
(Straub, Darai, Subak-Sharpe).

As a general conclusion, it should always be kept in
mind, that from a biological standpoint, latency ensures the
durability of BHV-1 infection.

Part 2 of session II covered several animal
herpesviruses each with their own latency characteristics.
Thus for bovid herpesvirus 2, evidence was presented to
suggest that it may persist as a latent infection in
recovered animals in skin lesions whereas in the acute phase
of the disease it is also present in nervous tissue (Scott).
These findings were discussed in relation to skin and
ganglion trigger theories, and the work of Castrucci et al.
(Int. Workshop on Herpesviruses, Bologna, Italy 1981).

The epizootiology of the disease is still an enigma, but
it was hypothesized that outbreaks of the disease, which only
occur in Autumn, may be initiated by immunological changes in
latently infected cattle following calving.

Bovid herpesvirus 5 (BHV 5) (Scott), felid herpesvirus 1
(FHV 1) (Gaskell), and equid herpesvirus 1 and 3 (EHV 1 and
3) (Burrows) also appear to have a similar latent phase in
persistently infected, recovered animals. Virus may be

reactivated either by corticosteroid treatment or by natural stress situations, and apparently spontaneous episodes of shedding may also occur. The site or sites of latency for these viruses are unclear, though for FHV 1 there is limited evidence that the trigeminal ganglia may be involved.

It was discussed that although BHV 5 was originally thought to be the cause of pulmonary adenomatosis (Jaagsiekte) in sheep, the recent finding of a reverse transcriptase and a retrovirus in association with this tumour has led to the suggestion that CHV 1 may only be a passenger virus and undergoes reactivation as a result of immunosuppression induced by the tumour. The new agent has been purified on gradients and apparently induces the disease; however, whether or not the preparation was entirely free from the herpesvirus is not known.

FHV 1 (Gaskell) and EHV 1 (Burrows) both cause acute upper respiratory tract infections in their respective species and EHV 1 particularly may also induce abortions; EHV 3 induces coital exanthema. The characteristics of the feline virus carrier state (Gaskell) have been well defined in terms of reactivation stimuli and shedding patterns and studies are now in regress to examine such animals immunologically (Goddard). Similar attempts have also been made to study latent infections with the equine viruses (Burrows).

Another herpesvirus described in this session was malignant catarrhal fever (MCF) virus, the only known lymphotrophic herpesvirus to infect the larger domestic animals. (Plowright) Cattle are the indicator hosts and suffer a low morbidity but high mortality; a cell associated viraemia may persist intermittently in survivors for up to 5-6 months. The reservoir of infection for this and other similar viruses is in wild ungulates, such as wildebeest. Infection in these animals is probably inapparent and recovered animals remain persistently infected. The disease may be reproduced in rabbits and this could be a useful model for the study of lymphotrophic herpesviruses.

SESSION III :   PORCINE HERPESVIRUSES
                 (AUJESZKY'S DISEASE VIRUS)

Summarized by Tamar Ben-Porat, J.B. McFerran and H.-J. Rziha

This session was concerned with the latent infection of
suid herpesvirus 1, known as pseudorabiesvirus (PsR), the
causative agent of Aujeszky's disease. Papers were presented
dealing with production and detection of PsR latency in pigs,
including some molecular biological aspects.

Two of the papers dealt with differences in restriction
enzyme patterns of the genome of field isolates (Ben-Porat,
Herrmann). Isolates obtained from different epidemics can be
distinguished from one another on that basis. Obviously the
differences observed reflect deletions and/or insertions of
DNA gequences which are predominantly confined to 2 varable
regions of the PsR genome (Ben-Porat). However, isolates
obtained from different areas share similiarities in their
DNA cleavage patterns. According to these data a subdivision
of virus isolates into 4 groups is proposed (Herrmann). The
results obtained in several laboratories showed that the
restriction enzyme patterns of a given isolate remain stable
upon in vitro passage in cell culture or upon in vivo passage
in swine (Ben-Porat, Gielkens). But changes in the cleavage
patterns of the genomes of the virus were observed after
virus stocks were mutagenized (Ben-Porat).

Three papers showed that following challenge with 3
different virus strains serologically negative pigs, pigs
with maternally derived antibodies, pigs vaccinated either
parenterally with inactivated vaccine and/or intranasally
with attenuated vaccine all became latently infected
(McFerran, Van Oirschot, Wittmann). Virus could be unmasked
by immunosuppression (Van Oirschot, Wittmann) or by infection
by Salmonella cholera-suis (McFerran), and in addition
spontaneous breakdown occurred. PsR was reisolated by
co-cultivation of lungs, tonsils, and brain up to 18 months
after infection (Wittmann). In contrast, others only could

detect virus in the trigeminal ganglia of the latently
infected animals (Ben-Porat, Van Oirschot). In all cases
sufficient virus was shed following immunosuppression to
infect in-contact pigs. However, the frequency of virus
recovery decreases with prolonged time after infection
(Wittmann), and the efficiency of virus excretion is low
(McFerran). The presented data indicate that the titre of the
infecting virus in addition to the virus strain is important
in disease manifestation.

One set of studies with pigs either non-vaccinated or
vaccinated with inactivated vaccine showed that following
virus challenge high titres of neutralizing antibodies are
present up to 22.5 months after infection, which do not
prevent a virus reactivation (Wittmann). Additionally these
experiments revealed no significantly altered reactions in
cell-mediated immunity of non-vaccinated and vaccinated pigs,
or during different phases of virus latency.

Two interesting results were obtained in experiments by
superinfecting pigs, which were previously infected with
another PsR virus strain (Ben-Porat). Both virus strains were
readily discernible by their DNA restriction enzyme patterns.
These studies showed that (i) only the virus strain used for
the first infection can be recovered from the ganglia of the
superinfected pigs, and that (ii) the superinfecting virus
does not colonize the ganglia of the pre-immunized animals.

Similiar studies were done with pigs vaccinated with a
live vaccine virus (Bartha's K strain). They showed that the
challenge-exposed animals become infected, displaying only
mild signs of the disease (Van Oirschot). However, there was
no evidence for the excretion of the vaccine virus
(Gielkens).

Results of studies dealing with the presence and the
state of the viral genome in the trigeminal ganglia of
latently infected pigs using different methods (in situ
cytohybridization, as well as Southern and Northern blotting)
were presented. Homologies between nucleotide sequences
present in PsR DNA and in swine cellular DNA were noted

(Ben-Porat). The results of one set of studies indicate that
the ganglia of the swine that were probed carried a
relatively heavy load of viral genome equivalents per cell
(Rziha). By in situ hybridization it was shown that some of
the cells in these ganglia and in other neural tissues
contained many copies of the viral genome (Rziha). In
addition, the presence of viral DNA was suggested in white
blood cells of latently infected pigs (Rziha). In another set
of studies no viral DNA was detectable by methods that should
have revealed one genome equivalent per 30 cells. Also, no
virale RNA was detected in these ganglia.

SESSION IV :   AVIAN HERPESVIRUSES

Summarized by L.N. Payne and H.-J. Rziha

Vindevogel reviewed the extensive studies by his group
on infection of pigeons by the pigeon herpesvirus 1 (PHV-1).
Primary infection by inoculation of PHV-1 onto the pharynx is
followed by the development of lesions in the upper digestive
and respiratory tracts within 3 days, accompanied by maximum
excretion of virus between 2-4 days, with persistence of
excretion for 7-10 days. The virus then becomes latent, but
mild episodes of virus excretion, without clinical signs, may
occur spontaneously. This recurrence is unrelated to antibody
levels. Asymptomatic carriers also occur in naturally
infected pigeons, and occasional shedding of virus is
responsible for spread of infection to their offspring. The
squabs are, however, provided with a degree of immunity by
passive antibodies transferred through the yolk, and they
also may become carriers.
      Treatment of latently infected pigeons with
cyclophosphamide causes the development of pharyngeal
lesions, and birds may die. Virus is re-excreted from 1-10
days after the beginning of this treatment. This drug may

also be used to modify the response of pigeons to primary
infection. Treated pigeons show a more severe and acute
clinical disease, and antibody responses are weaker.

Latently infected pigeons are protected against symptoms
following challenge with virulent virus, and viral
replication can be inhibited. A tissue culture attenuated
strain of PHV-1 also becomes latent following primary
infection, but can be activated by cyclophosphamide
treatment.

Vaccination of uninfected pigeons with both attenuated
PHV-1 or inactivated PHV-1 in oil adjuvant conferred
resistance to replication of challenge virus, reduced signs
of infection and prevented spontaneous re-excretion. Latent
infection was not prevented but virus excretion was reduced
following cyclophosphamide treatment. Vaccination with
inactivated virus after a primary infection also causes less
re-excretion following the drug treatment. The location and
state of the PHV-1 during latency was not reported.

The remaining papers were devoted to Marek's disease
virus (MDV). Rziha and Bauer reported on the state of the MDV
genome in latently infected lymphoblastoid cell lines derived
from MD lymphomas in chickens. In the producer line
MDCC-MSB1, and the non-producer line MDCC-HP2 (formerly an
producer line), viral DNA sequences banded in neutral CsCl
gradients at the density of purified virion DNA, indicating
the presence of free MDV DNA. Evidence for viral DNA closely
associated with cellular DNA from these lines was also
obtained. In contrast, in the MDCC-RP1 cell line, the
majority of the viral DNA was detected in the cellular DNA
range, suggesting an association, and possibly integration,
with host cell DNA. About 30% of the free viral DNA from the
MSB1 and HP2 lines analyzed by glycerol gradient centrifugation banded in the region expected for covalently closed
circular molecules, and the presence of circular molecules
was confirmed in this material by centrifugation on ethidium
bromide-CsCl-density gradients.

Attempts were made to induce virus production, viral

antigen, and DNA synthesis in the three cell lines by treatment with the phorbol ester TPA. Enhancement of viral antigen and DNA production was observed for the MSB1 producer line, but not for the two non-producer lines.

These studies thus demonstrate the presence of circular plasmid viral DNA in two of three MD cell lines examined, as has been shown for cell lines transformed by EBV and herpesvirus saimiri. The authors speculate that circular viral DNA may be mandatory for herpesvirus-induced transformation.

Bumstead, Payne, Howes, Lawn and Ross described the spontaneous development of lymphoblastoid cell lines in cultures of spleens and other tissues of hatched and embryonic chickens from the B-S and several other strains of fowl maintained under specific pathogen-free conditions. The cell lines expresed T-cell antigen, embryonic antigen, MD tumour-associated surface antigen (MATSA) and, in low frequency, MD viral membrane antigen. Infectious pathogenic, MDV could be rescued in vitro and in vivo from the lines derived from young chickens, but not from embryo-derived lines. DNA hybridization studies revealed the presence of MDV genome in all the cell lines, and also in lymphoid and other tissues from normal B-S line embryos. These findings suggest, contrary to current opinion, that vertical transmission of MDV in a latent state can occur. The viral genome may exist in an endogenous, integrated state, since it could not be rescued from the embryo-derived lines. Experience with isolation-rearing of infection-free chickens derived from MDV-infected breeder flocks suggests that if vertical transmission does occur it seems to do so in a state of latency which does not normally lead to active infection.

Aspects of the induction of MD in turkeys were discussed by Powell, Payne, Howes, Mustill, Rennie and Thompson. Large doses of the GA strain of MDV induced lymphoma and lymphatic leukemia in young turkeys which, in contrast to chickens, showed very limited evidence of semi-productive or productive virus infection during the development of the lymphoproliferative disease. No lymphoproliferative changes were observed in peripheral nerves or around feather follicles. Leukaemic blood contained on average 68% T-cells and 13% B-cells, suggesting an increase in the number of null cells. MATSA-bearing cells were increased in the blood of leukemic turkeys. Depression of humoral antibody responses were observed in affected turkeys. These findings suggest that in the turkey strain studied MDV may commonly exist in a latent state following exogenous infection. Eight lymphoid cell lines were developed from spleen of buffy coat cells from diseased turkeys. These lines expressed MATSA and, like chicken MD-derived cell lines, were characterised a T-cells.

The persistence of MDV in long-term explant cultures of lymphomatous and non-lymphomatous tissues from infected chickens was reported by Coudert and Cauchy. Thirteen of 20 cultured tissues revealed herpesvirions under the electron microscope, and infectious viruses could be isolated from cells migrating from most of the explants, but not from the explants themselves. It was suggested that the persistently-infected cell in culture could have a counterpart in vivo which was responsible for the maintenance of viraemia in infected chickens.

LIST OF PARTICIPANTS

AUSTRIA

Dr. Marianne Scriba
Sandoz Forschungsinstitut
Brunnerstr. 59
A-1235 Wien

BELGIUM

Dr. P.-P. Pastoret
Faculté de Médecine vétérinaire
Université de Liège
Service de Virologie
45, rue des vétérinaires
B-1070 Bruxelles

Dr. E. Thiry
Faculté de Médecine vétérinaire
Université de Liège
Service de Virologie
45, rue des vétérinaires
B-1070 Bruxelles

Dr. H. Vindevogel
Faculté de Médecine vétérinaire
Université de Liège
Service de Virologie
45, rue des vétérinaires
B-1070 Bruxelles

CANADA

Dr. J.B. Hudson
The University of British
Columbia, Faculty of Medicine
Division of Med. Microbiology
2075 Wesbrook Place
Vancouver, B.C. V6T 1W5

DENMARK

Dr. V. Bitsch
Statens veterinaere
Serumlaboratorium
Bülowsvej 27
DK-1870 København V

FEDERAL REPUBLIC OF GERMANY

Dr. G. Bayliss
Max v. Pettenkofer-Institut
für Hygiene u. Mikrobiologie
Pettenkofer Str. 9a
D-8000 München 2

Dr. G. Darai
Institut für Medizinische
Mikrobiologie am Hygiene-
Institut der Universität
Im Neuenheimer Feld 324
D-6900 Heidelberg

Angelika Ebeling
Bundesforschungsanstalt für
Viruskrankheiten der Tiere
Paul-Ehrlich-Str. 28
D-7400 Tübingen

Dr. P.-J. Enzmann
Bundesforschungsanstalt für
Viruskrankheiten der Tiere
Paul-Ehrlich-Str. 28
D-7400 Tübingen

Dr. B. Fleckenstein
Institut für Klinische
Virologie der Universität
Erlangen-Nürnberg
Loschgestr. 7
D-8520 Erlangen

Dr. G. Keil
Bundesforschungsanstalt für
Viruskrankheiten der Tiere
Paul-Ehrlich-Str. 28
D-7400 Tübingen

Dr. U. Koszinowski
Bundesforschungsanstalt für
Viruskrankheiten der Tiere
Paul-Ehrlich-Str. 28
D-7400 Tübingen

Dr. R.J. Lorenz
Bundesforschungsanstalt für
Viruskrankheiten der Tiere
Paul-Ehrlich-Str. 28
D-7400 Tübingen

Dr. H. Ludwig
Institut für Virologie
Fachbereich Veterinärmedizin
Freie Universität Berlin
Nordufer 20
(im Robert Koch-Institut)
D-1000 Berlin 65

Dr. Noemi Lukacs
Bundesforschungsanstalt für
Viruskrankheiten der Tiere
Paul-Ehrlich-Str. 28
D-7400 Tübingen

T. Mettenleiter
Bundesforschungsanstalt für
Viruskrankheiten der Tiere
Paul-Ehrlich-Str. 28
D-7400 Tübingen

Dr. Susanne Modrow
Max v. Pettenkofer-Institut
für Hygiene und Mikrobiologie
Pettenkofer Str. 9a
D-8000 München 2

Dr. V. Ohlinger
Bundesforschungsanstalt für
Viruskrankheiten der Tiere
Paul-Ehrlich-Str. 28
D-7400 Tübingen

Dr. G. Pauli
Institut für Virologie
Fachbereich Veterinärmedizin
Freie Universität Berlin
Nordufer 20
(im Robert Koch-Institut)
D-1000 Berlin 65

M.J. Reddehase
Bundesforschungsanstalt für
Viruskrankheiten der Tiere
Paul-Ehrlich-Str. 28
D-7400 Tübingen

Dr. H.-J. Rziha
Bundesforschungsanstalt für
Viruskrankheiten der Tiere
Paul-Ehrlich-Str. 28
D-7400 Tübingen

Dr. K.E. Schneweis
Institut Med.Mikrobiologie
und Immunologie der
Universität Bonn
Venusberg
D-5300 Bonn

Dr. W. Schwöbel
Bundesforschungsanstalt für
Viruskrankheiten der Tiere
Paul-Ehrlich-Str. 28
D-7400 Tübingen

Dr. O.C. Straub
Bundesforschungsanstalt für
Viruskrankheiten der Tiere
Paul-Ehrlich-Str. 28
D-7400 Tübingen

Dr. H.-J. Thiel
Bundesforschungsanstalt für
Viruskrankheiten der Tiere
Paul-Ehrlich-Str. 28
D-7400 Tübingen

Dr. Emilie Weiland
Bundesforschungsanstalt für
Viruskrankheiten der Tiere
Paul-Ehrlich-Str. 28
D-7400 Tübingen

Dr. F. Weiland
Bundesforschungsanstalt für
Viruskrankheiten der Tiere
Paul-Ehrlichstr. 28
D-7400 Tübingen

Dr. G. Wittmann
Bundesforschungsanstalt für
Viruskrankheiten der Tiere
Paul-Ehrlich-Str. 28
D-7400 Tübingen

FRANCE

Dr. L. Cauchy
Institut National de la
Recherche Agronomique
Station de Pathologie
Aviaire et de Parasitologie
C.R. Tours-Nouzilly
F-37380 Monnaie

ISRAEL
Dr. Y. Becker
Dept. of Molecular Virology
The Hebrew University -
Hadassah Medical School
P.O. Box 1172
91010 Jerusalem

NETHERLANDS

Dr. A.L.J. Gielkens
Centraal Diergeneeskundig
Instituut
Houtribweg 39
8221 RA Lelystad

Dr. J.T. van Oirschot
Centraal Diergeneeskundig
Instituut
Houtribweg 39
8221 RA Lelystad

UNITED KINGDOM

Dr. Janene M. Bumstead
Houghton Poultry Research
Station
Houghton
Huntingdon, Cambs. PE17 2DA

Dr. R. Burrows
Animal Virus Research Institute
Pirbright
Woking, Surrey GU24 ONF

Dr. Rosalind M. Gaskell
University of Bristol
Dept. of Veterinary Medicine
Langford House
Langford
Bristol BS18 7DU

Dr. Loraine Goddard
University of Bristol
Dept. of Veterinary Medicine
Langford House
Langford
Bristol BS18 7DU

Dr. J.B. McFerran
Department of Agriculture
Veterinary Research
Laboratories
Stormont
Belfast BT4 3SD

Dr. P.F. Nettleton
Animal Diseases Research
Association
Moredun Institute
408 Gilmerton Road
Edinburgh EH17 7JH

Dr. L.N. Payne
Houghton Poultry Research
Station
Houghton
Huntingdon, Cambs. PE17 2DA

Dr. W. Plowright
Institute for Research on
Animal Diseases
Compton, Nr Newbury,
Berkshire RG16 ONN

Dr. F.M.M. Scott
Animal Diseases Research
Association
Moredun Institute
408 Gilmerton Road
Edinburgh EH17 7 JH

Dr. J.H. Subak-Sharpe
Institute of Virology
University of Glasgow
Church Street
Glasgow G11 5JR

UNITED STATES OF AMERICA

Dr. Tamar Ben-Porat
Department of Microbiology
Vanderbilt University
School of Medicine
Nashville, Tennessee 37232

Dr. A.S. Kaplan
Department of Microbiology
Vanderbilt University
School of Medicine
Nashville, Tennessee 37232

Dr. H. Openshaw
Department of Neurology
University of California
Professional Building
4301 X Street, Room 210
Sacramento, California 95817

SWITZERLAND

Dr. M. Ackermann
Institut für Virologie
der Universität Zürich
Winterthurerstr. 266a
CH-8057 Zürich

Dr. R. Wyler
Institut für Virologie
der Universität Zürich
Winterthurerstr. 266a
CH-8057 Zürich

CEC

Dr. J. Connell
rue de la Loi 200
B-1049 Bruxelles